THE ENCYCLOPEDIA OF

COMPLEMENTARY AND ALTERNATIVE MEDICINE

Tova Navarra, B.A., R.N.

Foreword by
Adam Perlman, M.D., M.P.H.
Siegler Center for Integrative Medicine
St. Barnabas Health Care System, Livingston, NJ

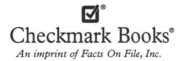

Checkmark Books®

An imprint of Facts On File, Inc.

The Encyclopedia of Complementary and Alternative Medicine

Checkmark Books
An imprint of Facts On File, Inc.
132 West 31st Street
New York NY 10001

Library of Congress Cataloging-in-Publication Data

Navarra, Tova
The encyclopedia of complementary and alternative medicine / Tova Navarra; foreword by Adam Perlman.
p.cm.
Includes bibliographical references and index.

ISBN 0-8160-4997-1(hc: alk. paper)—ISBN 0-8160-6226-9 (pb: alk. paper)
1. Alternative medicine—Encyclopedias. I. Title.
R733. N38 2004
615.5'03—dc21   2003043415

Checkmark Books are available at special discounts when purchased in bulk quantities for businesses, associations, institutions, or sales promotions. Please call our Special Sales Department in New York at (212) 967-8800 or (800) 322-8755.

You can find Facts On File on the World Wide Web at http://www.factsonfile.com

Text design by Cathy Rincon
Cover design by Pehrsson Design

Printed in the United States of America

VB FOF 10 9 8 7 6 5 4 3 2 1

This book is printed on acid-free paper.

COMPLEMENTARY AND ALTERNATIVE MEDICINE

For Frederic

CONTENTS

Foreword   ix

Preface   xiii

Acknowledgments   xv

Introduction   xvii

Entries A–Z   1

Appendixes   175

Bibliography   251

Index   255

FOREWORD

At the age of 16 I began training in martial arts. What started as a hobby, a way to get in shape and increase my self-confidence, soon turned into a passion. I unexpectedly found myself on a path. This path was one of self-exploration and development. As I progressed in rank and understanding and began to appreciate the benefits of improved health, discipline, and self-esteem, as did so many students before me, I developed a desire to teach and pass on what I had been taught. After a number of years of assisting, several fellow instructors and I opened up a martial arts school. I was in college at the time and frequently finished classes and immediately raced down to the school to teach or train. I found those days extremely challenging and rewarding.

However, I soon discovered that my parents and family did not fully appreciate my vision of my life as a martial arts instructor. Although they were always supportive, they encouraged me to consider other avenues of employment. Given that my father was a lawyer and I was a history major, law seemed a reasonable way to make a living while continuing my career as a martial artist. After going through the application process, I was fortunate enough to be accepted for admission. As I began to contemplate graduation from college and the prospect of the first year of law school, I began to question my decision. I simply did not feel passionate about becoming a lawyer. I began to reevaluate what I did feel passionate about. What was it about teaching martial arts that made me feel so fulfilled?

What I soon concluded was that I enjoyed teaching and I enjoyed helping people improve their health and well-being. Although a number of careers would have afforded me the opportunity to teach and promote health, I decided to become a physician. For is not the essence of medicine to teach people to improve and maintain their health? In fact, the Latin root for *doctor, docere,* means "to teach." I can still remember the phone call to my parents when I informed them that I was deferring my law school entrance and planned to start premed classes in summer school less than a week after graduation.

Over the next year and a half, I completed the premed requirements and was ultimately accepted to Boston University School of Medicine. During that time, I continued on my path of self-exploration. I continued teaching martial arts and began to question why conventional medicine did not often utilize methods from other healing traditions. I had seen multiple examples of problems, such as back pain, improved through the use of t'ai ch'i, or asthma through the use of various breathing exercises. I had seen multiple students lose weight, improve their control of stress, and in general improve their quality of life. To me a martial arts instructor, nothing felt more meaningful and rewarding. To me, this was the essence of good medicine.

As I began my formal medical training, I quickly realized that teaching patients to improve or maintain their health was a part of medicine that often got lost in trying to provide patients with the latest advancements in order to diagnose, treat, or cure disease. I also realized that others were less than understanding of my desire to expand the usual treatment options to include "alternative" methods. One day, during my second year of residency, the chairman of medicine asked me what I planned to do when I finished training. I told him that I was interested in alternative medicine, to which he responded, "Show me the evidence," and quickly changed the subject.

Although I was somewhat disappointed by this reaction, his statement ultimately turned out to be one of those seemingly innocent comments that unintentionally have a profound effect. I began pondering the challenge of integrating alternative medicine into conventional medicine and the conventional medical establishment. I began to appreciate more fully the need for additional research on alternative medicine. Only through that research can conventional medical providers know which therapies to recommend to their patients. Only through that research can the public truly know which treatments are safe and effective.

Ultimately I decided to pursue a two-year research fellowship and a master's degree in public health with the goal of obtaining the skills necessary to do research and further the integration of nonconventional and conventional medicine. Unfortunately I soon realized that it was not quite that easy. Good research takes years and costs significant amounts of money. Clearly, multiple agencies are funding research on alternative medicine. Congress has established the National Center for the Study of Complementary and Alternative Medicine under the National Institutes of Health, and the amount and quality of research on alternative treatments are increasing exponentially. However, the various types of alternative treatments available are also increasing. No matter how much research is conducted, there will always be numerous treatment options available that have little or no data beyond anecdotal evidence to support their use. There will always be treatments being utilized that will ultimately be shown to be safe and effective as well as ones that will be harmful and futile.

Many treatments are from healing traditions that have developed over hundreds, if not thousands, of years through a process of trial and error on thousands of patients. Acupuncture, a traditional Chinese medicine utilized for thousands of years, is an example of an alternative medicine that is just now being researched and shown to be effective for many ailments, such as nausea caused by chemotherapy or pregnancy. Other treatments such as *ma huang* (or ephedra) to assist with weight loss *may* be efficacious but when used improperly are potentially dangerous (there have been more than 50 reported deaths). Other treatments are newly invented or conceived. Although some of these treatments will ultimately be shown to be of value, individuals who seek to take advantage of a vulnerable public are often marketing fraudulent products or interventions. The Internet has led to increased empowerment of the public through access to an endless amount of medical information. Unfortunately it has also led to access to a seemingly endless amount of inaccurate or potentially misleading health information.

Traditionally the public has turned to physicians and other health care providers for reliable information on health-related matters. But multiple studies have shown that the majority of people who use alternative medicine do so without telling their physicians or other health care providers. This occurs for many reasons. Most health care providers do not ask about alternative medicine use, perhaps because of a lack of knowledge about the subject matter and a desire not to appear uninformed. This omission often gives the impression that the subject is not important or they simply do not wish to know. At times physicians may be dismissive of such therapies because of a perception that there is a lack of credible and authoritative evidence of their effectiveness.

Patients, on the other hand, tend to believe that it is unimportant for health care providers to know about their use of alternative treatments. They often believe that the alternative therapy is irrelevant to the biomedical treatment course. They may think that a decision to pursue an alternative treatment does not require input from the conventional medical establishment, since they believe these therapies are not truly harmful. Still others hesitate to speak openly about their use of or desire to use alternative medicine because of concern that their questions may be dismissed or they may be viewed as ungrateful, unrealistic, or gullible.

Regardless of the reason, lack of communication about alternative medicine is yet another obstacle to a strong doctor-patient relationship, in this era of managed care and the seven-minute office visit. If the public cannot turn to the conventional medical establishment, turn to their own physicians or other health care providers for reliable information and open discussion about alternative medicine, then to whom? The conventional medical establishment has an obligation to protect the public from harm without limiting access to potentially beneficial alternative treatment options.

Clearly the public's desire for and utilization of alternative medicine are increasing. In 1997 there were 629 million visits to alternative medicine practitioners, a 20 percent increase from seven years earlier, and more visits than to U.S. primary care physicians during the same year. In the United States, more than $27 billion is spent annually on alternative medicine. The public has the freedom of choice to pursue alternative treatments. However, without reliable, credible sources of information, it is challenging for the individual to make informed health care decisions. Discussing one's use of alternative medicine with one's health care provider is an opportunity to share values, explanatory models, lifestyle, health beliefs, and goals for care, all of which not only are clinically relevant but also contribute to strengthening the health care provider–patient relationship.

Many conventional practitioners, medical centers, health care systems, and universities are beginning to recognize the public's desire for information about and increased access to alternative medicine. In 1998, after finishing my training, I was fortunate enough to have the opportunity to pursue my dream of a more integrated health care system and was hired to develop a program in alternative medicine for the Saint Barnabas Health Care System in New Jersey. After much consideration, we chose to call the clinical center the Siegler Center for Integrative Medicine, as opposed to Alternative or Complementary Medicine. More than just a matter of semantics, unlike *alternative*, *integrative* implies the combination of conventional medicine or biomedicine with certain validated alternative treatments through an evidence-based approach.

Although the center is involved in research and education to a limited degree, the primary focus is on providing integrative medicine. Patients can undergo a conventional medical evaluation as well as see an acupuncturist, nutritionist, massage therapist, clinical herbalist, or mind-body practitioner (licensed clinical social worker or Ph.D. psychologist). The more I practice medicine in this setting, the more I find myself returning to the principles I found to be most effective in maintaining my own health and quality of life. Namely I focus on trying to help people find their path. That path always tends to have physical, mental, and spiritual components.

Of course at times a patient enters my office with tennis elbow and is quickly referred for a trial of acupuncture. However, it is more common that I will see someone with low back pain who not only gets a referral for acupuncture, but also is sent to the nutritionist because of obesity and unhealthy eating habits, to the Wellness Center to address deconditioning and a sedentary lifestyle, and to the mind-body practitioner to learn meditation or guided visualization to address poorly managed stress. I ask patients to ask themselves, "What gives my life meaning? What gives my life purpose?" Without taking this "holistic" approach, it is difficult to find true health and wellness. The answer for most people is not solely contained in a bottle, whether that bottle contains a medication or an herb.

I find practicing in this fashion to give me the same sense of fulfillment that I had when I was teaching martial arts. I also found myself longing for a more academic environment, where I could focus on teaching not only patients, but also health care providers. I found myself eager to get involved in the research that will provide the evidence-based framework for integrative medicine to grow upon. Therefore, in July 2002 I accepted the position of executive director for the Center for the Study of Alternative and Complementary Medicine (CSACM) at the University of Medicine and Dentistry of New Jersey. CSACM is just one example of a university-based center committed to research and education in the area of alternative medicine.

The more centers like the Siegler Center and CSACM open and are successful, the more the conventional medical community is able to accept and even embrace new ideas about how to care for patients. Conventional medicine is going through a transition. A more humane physician who respects patient autonomy is replacing the paternalistic, all-knowing physician. As science increases our understanding and our ability to treat disease as never before, we continue to be forced to reconsider that science. The hormone replacement controversy is one example of this. We continue to struggle with finding a balance among science, economics, and patient-centered humanistic care.

This transition, like most change, is neither all good nor all bad. Few would argue that a more patient-centered health care system in which patients have autonomy is a bad thing, but patient autonomy has a price. For the individual to make health care decisions that he or she feels are in his or her best interest, that individual must take the responsibility of being fully informed. This applies whether the treatment is conventional or alternative. It is through comprehensive, reliable information that one is able to begin to find the correct path.

It is for that reason that I am honored to be able to write this Foreword. It is my hope that this reference will be used as a tool to help people inform themselves and get onto the right path: a tool that health care providers can use to educate themselves, a tool that will help foster communication about alternative medicine between health care providers and the public.

—Adam Perlman, M.D., M.P.H.
Executive Director, Institute for
Complementary and Alternative
Medicine; Assistant Professor,
UMDNJ-School of Health Related
Professions, Newark, New Jersey

PREFACE

Shortly before I began research for this book on alternative and complementary medicine, I informed a dear friend of the pending task. His first comment was "How many volumes?"

Those three words would haunt me throughout the project. One book hardly scratches the surface; therefore my objectives were to compile up-to-date information on and explanations of as many alternative, complementary, or integrative healing methods as possible and to present them in an unbiased and accessible A-to-Z format. That numerous books on the subject—from single topics to comprehensive references—already existed, was intimidating in itself, so my contribution became embracing them all. In the precise spirit of alternative medicine, I wished to offer readable entries that would not only inform, but perhaps also inspire people to have a go at a healing method that might turn out to be effective for them but that they had never heard of before. I also wished to present the seemingly infinite possibilities for healing treatments to physicians and other healers, and introduce the diverse healers to one another.

I also hoped to create something of a "botanical-garden" effect by gathering in one book a multitude of ideas and disciplines that have been established by great thinkers past and present. In the course of such gathering I found myself riveted, fascinated by the breadth and depth of healing as it has evolved throughout the history of humankind. From the most preposterous to the most solid, practical concepts, healing has always been a fundamental aspect of life. We learn in our high school sociology classes that self-preservation is a primary human drive, and today we add to our efforts for self-preservation what has become universally known as the connection between mind and body. The mind-body connection, then, plays a huge part in the whole of alternative medicine. In fact, any method involving mind-body-spirit is often the alternative.

As I see it, ideal medicine is a combination of whatever treatments work for an individual, a healer who accurately perceives and offers those particular treatments, and the willingness of both healer and patient to supplant illness with wellness. All over the country, new versions of and combinations of healing/wellness methods are forming—yoga/pilates (at times I've heard it called "yogalates,") for example. "Mommy and Me" yoga, meditation, tai chi, martial arts, and other types of classes are cropping up at specialized schools, preschools, day-care centers, community fitness and wellness centers and after-school programs. One of my personal dreams as a health care professional is that one day, yoga—not to be confused with any religious affiliation—will be taught as part of every core curriculum in our schools on every educational level. More new ideas for relieving and managing stress and for strengthening our immune systems have developed since this book was first published. New findings come out almost daily in the media about new and established treatment or wellness methods. It's almost impossible to keep up, but happily I contribute as best I can to helping people open their minds to a significant road they may not have taken. And I offer heartfelt praises to others who contribute to the proactive, preventive "combination" philosophy as well. As Norman Cousins wrote in *Anatomy of an Illness:* "Your heaviest artillery will be your will to live. Keep the big gun going."

This book's approach aspires to the celebrated manner and philosophy of William Osler, a physician who would go "unsolicited and unsparingly" to help anyone ill or in distress of any kind. From here, I would like to think at least one reader might invent yet another effective healing method and make certain to let me know about it for the next edition.

ACKNOWLEDGMENTS

I could not have written this volume without the precious support and cooperation of my family, especially Yolanda and Guy Fleming; Johnny and Mitzi Navarra; Tony and Jacquie Munoz; Joe and Rose Treihart, R.N., M.S.; and Dorothy Fox, R.N., Ed.D.; Dr. Andrea Campbell; Sarita ("Bunny") Schuler, M.S.W.; Dr. Donald Gill; Dr. Kenneth Titian; Mary Jo Alburtus, L.C.S.W.; Dr. Arlene Thoma; and all the physicians, nurses, and other health care givers who share their knowledge and experience through books, interviews, and articles; the Facts On File, Inc., editor James Chambers; special thanks to my long-time agent, Faith Hamlin; Dr. Adam Perlman, who so graciously wrote the Foreword; Frederic C. Pachman, Academy of Health Information Professionals, (AHIP), director of Monmouth Medical Center's Medical Library, Long Branch, New Jersey; Victor Zak; Paul Boyd; Donald Bridge, of Savannah, Georgia; Betty Sorrentino, Mona Wichman, Sallie and Stan Tillman, Denise Walker, Trista Clayton, Chris and Vicki Reidemeister, Lee and Diane West, Tommy Noble, Charlotte Yingling, and Jim and Teresa Sanford—my beloved "Rumson gang"; Dorie Leonardi; Cynthia Schooley, and Reba Justice, of Cumming, Georgia. I also respectfully acknowledge my late mentors Sal Foderaro, Clarence Holbrook Carter, and Dr. Myron A. Lipkowitz, because every principle they represented continues to bestow a positive effect on me, particularly Sal's motto: *pazienza e coraggio*. Most definitely patience and courage loom large when one applies the mind-body concept to daily life. I also wish to extend love and a unique gratitude to my husband, Robert Kern. Thank you, all.

INTRODUCTION

D.H. Lawrence wrote in his poem "Healing," "I am not a mechanism, an assembly of various sections. And it is not because the mechanism is working wrongly, that I am ill. I am ill because of wounds to the soul, to the deep emotional self" (*The Complete Poems of D. H. Lawrence.* New York: Penguin, 1914–1977).

This is testimony to what a good portion of the population now refers to as "the mind-body connection." Although Hippocrates, considered to be the "father of medicine," said, "I would rather know what kind of person has a disease than what kind of disease a person has," the medical community had long pooh-poohed anything but traditional Western practices that have been traditionally and largely based on prescription drugs, surgery, chemotherapy, and other treatments developed from scientific research.

Traditional medicine has accomplished and continues to accomplish phenomenal strides in all aspects of medicine. However, many patients who found no relief from traditional treatment began to seek help elsewhere—that is, in modalities that claimed no hard and fast scientific proof, but only a huge sweep of anecdotal success. After being generally shunned as quacks for decades, chiropractic physicians suddenly came into their own because people reported that after the hands-on treatment, their symptoms subsided or disappeared. Word spread, and now visits to a chiropractor are covered by most leading health insurance companies. In other words, chiropractic entered and took root in the mainstream, as have acupuncture, acupressure, and other Asian methods of healing, along with massage, hydrotherapy, therapeutic touch, nutritional therapy, hypnosis, osteopathy, relaxation techniques, guided imagery and visualization, aromatherapy, homeopathy, meditation, yoga, and hundreds of other approaches to combating disease and promoting well-being. The public calls these "alternative medicines," resonating with the part of the Constitution of the World Health Organization (WHO) that says, "Health is a state of complete physical, mental and social well-being, and not merely the absence of disease or infirmity."

In *Taber's Cyclopedic Medical Dictionary*, a widely respected reference, alternative medicine is defined as "approaches to medical diagnosis and therapy that have not been developed by use of generally accepted methods of validating their effectiveness. Included are a great number of 'systems,' including manipulative medicine, ayurveda, shiatsu, hypnosis, biofeedback, acupuncture, acupressure, holistic medicine, macrobiotics, rolfing, Christian Science, reflexotherapy, homeopathy, aroma therapy, and faith healing. This is not to say that, were these methods subjected to scientific study, all of them would be found to be ineffective." According to the American Cancer Society website on complementary and alternative therapies, June 18, 2002, *alternative* refers to "treatments promoted as cancer 'cures' but still unproven because they haven't been scientifically tested or because tests show they're ineffective or harmful," and *complementary* to "treatments used to support other evidence-based therapies. Instead of curing cancer, complementary treatments help control symptoms, reduce stress, or improve well-being." Furthermore the term *integrative medicine* refers to "combinations of complementary and evidence-based treatment." (www.cancer.org/eprise/main/docroot/ETO/content/ETO_5_1_Introduction).

A recent U.S. Senate hearing was held on alternative medicine practices, many of which are still resented or denounced by the American Medical Association. But many medical schools throughout the country now see fit to include courses on patients' emotional issues, nutrition (not historically a standard medical-school course), and the like, and acknowledge that, indeed, there is a mind-body connection working at top speed. Many physicians have produced books and articles on alternative, complementary, and integrative practice in the name of "medical freedom," as Burton Goldberg, editor of *Alternative Medicine: A Definitive Guide* (Celestial Arts, Berkeley, Calif., 2002), put it, and many have acquired additional degrees and certification in alternative methods. Dr. Bernie Siegel, a renowned oncologist and best-selling author, documented his experiences with what he says is obviously a connection between the palpable, visible, audible human body and mysterious forces and mechanisms interpreted as "mind." Other physicians who have had the courage to come forward and report their findings that support this concept include Dr. Deepak Chopra, Dr. Larry Dossey, Dr. Andrew Weil, Dr. Brian Weiss, Dr. Elisabeth Kübler-Ross, Dr. Wayne Dyer, Dr. Dean Ornish, Dr. C. Norman Shealy, and hundreds of others. Finally, in the 21st century, mind-body ideas not only have resurfaced, but also have established themselves much as they were set forth by the ancients— Imhotep, Galen, Plato, Aristotle, to name a few— and by prominent figures such as Florence Nightingale, who wrote that health is a balance of body, mind, and spirit, and that illness may as easily be caused by emotional needs as by a disease.

Richard Gerber, M.D., author of *A Practical Guide to Vibrational Medicine* (Quill / HarperCollins Publishers, New York, 2000), brings Nightingale's ideas to the fore not only in terms of holism, but in terms of the latest scientific thinking. "According to the new perspective of Einsteinian and quantum physics, the biochemical molecules that make up the physical body are actually a form of vibrating energy," Gerber wrote. "During the early part of the twentieth century, Albert Einstein came up to the startling conclusion that matter and energy were actually interconvertible and interchangeable. His famous $E = mc_2$ mathematically described how matter and energy were interrelated. Einstein said matter and energy were, in fact, two different forms of the same thing. At the time Einstein came up with this conclusion, few scientists could entirely understand its magnitude. . . . Since all energy vibrates and oscillates at different rates, then, at least at the atomic level, the human body is really composed of different kinds of vibrating energy. . . . [V]ibrational medicine is an approach to the diagnosis and treatment of illness based upon the idea that we are all unique energy systems. . . . The concept of the body as a complex energetic system is part of a new scientific worldview gradually gaining acceptance in the eyes of modern medicine."

And in the eyes of mainstream America as well. In the spirit of Frank Sinatra's affable remark, "I'm for whatever gets you through the night," it has been reported that eight of 10 patients have tried alternative treatments, and of those, three-quarters reported success. Given the thousands upon thousands of alternative practitioners, Americans seem more than willing to try "whatever works." Often this means combining traditional Western medicine with alternatives. In his book, *Radical Healing: Integrating the World's Great Therapeutic Traditions to Create a New Transformative Medicine,* Rudolph Ballentine, M.D., says that the integration and interaction of Western and Eastern medicines make for an exciting path: " 'Radical Healing' is built on these unifying concepts; they are the practical essence of a medicine that is simple and universal, rooted in the perennial principle of healing as personal evolution," Ballentine wrote. "Each of the great healing traditions has arisen in its own culture to help resolve problems peculiar to that setting, so each—e.g., Ayurveda, homeopathy, Traditional Chinese Medicine, European and Native American herbology, nutrition, and psychotherapeutic bodywork—has its weaknesses as well as strengths. By integrating them, superimposing one upon another in layer after layer of complementary perspectives and techniques, we can arrive at an amalgam that is far more potent and thorough than any one of them taken alone."

The former president of the American Holistic Nursing Association, Veda Andrus, said resistance to alternative medicine in part is related to the "set ways" of the American health care system and lack of education. But those set ways are changing as the concept of mind-body connection grows stronger; even West Point "plebes" are instructed in *The West Point Candidate Book,* by William L. Smallwood (Beacon Books, Ariz., 1990), to realize that academic, military, and virtually any success evolves from a positive mindset in the face of difficulty and daunting challenge. Chapter 3 is entitled "Mental Preparation Is Most Important."

One of the most influential and beloved proponents of positive life change based on a better-educated attitude is the author and television personality Dr. Phillip C. McGraw, Ph.D. In *Self Matters: Creating Your Life from the Inside Out* (Simon and Schuster Source, New York, 2001), McGraw gives the basis for a self-improvement strategy that easily applies to choosing health care: "Trust that you are the best judge, by far, of what is best for you. At the same time, be ruthless about testing your thoughts. Verify that your own internal responses and interpretations will stand up to the test of authenticity. . . . Give yourself permission to generate as many alternative responses as possible. . . . Pursue only those that are Triple-A (Authentically Accurate Alternative). Replace any response that causes you trouble and pain with one that moves you toward what you want, need, and deserve." With all that is available to us in our hungry-for-information culture, McGraw advocates accountability and the courage to identify and evaluate options. "Insight without action," he wrote, "is worse than being totally asleep at the switch."

As an antidote for lack of awareness or information, the present *Encyclopedia of Complementary and Alternative Medicine* provides a comprehensive source of definitions, explanations, and perspectives from ancient to modern in an accessible for-

mat. If you come across an isolated term pertaining to alternative or complementary medicine, you can look it up within these pages for identification and cross-reference. The Appendixes also provide at-a-glance information guides on various aspects of the integrative approach to both wellness and illness.

Part of gaining perspective on the current American view of alternative medicines lies in a glimpse at some pertinent statistics provided by the Foundation for the Advancement of Innovative Medicine (FAIM):

- Sixty-nine percent of Americans use unconventional medical therapies (Stanford University National Survey, 1998).
- Sixty-seven percent of health maintenance organizations (HMOs) offer at least one form of complementary alternative care.
- Sixty percent of physicians have referred patients to complementary care practitioners.
- Twenty-nine health insurers and HMOs cover alternative therapies, including Blue Cross of Washington and Alaska, Blue Cross of California, California Pacific, Catholic HealthCare West, HealthNet, Kaiser Permanente, Mutual of Omaha, Oxford Health Plans, and Prudential. There is also an organization called Alternative Health Benefit Services, based in California, that is geared toward creating greater credibility and access for less invasive, more natural health care, and to enable all Americans to select the type of medical care and physician/medical provider of their choice. The group is also parent to Holistic Health Insurance & Financial Services, Alternative Health Insurance Administrators, the National Marketing Association, Alliance for Alternatives in Healthcare, Alliance for Natural Health, Actuarially Sound Benefit Consultants, and the Holistic Health Network.
- Chiropractors are licensed in all 50 states, and 11 states mandate that health plans include chiropractic benefits.
- Sixty-four percent of all medical schools offer courses in alternative medicines.
- Eighty percent of medical students want training in alternative medicines.

- Fifty-six percent of Americans surveyed believe their health plans should cover alternative therapies.
- The alternative medicine marketplace is currently valued at more than $24 billion, with a growth rate of close to 15 percent per year (Rauber, *Modern Healthcare*, September 1998).
- Acupuncturists are licensed in 34 states.
- Fifty percent of physicians surveyed expect to begin or increase usage of homeopathic and holistic recommendations over the next year; because patient acceptance is greater for these therapies, better compliance results (Health Products Research, Inc., Aug. 11, 2000 survey of 3200 physicians).
- Seventy percent of family physicians want training in alternative therapies.
- Eight states have passed health freedom (practice protection) bills for M.D.s and D.O.s.
- Naturopaths are licensed in 11 states.
- There are 17 student chapters of the American Holistic Veterinary Medical Association among the 27 U.S. veterinary schools.

In addition, in December 1995, the American Medical Association passed the following resolution: "Unconventional Medical Care in the U.S." The AMA encourages the Office of Alternative Medicine of the National Institutes of Health to determine by objective scientific evaluation the efficacy and safety of practices and procedures of unconventional medicine; and encourages its members to become better informed regarding the practices and techniques of alternative or unconventional medicine (Policies of House of Delegates—1-95; H-480.973; BOT Rep. 15-A-94, Reaffirmed and Modified by Sub. Res. 514, 1-95).

In *Timeless Healing: The Power and Biology of Belief*, by Dr. Herbert Benson (Scribner, New York, 1996), alternative medicine is given serious due in light of the traditional practice of Western medicine: "Writer Luigi Barzini suggests that Americans are compelled to act because we believe 'the main purpose of a man's life is to solve problems.' Despite the fact that the body is the grandest problem-solver there is, quietly and perpetually sustaining life, overcoming billions of obstacles without our conscious imperatives for it to do so,

we don't trust it. Instead we turn to our medicine cabinets. Our doctors' first impulse is to prescribe something for us, and we fully expect to emerge from these visits with a prescription in hand. But at the same time, record numbers of Americans are spending record numbers of their health care dollars on unconventional healers—chiropractors, acupuncturists, herbalists, and so on—who they trust will care more about them as individuals than as sums of parts. While some studies show that patients are generally happy with their own doctors, managed care, with its provider lists and required numbers of patients a doctor must see each day, makes this relationship between doctor and patient harder to preserve."

C. Norman Shealy, M.D., Ph.D., author of *The Illustrated Encyclopedia of Natural Remedies*, pointed out that the physician's role is to be a "triage officer," one who quickly assesses the status of patients and what immediate treatment they need. Triage is usually associated with victims of accidents, war, or natural disaster and is geared to saving as many people as possible. "A triage officer would stand at the door when a patient was significantly ill and advise when medicine or surgery was truly needed to save life or function," stated Eugene A. Stead, Jr., Shealy's professor of medicine. "Dr. Stead advised that when life and function are not at risk, as in the vast majority of symptomatic illnesses, the patient should 'go into the department stores and choose that which most appeals.'" The "department store," of course, is his analogy for all the alternative methods of healing that are now available to us.

Bolstering that "department store" is the National Center for Complementary and Alternative Medicine (NCCAM) at the National Institutes of Health (NIH), formerly known as the Office of Alternative Medicine (OAM), dating to 1992. The NCCAM was established by Congress in 1998 to stimulate, develop, and support research on complementary and alternative medicines for the benefit of the public. According to NCCAM's website, the organization's objectives include research (collaborating with other NIH and federal agencies to advance the scientific study of alternative medicine, identifying and investigating promising understudied areas, and establishing a global network for research); research training (implementing a comprehensive research training plan, providing research training and clinical fellowships, educating complementary/alternative medicine scientists about biomedical research methods, and educating conventional researchers about the nature and principles of alternative medicines), and communications (establishing effective partnerships with complementary/alternative medicine researchers, health professionals, and the public; disseminating information along with other federal agencies; and distributing scientifically based information about research, practices, and findings to health care providers and consumers).

A well-known and respected neurosurgeon from Springfield, Missouri, Shealy founded the American Holistic Medical Association (AHMA) in 1978, with the mission to provide a "common community" for medical doctors who embrace the philosophy of treating the whole biopsychosocial person. The following are the 12 principles of the AHMA: (1) to use safe, effective diagnostic and treatment options; (2) search for underlying causes of disease, as is preferable to treating only symptoms; (3) use the Hippocratic idea (including that the life forces pervade all of nature) of finding out what kind of person has a disease; (4) evoke the patient's innate ability to heal and promote prevention; (5) view illness not as an isolated event but as a dysfunction of the whole person; (6) establish a high-quality relationship with the patient and encourage the patient to take responsibility for his or her health; (7) consider the needs, desires, awareness, and insight of both patient and physician; (8) influence patients by setting an example; (9) view illness, pain, and dying as learning opportunities for both patients and doctors; (10) promote love, hope, humor, and enthusiasm and release fear, anger, grief, hostility, shame, greed, and depression; (11) adopt an attitude of unconditional love for all; and (12) pursue the highest qualities of the physical, environmental, mental, emotional, spiritual, and social aspects of being human.

The establishment of this and other organizations promoting alternative and complementary medicine would have likely been a source of personal satisfaction to the late author Norman Cousins, well known for books such as *Anatomy of an Illness* (New York: Norton, 1979) and *Head First: The Biology of Hope and the Healing Power of the Human Spirit* (New York: Dutton, 1989). A teacher at the UCLA School of Medicine and contributing essayist for *The Power to Heal: Ancient Arts & Modern Medicine* (New York: Prentice Hall, 1990), Cousins explained, "Clearly, in our modern age, treatment for any disease requires the best that medical science has to offer; all the emotional determination in the world usually falls short without prompt and consistent medical intervention. But just as clearly, treating physical illness without paying corresponding attention to emotional needs can have only a partial effect. More than 2,000 years after the death of Hippocrates, we are coming back to the original Hippocratic ideal of the patient not as a passive vessel into which the physician pours therapeutic skills and medicaments, but as a sovereign human being capable of generating powerful responses to disease. These powerful responses won't reverse every incidence of disease or illness; otherwise, we would live forever. But by beginning to recognize these powers, we are enhancing vital elements of the recovery process."

Cousins was a high-profile American proponent of combining conventional and alternative medicines for years before his death in 1990 at age 78. When in the 1970s he was afflicted with ankylosing spondylitis, a life-threatening degenerative spinal disease, and given a dim prognosis, he decided to take massive doses of vitamin C in addition to his physician's treatments and introduced laughter as the best medicine of all. He deluged his days with Marx Brothers films, *Candid Camera* episodes, humorous books—anything and everything funny that elicited belly laughter for at least 10 minutes at a time. After each laugh session, his doctor tested Cousins's blood sedimentation rate (an indicator of the status of inflammation in the body) and found that it dropped consistently, until, in 1976, Cousins recovered from the disease. The first published account of this experience appeared in the *New England Journal of Medicine*, and Cousins received an honorary degree in medicine from

Yale University. Since then, laughter has actually been scientifically measured and shown to reduce stress and pain by creating changes in certain hormonal and immune system levels. In addition, increased antibody production in the upper respiratory tract; an increase of lymphocytes, cells that fight tumors and viruses; and the lung-expanding, heart rate–increasing exercise of laughing all serve to encourage people to heed Proverbs 17:22: "A merry heart doeth good like a medicine."

Other respected figures in our society also contribute admirably to a more global view of healing. The Harvard-educated novelist and filmmaker Michael Crichton, M.D., also a guest essayist in *The Power to Heal*, wrote:

> Accompanying the use of more refined technology to prevent and treat illness, psychoimmunology, the science that deals with the mind's role in helping the immune system to fight disease, will become a vitally important clinical field in the years to come—perhaps the most important medical field in the twenty-first century, supplanting our present emphasis on oncology and cardiology. The encouragement of healthy thinking may eventually become an integral aspect of treatment for everything from allergies to liver transplants. What all this means is that our present concept of medicine will disappear. Pressed both by patients and its own advancing technology, medicine will change to focus from treatment to enhancement, from repair to improvement, from diminished sickness to increased performance.

For all its seemingly newfound accolades and anecdotal successes, what we call alternative medicine really began when humankind first recognized the need to deal with and counteract abnormalities and ailments that emerged in their lives. The ancients developed their own medicines, treatments that ultimately involved acknowledgment of a mind-body connection, from whatever nature provided.

In 1933, the editor-in-chief Bernarr McFadden wrote in his foreword to the *Encyclopedia of Health* (McFadden Book Company, Inc., New York): "Only recently has it begun to dawn on the world that health is something within the control of the individual, and with it vitality of mind and heart and all the personal attraction that goes with them. People in general have given little attention to health until it was destroyed. Men and women waited until they were ill before they thought of the proper care of their bodies. Then they called in a doctor and there ended their responsibility, or at least so they thought. The idea that they alone might be responsible for their health or disease and that responsibility for their recovery rested on them and not on the doctor was foreign to their thought. To them health and disease were largely matters of chance. All this has passed, or is rapidly passing. Health and disease are now known to be subject to laws eternal and unchangeable, as are all laws of Nature. Individual responsibility for one's own health or disease is coming to be generally recognized. With the generally growing recognition of this responsibility has come an increasing interest in ways and means of preserving and restoring health. People are interested in learning how to care for their own health. They are no longer content to place an almost unlimited faith in potions and pills."

It is somewhat mind-boggling to find literature dating back so many years that pinpoints the medical climate of today. Does it imply that we have stagnated to a certain degree in our thinking on the logic of integrative methods? Or does it grant that perhaps this "New Age" simply means we are at last opening our arms in a more unified, consistent way to all the healing methods available on our planet since the beginning of time? Alternative and complementary medicine need not be "on the fringe" but rather a meritorious component among a staggering array of modern comforts and conveniences. Finally a visible force in the mainstream, the field of alternative therapies pours into American homes by way of television and other broadcast media, newspapers, books, and magazines, including *Alternative Therapies in Health and Medicine*, a peer-reviewed journal edited by Larry Dossey, M.D., and *Alternative Medicine*, a consumer publication of AlternativeMedicine.com. Both magazines have impressive advisory boards, an undeniable proclamation of support for the universal mission—well-being, however we choose to accomplish it. The American psychologist and philosopher William James

(1842–1910) summed it up so many years ago: "The great revolution of our generation is the discovery that human beings, by changing the inner attitudes of their minds, can change the outer aspects of their lives." So be it, even as we beckon alternative and complementary options with "Show me!" as though we were all diehard Missourians. Although Albert Einstein observed, "Few are those who see with their own eyes and feel with their own hearts," many of us have in fact grown willing to accept and choose options that defy specific explanation, and still more are beginning to follow that lead. Perhaps in light of this en masse acceptance—this breakthrough surrender—we will create a climate that lends itself to our finding the answers and the improvements we want. Now, at last, ours is a relentless, all-embracing quest for healing and flourishing.

ENTRIES A–Z

aama A term in Ayurvedic medicine, also known as *aamdosh*, which refers to the accumulation of undigested or incompletely digested food—by-products of metabolism—which in turn may possibly act as antigens, or foreign substances, in the body. *Aama* is said to cause indigestion, bad breath, a coated tongue, and other gastrointestinal problems. The accumulation of these unusable "remains" in the body is also said to instigate an immune-system problem, in which they may be attacked by antibodies, thus causing the *aama* sites to swell, lodge themselves in body tissues, and create dysfunction. For example, one Ayurvedic belief is that *aama* harbored in the joints induces arthritic symptoms. Ayurvedic cleansing techniques may provide an antidote. A homeopathic belief relates physical *aama* to psychological *aama*, involving stress or any type of mental "overload," as a possible cause of physical symptoms.

See also AYURVEDA; HOMEOPATHY.

abortifacient Any agent, substance, or method intended to induce an abortion, that is, deliberate termination of a pregnancy, usually during the earliest stage. The drug RU486 (Mifepristone), for example, which is used in some countries, may be administered in conjunction with a prostaglandin suppository or injection before 47 days have elapsed since a woman's last menstrual period if abortion is desired.

However, various methods of alternative medicine attempt to treat miscarriage, the unexplained, spontaneous, and undesired loss of an embryo or fetus. For symptoms of distress, shock, bleeding, and pain, practitioners of alternative medicine may employ astringent remedies to discourage bleeding, herbal sedatives, aromatherapy, Bach Flower Remedies, the homeopathic substances ignatia and staphisagria, massage, color therapy, and other methods believed to have a healing effect.

Accreditation Commission for Acupuncture and Oriental Medicine See Appendix I.

acupoints Also called acupuncture points or trigger points, specific places along a network of nerves and other bodily structures used as landmarks over which to apply pressure, as in acupressure; insert acupuncture needles; or apply other methods to the skin in order to release the flow of energy so an ailing or dysfunctional organ or body part may heal.

See also ACUPRESSURE; ACUPUNCTURE.

acupressure An ancient Asian technique of natural healing, at least 5000 years old, involving the use of the hands and fingers to apply pressure on or to massage body certain meridians in order to unblock stagnant energy that may be causing pain. The third most popular method for treating pain and illness in the world and considered a painless, nontoxic method for redirecting *ch'i*, the Chinese word for energy, acupressure (and its close associate acupuncture) draws upon the body meridians, also known as energy pathways, as connections or correlations with body organs and functions. When *ch'i* flows unimpeded throughout the body, well-being results. If the energy is thwarted for any reason, illness results. Related to acupuncture without the use of needles, acupressure is said to be effective as disease prevention as well as a component of traditional treatments for arthritis, carpal tunnel syndrome, chronic pain, symptoms of addiction withdrawal, motion sickness, multiple sclerosis, insomnia, fatigue, bronchitis, colds and flu, arthritis, allergies, pneumonia, toothache, sinusitis, sciatica, nausea, hemorrhoids, ear infection, diarrhea, fever, indigestion—approximately 3,000 maladies altogether.

According to the Complementary Wellness Professional Association (http://www.compwellness.com/eGuide/acupre.htm), "There is a natural source of healing power in everyone. When this healing power is activated, it triggers a series of complicated internal processes producing a healing response. Pain or injury acts to alert the body that damage control is needed, at which point the healing response begins and endorphins are generated to repair the affected area. This increases the heart rate and alters the blood pressure to speed up the elimination of toxins from the damaged area. . . . When applied to specific sore points along the meridians at different points for different conditions, the pressure tricks the body into thinking it has been damaged. The body then produces endorphins to relieve distress in the organs and systems corresponding to the acupressure point . . . and produces a healing response all along the meridian."

The association says that regular, systematic treatment usually gets the best results. Treatment three times each day for five to 10 minutes, or every two hours if necessary, reflects the concept that acupressure's positive effects are cumulative—one cannot overdose because the treatments are safe. However, they are not recommended for administration directly after a meal, and pregnant women should avoid pressure at certain points known as SP 6, Li 4, and St 36. (Pressure points are coded.) *Tui na* is a needleless form of acupressure used particularly for very young children and for those suffering from musculoskeletal distress.

According to *The One Spirit Encyclopedia of Complementary Health* (Hamlyn, London, 2000), acupressure is similar to shiatsu, which means "finger pressure" in Japanese, in that it is meant to trigger the release of *ch'i* along the meridians. It branches off from shiatsu, which includes massage, in that acupressure mostly employs thumb and fingertip pressure on acupuncture points. In clinical studies, acupressure was successfully used to treat morning sickness in 350 women at the Royal Maternity Hospital in Belfast, Ireland, in 1988. "In 1986," the text described, "car factory workers were screened in a study to exclude any with organic disease or infection, and 142 workers with chronic lumbar pain were treated with acupressure daily for 21 days on points along the spine, back and front of legs. A marked improvement was found in 29 percent of patients, 68 patients were cured, while 3.5 percent had no noticeable change. Additional benefits reported included improved sleep." Practitioners of shiatsu and acupressure may also use fingers, palms, elbows, arms, knees, and feet in lieu of the needles used in acupuncture.

Acupressure is also used for animals, particularly for arthritis and hip dysplasia.

See also ACUPUNCTURE.

acupuncture A component of traditional Chinese medicine (TCM) in which extremely fine long needles are inserted into the skin over points corresponding to parts and functions of the body mapped out in a system of meridians. (For example, a point near the wrist is associated with respiration.) The technique is used to reduce pain and promote restoration and bodily well-being. Acupuncture is reported to relieve blockage, pressure, or other ill effects from the body's 14 major meridians, or energy channels. Rendered as *qi* or *ch'i* (pronounced "chee"), the flow of this energy or life force is essential to health. Given a new credibility and acknowledgment by Western practitioners, acupuncture studies suggest that the technique stimulates the release of the body's natural, opiate-like substances called endorphins. Polypeptides produced in the brain, endorphins act as painkillers, at times as effective as morphine or anesthetics, because they bind to opiate receptor sites that involve the perception of pain and increase the threshold for pain. Endorphins and enkephalins, also polypeptides that work as endorphins do, are thought also to contribute to a feeling of well-being.

The author and physician Richard Gerber explained the 12-pathway acupuncture-meridian system as "the body's biocircuitry," through which more than 1,000 acupoints carry the environmental life energy *ch'i*. "This special type of life energy is said to come from three primary sources. Part of our *ch'i* energy comes from the vital-energy reserve we inherit from our parents. This type of 'inherited' life energy is referred to as ancestral *ch'i*. The second source of *ch'i* is absorbed (and produced) from the foods we eat. The third (and possibly the most important) source of *ch'i* comes directly from the environment. A certain amount of *ch'i* is absorbed from our surroundings and taken into the body and the meridian system via the acupuncture points themselves. Acupoints appear to function like tiny energy pores in the skin that absorb this unique environmental subtle energy directly into the meridians, where it is then distributed to the organs of the body." Gerber further explains that the perspective of traditional Chinese medicine on illness is that *ch'i* becomes imbalanced, and acupuncture is one way to rebalance the flow of ch'i energy to whatever organ or bodily structure is dysfunctional.

"The acupuncture points located on the skin also seem to function like miniature electrical relay stations along a vast power line, helping to maintain the flow of energy along each meridian," Gerber wrote; that concept, he believes, requires "a great leap in thinking beyond the limited biomechanistic paradigm of traditional medicine."

Although many traditional practitioners argue that acupuncture treatment for pain, despite its anecdotal success, has more of a placebo effect (which can be extremely powerful) than an actual physical repair result, an expert consensus panel of the National Institutes of Health (NIH) in 1997 agreed from certain studies that acupuncture treatments did relieve nausea and vomiting associated with pregnancy, chemotherapy, and anesthesia; reduced pain after dental surgery; and helped alleviate pain caused by osteoarthritis, headache, carpal tunnel syndrome, fibromyalgia, asthma, and other conditions. Acupuncture is also reported to have positive results in the treatment of addiction withdrawal and in the course of rehabilitation for stroke patients. In addition, the World Health Organization (WHO) reported that sinusitis, the common cold, tonsillitis, eye inflammation, nearsightedness, duodenal ulcer and other gastrointestinal disorders, trigeminal neuralgia, Ménière's disease, tennis elbow, sciatica, rheumatoid conditions, menstrual cramps, radiation illness and other types of environmental poisoning, and speech aphasia may also be treated with acupuncture.

The book *Alternative Medicine: The Definitive Guide* (Celestial Arts, Berkeley, Calif., 2002), says that in 1997, "acupuncture's credibility as a viable medical treatment was bolstered by the U.S. Food and Drug Administration (FDA), which reclassified the acupuncture needle from 'experimental' to 'medical device' status, thereby acknowledging that the acupuncture needle is a safe and effective medical instrument. . . . The FDA estimates that Americans make 9–12 million visits per year to acupuncturists and spend as much as $500 million on acupuncture treatments annually. . . . In the 1970s, under a grant from the NIH, Robert O. Becker, M.D., and the biophysicist Maria Reichmanis were able to prove that electrical currents did indeed flow along the ancient Chinese meridians and that 25% of the acupuncture points existed along those scientifically measurable lines. They reasoned that these points acted as amplifiers to boost the minute electrical signals as they traveled along the body, and that the insertion of a needle could interfere with that flow and thus block the stimulus of pain."

The volume also cited acupuncture as an effective treatment for neck pain, and that a study was conducted with nearly 200 patients suffering from chronic neck pain. Each patient received a half-hour acupuncture treatment five times a week for three weeks; acupuncture proved effective, especially for those who had experienced neck pain for more than five years or who had myofascial pain syndrome (caused by tension in the muscles). Another study, of more than 20,000 patients at the University of California at Los Angeles, indicated that acupuncture lessened the frequency and intensity of migraine and tension headaches.

In general, there are no medical conditions that would preclude the use of acupuncture as a treatment modality, and no known side effects, with the exception of infection resulting from improperly sterilized needles or treatment by an incompetent practitioner. Patients may request disposable needles to eliminate the sterilization issue. For individuals who have a fear of needles, there are laser acupuncture, which uses laser beams instead of needles; ultrasound and light-therapy acupuncture, which use sound waves and light waves in lieu of needles; and electroacupuncture, which uses small electrical currents to stimulate acupoints. An additional technique, called cupping, involves the use of glass, metal, wood, or bamboo cups of varying size. The cups are warmed and placed top-down on an acupoint or any flat area such as the back, abdomen, or legs. The vacuum created by the cups "sucks" the skin so that blood rushes to the point and rebalances the flow of energy. Cupping is said to be most effective for treating bronchitis, colds, and arthritis.

Moxibustion, a term derived from the Japanese word *mokusa*, or "burning herb," is a technique of acupuncture that employs needles to which the heat of a dried herb (moxa) is attached. A tiny stick, roll, or cone-shaped amount of moxa, from the herb mugwort, burns on the head of the needle to send warmth to the acupoint. The moxa, which may also be used without needles but with a small tip, does not touch the skin directly and is reported to be aromatic and a pleasant treatment.

Auricular therapy, revived and improved in the 1960s by the French acupuncturist Dr. Paul Nogier, is a type of acupuncture that focuses exclusively on the ear for pain management and the treatment of migraines, arthritis, and stomach ailments. When Nogier treated patients with sciatica by cauterizing part of their earlobes, he discovered after they reported relief that the technique dated back to ancient Egypt. He also developed an electrical device called a Punctoscope so needles were not required. Also, while small acupuncture needles may be used in the ear, electrotherapy, light therapy, and small, magnetically charged ball bearings (which can be taped over acupoints for long-term, or semipermanent, therapy) may be preferred methods. Auricular therapists, popular in France, say this type of acupuncture helps provide diagnostic information; is less invasive than regular acupuncture, particularly for anxious patients; and is calming and effective against pain.

The theory is that the ear, with its approximately 200–300 acupoints, has the shape of a fetus in the womb and therefore relates to the acupoints in the adult body. The measurable electrical properties of acupuncture points allow practitioners to diagnose problems, and auricular therapy is said to relieve addictions, certain respiratory disorders, labor pains, and pain related to terminal illnesses.

To date, approximately 10,000 acupuncturists in the United States are licensed, registered, or certified, and approximately 3000 medical doctors, both M.D.s and D.O.s, who practice acupuncture. Organizations that set standards and certify practitioners include the Accreditation Commission for Acupuncture and Oriental Medicine and the National Certification Commission for Acupuncture and Oriental Medicine (NCCAOM). (See Appendix I.) Every practitioner has an individual approach, and it is possible that one practitioner, as with any health care provider, may be more suited to a particular patient than another. The NIH suggests that the typical gauge for effectiveness is 10 sessions, and chronic pain relief should be experienced from acupuncture after six treatments. Some conditions such as asthma may require months of acupuncture before a patient perceives relief. Acupuncture may be combined with other conventional or alternative treatments.

"Many unconventional treatments have been around for a very long time," writes Dr. Herbert Benson in *Timeless Healing* (Scribner, New York, 1996), "but their positive effects, if present and above those of remembered wellness, are still questionable. Acupuncture is a case in point. If its inherent healing effects were equivalent to those of proven scientific remedies, they would already have been recognized by Western scientific medicine."

The licensed acupuncturist and author Harriet Beinfield, and her coauthor Efrem Korngold, also a licensed acupuncturist and practitioner of osteopathic manipulative medicine, wrote in *Between Heaven and Earth: A Guide to Chinese Medicine* (Ballantine Books, New York, 1991): "While neurological and hormonal hypotheses describe how acupuncture alleviates pain, they do not accurately explain its diverse therapeutic effects. . . . [E]xperiments, including the study of acupuncture-assisted surgery, have shown that acupuncture not only inhibits pain, but also directly affects peripheral microcirculation, rhythm and stroke volume of the heart, blood pressure, levels of circulating immunoglobulins, gastrointestinal peristalsis, secretion of hydrochloric acid, and the production of red and white blood cells. Acupuncture seems to adjust all the physiological processes of the organism, possibly through activation of the homeostatic function of the autonomic nervous system. . . . The central issue from the classical Chinese medical point of view is not why acupuncture works, but rather how and when to use it. The dynamic balance that Chinese medicine equates with health manifests as smooth and constant movement. When *Qi* and *Blood* stagnate, the processes of elimination and regeneration deteriorate, constituting the basic condition underlying many forms of illness. . . .

"Acupuncture is not like a drug that is supposed to produce a discrete and limited result. In Western medicine a given drug or procedure results in a limited, desired effect, plus so-called side effects, which are adverse changes in the organism as a whole. In Chinese medicine, this logic is reversed, so that global changes in the whole organism result in the disappearance of specific symptoms. In acupuncture 'secondary' effects are intended, all part of one continuous process of change."

See also RELAXATION.

affirmations Sentences, phrases, or words that are composed in order to emphasize and reinforce a certain belief, used as a therapeutic device for its emotional force or impact when they are spoken and repeated. According to the self-help author Stuart Wilde, there are four types of affirmations—word, thought, feeling, and action—and there are both positive and negative affirmations. Wilde wrote in his book *Affirmations* (Nacson & Sons PTY LTD, Australia, and White Dove International, Inc., Taos, N. Mex., 1993) that affirmations of word resemble a prayer or mantra, such as "I am the power, I am the light, I control my life." Affirmations of thought, such as Wilde's "I grant myself forgiveness and complete absolution. For my energy has now risen above and beyond any errors I may have made in the past," are geared to calming emotions and evoking the energetic, personal power to transcend difficulties. An example of a heart or feeling affirmation is "My life is heroic. I acknowledge and honor each step I take." Wilde says developing affirmations of feeling increases sensitivity and honesty, as affirmations of action help promote good choices and deeds, as in "In softness I have strength." The author and healer Louise Hay also provides affirmations for personal growth and self-esteem, including "I deserve love." Affirmations may be used as a component of self-healing, positive thinking, meditation, psychotherapy, relaxation, and other alternative techniques.

agni Ayurvedic term referring to the element of fire, the central bodily fire, the digestive fire, or the pitta temperament.

See also AYURVEDA.

ahara rasa The "nutrient plasma" that contains nutrition for all the *dhatus* (basic vital bodily structures) in Ayurvedic medicine.

See also AYURVEDA.

Alexander Technique A type of holistic training for stress reduction developed by the Australian actor Frederick Matthias Alexander (1869–1955, born in Tasmania), who believed that "every man, woman and child holds the possibility of physical perfection; it rests with each of us to attain it by personal understanding and effort." Also referred to at times as posture training, the Alexander Technique involves a process of mind-body connection and of reeducation of what Alexander determined to be the body's innate poise and grace in order to control posture, balance, and action. When a person's body does not move or rest harmoniously, he taught, stressors such as tension and emotional problems may become worse or evolve into more serious health problems.

As a result of a seemingly intractable laryngitis during his acting career, Alexander discovered that although he had lost his voice onstage, he was able to speak normally when not performing. Using several mirrors so he could observe any differences between his onstage and offstage experiences, he realized that as he gave a dramatic reading, he had the tendency to suck in air and pull his head down, actions that put pressure on his vocal cords and adversely affected his spine, back, and breathing pattern. As he spoke normally, he observed that his posture was similar, but significantly less tense. He concluded that undue tension in the head, neck, and back created an imbalance that could lead to physical ailments. After he developed specific ways to improve general body use, including the correlation between the head and neck and the rest of the body as a key principle that he called "The Primary Control," Alexander began to teach fellow performers and others. With his vocal cord problems eliminated, he felt inspired to go to London in 1901 and thereafter to America to develop further and teach his technique. Training courses on the Alexander Technique exist in many countries, and more than 2000 teachers are practicing throughout the world, according to Noel Kingsley, who offers more information by E-mail: noel@ale tech.co.uk. Other sources include http://www.alexandertechnique.com/at/ and Joan Arnold, a certified teacher of the Alexander Technique in New York City (E-mail: JoanArn@aol.com).

Arnold wrote, "We all have unconscious movement habits. Without realizing it, we put undue pressure on ourselves. We use more force than we need to lift a coffee pot or a weight bar. We slouch as we sit, unaware that our way of doing things gives out bodies a certain look. We blame body problems on activities—carpal tunnel syndrome on computer work, tennis elbow on tennis. But often it is how we do something that creates the problem, not the activity itself. An Alexander Technique teacher helps you see what in your movement style contributes to your recurring difficulties—whether it's a bad back, neck and shoulder pain, restricted breathing, perpetual exhaustion, or limitations in performing a task or sport. Analyzing your whole movement pattern—not just your symptom—the teacher alerts you to habits of compression in your characteristic way of sitting, standing and walking. He or she then guides you . . . to move in a freer, more integrated way." See Appendix I.

allopathy From the Greek words *allos*, meaning "other," and *pathos*, meaning "disease or suffering," methods for treatment of disease that attempt to counteract the disease or cause of the disease directly. According to *Taber's Cyclopedic Medical Dictionary*, *allopathy* or *allopathic medicine* is an incorrect term used to differentiate the traditional practice of Western medicine from alternative therapies, such as homeopathy. Rudolph Ballentine, M.D., defines *allopathic medicine* in *Radical Healing: Integrating the World's Great Therapeutic Traditions to Create a New Transformative Medicine* (Harmony Books, New York, 1999) as "operating according to the Law of Contraries or opposites, in contradistinction to those approaches that are based on the Law of Similars, which are referred to as *homeopathic*. Treating a fever with cold, for example, is allopathic."

alteratives Substances or agents that promote a gradual change in nutrition or in the body without creating a specific effect of their own.
See also AYURVEDA.

alternative medicine Any method, technique, or practice that promotes the restoration of health and well-being that is not included in conventional, or traditional, Western medicine. Alternative medicine as an entire field maintains there is a mind-body connection that has an important impact on one's ability to prevent illness, regain health, and create a biopsychosocial balance. Homeopathy, chiropractic, Ayurveda, herbal medicine, acupuncture, aromatherapy, and reflexology are among the numerous choices of alternative medicines available. A trend has begun to combine traditional Western medical modalities with one or more alternative treatments, depending upon the condition and needs of individual patients and the effectiveness of the treatments.

ama Ayurvedic term for toxins that affect weakened areas of the body.
See also AYURVEDA.

American Academy of Medical Acupuncture See Appendix I.

American Alliance of Aromatherapy See Appendix I.

American Apitherapy Society See APITHERAPY; Appendix I.

American Aromatherapy Association See Appendix I.

American Association of Acupuncture and Oriental Medicine See Appendix I.

American Center for the Alexander Technique See Appendix I.

American College of Acupuncture & Oriental Medicine See Appendix I.

amma   An ancient Japanese holistic therapy for treating mind, body, and spirit, now called shiatsu. *Amma* therapy schools combine the principles of Oriental medicine for deep tissue manipulation with the application of pressure, friction, and touch to specific joints, energy channels, muscles, ligaments, and joints. *Amma* therapy may also include dietary, detoxification, herbs and supplements, therapeutic exercise, stress, and emotional and spiritual counseling. The chief diagnostic technique of the *amma* therapist is palpation with the hands and fingers in areas where there is dysfunction or pain. Palpation may be performed through clothing. For additional information on *amma* education, you may log on to http://www.natural healers.com/qa/amma.shtml.

See also SHIATSU.

animal-assisted therapy   The technique of using dogs, cats, and other animals to cuddle and interact with traumatized or catastrophically ill patients of all ages in order to heighten emotional comfort and help people reconnect with normal activity after a significant event, such as natural disaster or war. The Delta Society, which is an organization that teaches how to use therapy dogs, may be contacted at 425-226-7357 or www.deltasociety.org.

antibiotics, herbal   Substances extracted from natural sources used for the treatment of infection or ailment caused by microbial invasion in the body. For example, antimicrobial properties are attributed to the Native American herbs echinacea, goldenseal, osha, *Lomatium dissectum*, usnea, and saw palmetto.

See also HOMEOPATHY.

anxiety   An emotional disorder that may include physiological symptoms or illness, usually affecting twice as many women as men. According to the National Center for Health Statistics, as of 1998, drugs prescribed for sufferers of anxiety rank among the 20 drugs most commonly prescribed overall. Some of the most common symptoms of anxiety are hyperventilation, chest tightness or pain, fainting, dizziness, nausea, vomiting, clammy skin, flushing, dry mouth, loss of appetite, headache, abdominal pain, diarrhea, insomnia, and a host of individualized manifestations of stress. Anxiety may also occur as a result of a physical problem, such as metabolic imbalance, hyperthyroidism, prostaglandin deficiency, poor nerve health, smoking, any catastrophic illness such as cancer, and many other diseases, or it may be secondary to posttraumatic stress, obsessive-compulsive, and other psychological disorders.

In the field of complementary medicine, the mind-body connection is taken into consideration when treating an individual presenting signs of panic attack or another stress-related condition regardless of its origin. Relaxation techniques; meditation; Ayurveda; massage; aromatherapy (particularly with essential oils of peppermint, lavender, geranium, bergamot, cinnamon, etc.); acupressure; acupuncture; homeopathic medicines such as aconite, arsenicum, calcarea, and ignatia; nutrition therapy (such as magnesium, calcium, B vitamins, sea minerals, brewer's yeast, sunflower seeds, molasses, carrot-celery juice, wheat germ oil, and garlic); psychotherapy; reflexology; and many other healing methods have been known anecdotally and shown in scientific studies to be effective treatments. Herbal therapies include chamomile, valerian, peppermint, hops, Chinese angelica, white peony root, lady's slipper, rosemary, skullcap, Reishi mushrooms, bee pollen, ginseng, gotu kola, lobelia, and catnip. Flower remedies include elm, aspen, red chestnut, Rescue Remedy, and Emergency Essence.

In her book *Healthy Healing: An Alternative Healing Reference* (Healthy Healing Publications, Carmel Valley, Calif., 1994), Linda G. Rector-Page, N.D., Ph.D., describes depression and anxiety as the mental and emotional state that can stem from as wide a range of causes as there are individuals. For the "inability to cope with prolonged and intense stress, excessive worry, anger and guilt, insomnia, and diminished ability to concentrate," she recommends (1) food therapy, including sufficient protein (about 15 percent of total calorie intake), carrot juice two to three times a week with a pinch of sage and a teaspoon of Bragg's Liquid Aminos, the elimination of sweets, alcohol, and drugs, drinking of bottled water, and a daily mix of lecithin granules, brewer's yeast, wheat germ, and pumpkin seeds; (2) brain oxygenators, including wheat germ oil capsules, glutamine, and germanium with suma; (3) herbal therapy, including royal jelly, evening primrose oil, Bach's Rescue Remedy, gingko biloba, and ginseng; (4) bodywork, including exercise, sunlight, yoga, shiatsu, and breathing exercises; (5) aromatherapy (particularly ylang ylang, basil, jasmine, and geranium); and (6) the cessation of smoking.

See also AUSTRALIAN BUSH FLOWER ESSENCES; BACH FLOWER REMEDIES.

apitherapy Treatment using bee products, including bee venom, royal jelly, bee pollen, raw honey, and propolis, for arthritis, desensitization of allergy to bee stings, chronic pain, back pain, migraines, hair loss, vision problems, gout, asthma, various skin conditions, memory loss, multiple sclerosis (MS), and urinary incontinence. According to The *PDR Family Guide to Natural Medicines & Healing Therapies* (Ballantine Books, New York, 1999), the Multiple Sclerosis Society has funded a study of bee venom as a treatment for MS, and the International Apiary Society is currently tracking 4500 individuals with MS as possible candidates for bee-venom remedies. Allegedly, bee venom injected into the joints eases the pain and inflammation of rheumatoid arthritis, as some patients have reported. Royal jelly, secreted by the salivary glands of worker bees to nourish the queen bee, is a source of vitamins, amino acids, minerals, and testosterone. Used for hundreds of years for its rejuvenating properties, royal jelly is also said to be antibacterial; reduce allergic reactions; boost the immune system compromised by chemotherapy and radiation; control cholesterol levels; treat subfertility, eczema, psoriasis, acne, muscular dystrophy, thrush, and athlete's foot; and possibly help prevent leukemia.

Bee pollen that is collected by bees contains vitamins, minerals, sugar, protein, and fat; its advocates believe it fights infection and inhibits aging. Raw honey is allegedly a source of B-complex vitamins, glucose, several other vitamins, and propolis, the substance bees collect from buds or tree bark (and then use to seal the interior of their hives); it is a combination of wax, resin, balsam oil, and propolis. Rich in bioflavonoids, bee propolis has antibiotic and bactericidal properties and may be used topically on wounds. As with any bee product, individuals must be cautioned that an allergic reaction may occur, and those who have cardiac problems, tuberculosis, or other infections or who are pregnant should probably avoid using bee remedies.

Apitherapists may be contacted through the American Apitherapy Society (AAS), P.O. Box 54, Hartland Four Corners, VT 05049, or at 800-823-3460.

applications, healing Any item or agent placed topically on the skin over an area of the body that requires healing. Among the types of applications are hot or cold, dry or moist compresses. Compresses have long been used to draw out waste and its residue, such as the contents of cysts or abscesses, through the skin, an organ of elimination and protection. Herbs may be applied to compresses; for example, cayenne, ginger, and lobelia may be added to a hot compress. Green clay compresses may be used for growths. Alternating hot and cold compresses is usually recommended. Herbal wraps are also healing applications and quick body-cleansing or conditioning techniques, which are reported to elasticize, tone, alkalize, and release body wastes. Spa herbal wraps may involve the use of seaweed or another natural substance with therapeutic qualities for balancing body minerals and enhancing metabolism. Other types of healing applications include mud, oatmeal, seaweed, and other baths.

See also FOLK REMEDIES.

applied kinesiology See KINESIOLOGY.

aquasonics A technique used by practitioners of cymatics involving the use of a heated pool for patients with arthritis, paralysis, and other physical disabilities. Various corrective sound frequencies are introduced into the water, which changes the water's molecular structure, thus providing a more effective "medium" for relaxation, stimulation, or whatever the patient's condition requires.

See also CYMATICS.

aromatherapy The use of appealing scents of essential oils extracted from various flowers and plants to induce relaxation and a sense of well-being. The ancient Greeks, Romans, and Egyptians recognized the beneficial effects of pleasantly scented baths, massages, steam inhalations, diffusers, and vaporizers. Hippocrates, the Greek known as the father of medicine, recommended aromatic fumigation for ridding Athens of the plague. Scents from essential oils were used throughout the world with some intention of a healing or therapeutic effect.

By the 1930s, the French chemist Dr. René-Maurice Gattefossé proposed the term and the basic principles of aromatherapy. Gattefossé began using lavender oil after he had burned his hand in his laboratory and quickly but inadvertently plunged it into a container of lavender oil. That his hand healed completely led him to think about and experiment with the possible benefits of essential oils in general. Gattefossé's further research on the effectiveness of essential oils led the French physician Jean Valnet to make therapeutic use of them during World War II as disinfectants and healing applications. Valnet went on in 1964 to write a *Aromatherapie, Traitement des maladies par les essences des plantes* (Aromatherapy, treatment of illnesses by the essences of plants), and to teach other physicians about essential oils.

Valnet's students Marguerite Maury and Micheline Arcier revived the use of essential oils in England, where there are now schools and clinics for aromatherapy. The Italian scientists Dr. Renato Cayola and Dr. Giovanni Garri also distinguished themselves with studies on the psychological effects of essential oils in the early 1920s, and Professor Paolo Rovesti, of the University of Milan, researched the effects and treated depressed patients with combinations of jasmine, sandalwood, orange blossom, verbena, and lemon oil. For treatment of anxiety disorders, he used bergamot, neroli, cypress, orange leaf, lime, rose, violet leaves, and marjoram. One contemporary physician helped a young girl with cancer to manage pain by administering a conventional pain medication accompanied by a whiff of rose oil with each dose. Eventually the girl needed only the fragrance to feel relief from the pain. Throughout the history of psychology, it has been known that an odor significant in the memory of an individual can trigger an array of somatic and emotional reactions.

According to Susanne Fischer-Rizzi, author of the *Complete Aromatherapy Handbook: Essential Oils for Radiant Health* (Sterling Publishing Company, New York, 1990), "Aromatherapy acts in accordance with holistic principles: it awakens and strengthens vital energies and self-healing capabilities of the patient. Essential oils can deeply influence our psychic equilibrium or psychological well-being and regulate physical imbalances—removing 'soil' on which illness flourish. . . . In addition, essential oils invite one to appreciate the beauty and wonders of creation, providing us inner contentment. . . . They have the ability to directly affect the brain and, from there, many psychological and physiological processes."

Aromatherapy enthusiasts and practitioners report that the cranial olfactory (odor-sensing) nerves act by transmitting impulses from odor molecules through the nasal passages to the limbic system, the seat of memory and emotion. Some claim certain aromas can trigger glandular stimulation, thus producing either calming or energizing results. For example, lavender is said to lower blood pressure; relieve headache, depression, inflammation, burns and cuts, menstrual cramps, and insect bites; and fight bacteria. Other aromas, such as peppermint, eucalyptus, tea tree, rosemary, chamomile, thyme, tarragon, and everlasting, allegedly help one deal with all manner of ailments and discomfort, including fungal infections, congestion, gas and liver problems, allergies, insomnia, digestive problems, stress, bronchitis, arthritis, muscle and other types of injuries, and skin problems such as boils and pimples. Aromatherapy may be administered via inhalation (usually in steam), diffusion (spraying into the air), massage (direct application to skin), bath water, and hot and cold compresses. Essential oils, which may be poisonous, are never to be taken internally.

Although aromatherapy is usually considered safe, precautions must be taken by those with asthma (many oils can set off bronchial spasms) or allergies, pregnant women (sage, rosemary, and juniper oils may trigger uterine contraction), and infants and young children, who may be hypersensitive to a potent essential oil. Also, the high concentration of essential oils may cause a toxic overdose, skin or eye irritation, hypersensitivity to sunlight, headache, fatigue, or a paradoxical effect (that is, an oil may cause a problem rather than help to relieve it). For aromatherapy organizations, see Appendix I.

Aromatherapy Seminars   See Appendix I.

aromatic   Any substance whose fragrance or agreeable odor acts as a relaxant or stimulant.
See also AROMATHERAPY.

artav   Reproductive tissue, one of the seven *dhatus* (basic vital bodily structures) in Ayurvedic medicine.
See also AYURVEDA.

art therapy   The technique of involving people in doing some form of artwork or working with art materials such as paints, crayons, or pastels, in order to achieve a therapeutic, nonverbal expression of feelings, particularly those related to bereavement, catastrophic illness, a disaster or public crisis, or personal psychogenic problems including depression. Art therapists believe that making art is a cathartic, healing experience, as well as an opportunity to release conscious or unconscious (and perhaps painful) feelings in an atmosphere of "play." The therapist and person discuss the painting, collage, drawing, or sculpture, for example, in a nonjudgmental, noncritical way, so the person derives the benefit of the therapist's assessment and guidance for the emotional problems that emerge from the art.

Art has been considered a valuable tool for rehabilitating those with mental or emotional illness since the 1940s, when artists who worked in psychiatric hospitals started to recognize the powerful messages in the artwork of patients. People of any age may participate in art therapy sessions, which are now integrated into the mainstream health delivery system and made available through local medical and health care centers.

One example of art therapy for mental patients is Rio de Janeiro's Museum of Images from the Unconscious. According to *The Power to Heal: Ancient Arts & Modern Medicine* (Prentice Hall Press, New York, 1990), "Art critics and psychotherapists

from around the world make pilgrimages to the Pedro II Psychiatric Center, which houses the museum's 250,000 pieces of patient-produced art. . . . Psychiatrists have long recognized the healing attributes of creating art, and the Museum of Images from the Unconscious helps scholars as well. Said the late British psychiatrist R. D. Laing, "This museum represents a major contribution to the scientific study of the psychotic process."

In *The Art Spirit* (Harper & Row Publishers, New York, 1923), the artist Robert Henri (1865–1929) wrote: "The more health we have in life the fewer laws we will have, for health makes for happiness and laws for the destruction of both. If as little children, we were enabled to find life so simple, so transparent that all the beautiful order of it were revealed to us, if we knew the rhythm of Wagner, the outline of Pericles, if color were all about us beautifully related, we should acquire this health and have the vision to translate our lives into the most perfect art of any age or generation." Bernie S. Siegel, M.D., quoted Henri further in his book *Love, Medicine & Miracles* (Harper & Row Publishers, New York, 1986): "When the artist is alive in any person, whatever his kind of work may be, he becomes an inventive, searching, daring, self-expressive creature. He becomes interesting to other people. He disturbs, upsets, enlightens, and opens ways for a better understanding. Where those who are not artists are trying to close the book, he opens it and shows there are still more pages possible." In his practice of oncology, Siegel is one of many proponents of using art as therapy. Art therapy programs, particularly for bereaved children, have cropped up in local medical centers as a service to the community and in connection with the treatment of patients with catastrophic illnesses.

asanas   Yoga postures or positions.
See also YOGA.

ascorbic acid flush   A procedure explained by Linda Rector-Page, N.D., Ph.D., as "accelerating detoxification, changing body chemistry to neutralize allergens and fight infections, promoting more rapid healing, and as a protective and preventive measure against illness" (from *Healthy Healing: An Alternative Healing Reference.* Carmel Valley, Calif.:

Health Healing Publications, 1994). The formula for the flush consists of ascorbate vitamin C or Ester powder with bioflavonoids, one-half teaspoon taken every 20 minutes to bowel tolerance (diarrhea results). Then reduce the amount taken to just below bowel tolerance until the stool is loose, but not diarrhea (which, medically, is considered to be watery). Continue for two days.

See also COLONICS.

ashtanga A school of yoga.

See also YOGA.

Association for Integrative Medicine (AIM) See Appendix I.

asthi Bone, one of the seven *dhatus* (basic vital tissues of the body) in Ayurvedic medicine.

See also AYURVEDA.

Aston-Patterning A type of bodywork, movement training, and massage geared to relieving muscle tension, pain, and stress and promoting healing from injuries. Developed by the dancer Judith Aston, who recovered from injuries sustained in two automobile accidents, Aston-Patterning is an extension of the deep massage therapy known as Rolfing. Specific techniques include "arcing," or the flexion and extension of the entire body, and "spiraling," which is geared toward relaxation of painful muscles and joints, as well as other movements and exercise drills. Aston-Patterning practitioners may also suggest that an individual make ergonomic changes in the home and workplace in order to increase comfort and relieve unconscious stress.

Although the goals of Aston-Patterning are to reduce stress, speed recovery from injury, and improve muscle tone, lightness of movement, and resiliency of the joints, it may not be recommended for those with osteoporosis, carpal tunnel syndrome, any disorder characterized by brittle bones, a bleeding disorder, or cardiac, circulatory, or respiratory problems. Nor is it recommended for those on long-term steroid or anticoagulant therapy. Some otherwise healthy people may experience fatigue and pain from the intense sessions or be emotionally resistant to the training. A competent practitioner

can adjust the massage and exercises according to the age and physical status of each client.

The Aston Training Center may be contacted at P.O. Box 3568, Inclined Village, NV 89450, or at 702-831-8228.

See also ROLFING.

Aston Training Center See Appendix I; ASTON-PATTERNING.

astringent A drying agent that reduces secretion of discharges from bodily tissues. Some of the major astringents are metal salts, such as ferric chloride, ferrous sulfate, and zinc oxide; alum; permanganates; and tannic acid. *Stypsis* is the Greek word meaning to "use an astringent," particularly to stop bleeding. In Ayurvedic medicine, astringency corresponds to one of the taste sensations; adding an astringent to a food creates a contraction that can have an effect upon hemorrhaging blood vessels or help dispel diarrhea.

See also AYURVEDA.

athma In Ayurvedic medicine, the soul or unique spirit that exists in the body and, after death, goes to another physical body.

See also AYURVEDA.

attunement An aspect of Reiki training, often called Reiki initiation, in which students are ceremonially brought into harmony, awareness, and responsiveness with the principles and techniques of Reiki practice.

See also REIKI.

aura From the Latin word meaning "breeze of puff of air," and perhaps derived from the Greek *aer* (air), a feeling one may get from a scent or any sensory stimulus, a feeling of a particular ambiance or atmosphere in a place, or a sensation that warns of or signals the exacerbation of a physical problem, such as a migraine or an epileptic seizure. Sensory hallucinations may accompany an aura in paroxysmal attacks; for example, the Dutch artist Vincent van Gogh was said to suffer from epilepsy or some sort of seizure disorder (which could have been linked to substance addiction and other problems), and he remembered after an attack was over that he had seen the color yellow, an image that stayed with him a long time.

In terms of alternative medicine, Therapeutic Touch, Reiki, and other practices rely on the premise that the body is surrounded by an electromagnetic field—also called an aura—that may be manipulated by hand in order to restore, direct, and balance healing energy for general well-being. In yoga philosophy, each chakra, or point of physical/spiritual energy, is associated with a color field emanating from the body that some people say they can "read" or actually see as illumination, such as a halo or source of light.

See also REIKI; THERAPEUTIC TOUCH; YOGA.

auricular therapy A branch of traditional Chinese medicine that includes acupuncture, this type geared solely to the ear in order to treat headaches, particularly migraines, arthritis, and stomach ailments, and for use as a pain-management option.

See also ACUPUNCTURE.

Australian Bush Flower Essences Infusions made from indigenous Australian flowers and plants that are used to strengthen the immune system and fight viruses. Developed by the herbalist Ian White, the essences include (1) Alpine mint bush—for revitalization from mental and emotional exhaustion; (2) Banksi Robur—for burnout, frustration, illness, and temporary loss of drive; (3) Bush Fuschia—for dyslexia, left/right brain imbalances, learning problems, stuttering, and promotion of keener intuition; (4) Crowea—for inner tension and worry; (5) Fringed Violet—for shock and trauma, damaged auric field, negative environmental energies, and effects of old traumas; (6) Isopogon—for poor memory, premature senility, stubborn, and controlling personality, and inability to learn from past experience; (7) She Oak—for infertility, premenstrual tension, hormonal imbalance, and fluid retention; (8) Spinifex—for oral and genital herpes, chlamydia, cuts, scrapes, and other skin conditions; (9) Sturt Desert Pea—for deep sorrow, emotional pain; (10) Sturt Desert Rose—for guilt, lack of self-esteem, lack of morality or conviction; (11) Radiation—a combination of essences to help combat the effects of radiation therapy for cancer, solar and nuclear radiation, electromagnetic energies; negative environmental energies, and

(12) Super Learning—a combination of essences to promote mental clarity, ability to concentrate, and learning skills, among other Australian essences.

See also BACH FLOWER REMEDIES; BELLHOUSE, ELIZABETH; FINDHORN ESSENCES; FLOWER ESSENCE SOCIETY; KORTE, ANDREAS; PERELANDRA ESSENCES.

autogenic training From the term that means "from within one's own self," a deep relaxation training that involves mental exercises for the reduction of both physical and mental stress and illness. Originated in Berlin, Germany, in the 1920s by the German psychiatrist and neurologist Dr. Johannes H. Schultz, autogenic training aims to help individuals deliberately control their autonomic nervous system, the part of the entire nervous system that focuses on involuntary bodily functioning—the heart, the smooth muscles, the adrenal medulla, and the salivary, gastric, and sweat glands, among other structures. The autonomic nervous system is divided into the sympathetic, or thoracolumbar, system, connected with thoracic and lumbar portions of the spinal nerve and other nerves, and the parasympathetic system, which consists of fibers of some of the cranial nerves and the nerves connected to the sacral portion of the spine. It is the sympathetic system that responds to stressors, and the parasympathetic system that induces relaxation.

When sympathetic fibers are stimulated by stress, fear, or a similar factor, the body's typical response includes vasoconstriction, increased blood pressure, "goose bumps," dilation of the pupils, thickened saliva, increase in heart rate, and other reactions related to the "fight or flight" syndrome. Stimulation of the parasympathetic nerves produces a reduction in blood pressure, vasodilation, pupillary contraction, thin saliva, and reduced heart rate.

The techniques of autogenic training resemble self-hypnosis and meditation. The series of mental exercises, performed three times daily for 15 minutes at a time, centers on certain words or phrases that, for the individual, will produce a relaxation response. There are two groups of autogenic exercises; the first group has six exercises that use phrases (an example is "My arms are warm and heavy") that prompt one's attention to physiological changes brought about by relaxation. The second group, known as intentional exercises, is geared to helping one release physical and emotional tension with activity such as crying, shouting, on punching pillows. Training sessions, private or in small groups, last an hour and continue for eight to 10 weeks. It has been reported that during the training some people experience an "autogenic discharge," a temporary exacerbation of symptoms, which is considered part of the healing process.

Autogenic training has been tested in several clinical experiments and is said to be beneficial for ailments that include anxiety and panic disorder, hypertension, and other stress-related problems.

Ayurveda Named from the Sanskrit word meaning "knowledge of life," a set of principles for healing based on the idea that three main types of energy form everything in the universe, including the human body, and as the rudiments of life itself must be considered in the cycle of growth, maintenance, and deterioration. Ayurveda, most commonly defined as the practice of ancient Hindu or Indian medicine, originates with the Vedas, the earliest Indian literature, dating from ca. 1500 B.C. In the Vedas are intricately described medical disorders and corresponding treatments, most of which are herbal but may also include simple surgical procedures. It is said that Vedic physicians invented prostheses—artificial limbs and eyes. By ca. 800 B.C., the Brahmans, the highest social caste, designated for the wisest persons, developed Ayurvedic practices and surgery, and by A.D. 500, Ayurveda evolved into a scientific system that included the herbal treatments.

Ayurveda has recently become the subject of studies conducted by its researchers and practitioners and collaboratively by those involved in traditional Western medicine.

The largest and most authentic resource of information on Ayurveda in America was established as the National Institute of Ayurvedic Medicine (NIAM) by the American physician Scott Gerson, in 1982. Gerson is reported to be the only physician in the United States who holds degrees in both traditional Western medicine and Ayurveda. NIAM is currently conducting research in conjunction with the National Cancer Institute in Bethesda, Maryland; the Central Council for Research in Ayurveda and Siddha Medicine in New Delhi, India; the Mount Sinai School of Med-

icine in New York; and the Richard and Hinda Rosenthal Center for Alternative and Complementary Medicine at Columbia University in New York City. Projects with the National Cancer Institute include an evaluation of antitumor effects of *Semicarpus anacardium* (an Ayurvedic phytomedicine, or plant extract). Initial reports over the last three years indicate that the growth of certain malignancies is thwarted by semicarpus. Further study seeks to determine whether semicarpus or other Ayurvedic medicine has the direct ability to kill cancer cells.

Asthma, immune diseases, and various diseases and conditions that affect women are the subjects of additional studies. A randomized, controlled cross-over-type study of an herbal-yoga treatment regimen to treat asthma is under way at the Central Council for Research in Ayurveda and Siddha Medicine, and Ayurvedic herbal treatments for perimenopausal symptoms, premenstrual syndrome, and dysmenorrhea (painful menstruation) are being researched at the Rosenthal Center. Ayurvedic herbal protocols are also under investigation for the treatment of hypertension, genital herpes, depression, adult-onset diabetes, obesity, uterine fibroid tumors, acne, irritable bowel syndrome, chronic constipation, and chronic fatigue syndrome. The effect of aromatherapy and meditation on brain wave patterns is being studied through the use of electroencephalography (EEG).

In addition, NIAM has nearly completed a four-year study to evaluate the effects of Panchakarma Therapies on the human immune system, and according to the NIAM website, updated 2/12/03, results are expected to be reported soon. See current research, http://niam.com/corp-web/current.htm.

Selected reading for additional information

Lad, Dr. Vasant, *Ayurveda: The Science of Self-Healing*. Twin Lakes, Wisc.: Lotus Press, 1984.

Rakel, David, M.D., *Intergrative Medicine*. New York:W.B. Saunders, 2003.

Sodhi, V., "Ayurveda: The Science of Life and Mother of the Healing Arts," in *A Textbook of Natural Medicine*, edited by J. E. Pizzorno and M. T. Murry. John Bastyr College Publications, Seattle, Wash., 1989.

Swami Sada Shiva Tirtha, *The Ayurveda Encyclopedia*. Bayville, N.Y.: Ayurveda Holistic Center Press, 1998.

Trivieri, Larry, *The American Holistic Medical Association Guide to Holistic Health*. New York: John Wiley & Sons, 2001.

Bach, Edward British bacteriologist, medical doctor, and homeopathic physician born in 1887 who worked at the London Homeopathic Hospital in England and who between 1928 and 1932 set forth the seven major negative human emotions that correspond with ill-being or illness and developed remedies (called nosodes, or homeopathic preparations) for them from specific flowers and plants.

At age 43 Bach (pronounced "Batch") became disillusioned with standard medical practice and decided to pursue his belief that healing involved more than traditional treatments. In tune with the homeopathic concept of vibrational healing, he discovered through his patients that grief, frustration, anxiety, fear, despair, loneliness, and uncertainty contributed significantly to their physical ailments. His training in homeopathy led him to the 38 natural remedies now known as Bach's Flower Remedies, which are usually sold over the counter in health food stores. At his home, Mount Vernon, in Oxfordshire, now known as the Bach Centre, he noticed that the habits and characteristics of flowers and plants related to human behavior. For example, the typical beech tree grows to approximately 100 feet tall and its branches span approximately 80 feet. Bach concluded from this and other growth habits and traits of the beech that its essence could encourage people who are intolerant, critical, and nonempathetic to open nonjudgmentally to the world's beauty. To create his remedy, he boiled leaves and twigs from the beech tree in water, let them simmer and cool thereafter, and then filtered them from the water. To that water Bach added a small amount of brandy (the standard mix per flower or plant substance is 50 milliliters (mL), or one-and-a-half fluid ounces, of the prepared water to 100 mL, or three fluid ounces, of brandy). Called a tincture, this remains

potent for many years. The typical dose of a Bach's flower tincture is four drops on or under the tongue as often as necessary. Another method for making flower tinctures is the sun method, in which harvested blooms or parts of the plant are floated on water in a glass bowl and placed in the sunshine for three hours, after which only the remaining filtered water is added to brandy.

Bach wrote extensively on his flower remedies, including the books *Heal Thyself* and *The Twelve Healers and Other Remedies* (both C. W. Daniel, 1931 and 1936). He also specified that after his death, no more essences were to be added to the 38 existing remedies for the purpose of keeping the system as simple as possible, so individuals would be able to diagnose their emotional problems and self-treat. The Bach Centre address is Mount Vernon, Sotwell, Wallingford, Oxfordshire, OX10 9PZ, UK. Also, one may contact the Dr. Edward Bach Healing Society, 644 Merrick Road, Lynbrook, NY 11563, and Ellon (Bach U.S.A.), Inc., P.O. Box 32, Woodmere, NY 11598.

See also BACH FLOWER REMEDIES.

Bach Flower Remedies In addition to being the inspiration for several other flower remedies made in Australia, California, Europe, and elsewhere, the original remedies that are believed to employ the life force, or vibrations, of each flower to help relieve negativity of varying nature, balance energy, and thereby encourage physical and emotional healing. The medical and homeopathic physician and author Rudolph M. Ballentine wrote of flower remedies: "If you have ever tried to pick blackberries, you know it's tricky. The vines are covered with sharp spines. The biggest and most succulent berries always seem to be a little deeper into the tangle of brambles. You work your way in edgewise so you can reach a bit further. Then suddenly you realize you can't move. The long branches of the blackberry plant are wrapped all about you, and each has thorns that curve back in toward the plant. No matter which way you move, some of those thorns dig in deeper. You are stuck. The essence of the blackberry flower is used as a remedy for those who are at a point in their lives where they feel stuck—unable to find a way to move. Whether it's a job or relationship one feels stuck in, the flower essence blackberry supports the effort to disentangle oneself from the situation. Perhaps the most valuable aspect of the homeopathic remedy is its ability to have a therapeutic effect on the mind and emotions, promoting the process of personal evolution" (*Radical Healing*, New York: Harmony Books, 1996).

Others believe the flower remedies and other natural medicinals may work as placebos, if they are effective at all. The 38 essences created by Bach derive from agrimony, aspen, beech, centaury, cerato, cherry plum, chestnut bud, chicory, clematis, crab apple, elm, gentian, gorse, heather, holly, honeysuckle, hornbeam, impatiens, larch, mimulus, mustard, oak, olive, pine, red chestnut, rock rose, rock water, scleranthus, star of Bethlehem, sweet chestnut, vervain, vine, walnut, water violet, white chestnut, wild oat, wild rose, and willow. Essences may be combined to treat more than one problem and are said to be therapeutic in producing support during a crisis, alteration of one's mental outlook during a chronic problem or disease or crisis state, and prevention of emotional imbalance attributable to common stress and individual circumstances. Flower remedies do not interfere with any other treatment, do not work in a biochemical way, are not addictive or dangerous, and may be taken safely by people of all ages, including babies. They may be given to animals and plants as well. (Bach tested all his remedies on himself.) However, people who are alcohol-intolerant or who are recovering from alcoholism should not take flower essence remedies with the alcohol in them. Used for preservation purposes, the alcohol may be removed from the remedy by putting the diluted drops of a remedy into a boiling hot drink

such as tea, so the steam can make the alcohol evaporate. When cool, the drink may be sipped throughout the day.

Essences—unlike herbal preparations, in that no actual part of the plant remains in the tincture—are to be taken until the patient feels relief and begins to notice the stimulus of his or her own healing mechanism. Each flower or plant addresses one or more emotional imbalances:

AGRIMONY: Hiding one's feelings by putting on a happy face; denying the existence of problems; lacking ability to express problems and feelings

ASPEN: Fear of the unknown or unexplained

BEECH: Perfectionism; intolerance of others' beliefs

CENTAURY: Over eagerness to please others; inability to say no

CERATO: Lack of self-confidence and trust in one's own judgment; constant seeking of advice from others

CHERRY PLUM: Fear of losing one's sanity; anxiety; inner turmoil

CHESTNUT BUD: Making the same mistake over and over; being unable to learn from past experiences

CHICORY: Overprotectiveness; possessiveness; inability to let go without feelings of rejection

CLEMATIS: Daydreaming; absentmindedness; inattention; boredom

CRAB APPLE: Feelings of being infected, unclean, impure either physically, emotionally, or spiritually

ELM: Feelings of inadequacy and of being overwhelmed by responsibilities or commitments

GENTIAN: Pessimism; loss of faith after a failure or setback; discouragement

GORSE: Feelings of being born to suffer; pessimism; feelings of hopelessness

HEATHER: Excessive talking about oneself; self-obsession; lack of listening skills

HOLLY: Feelings of hatred, jealousy, suspicion, resentment

HONEYSUCKLE: Excessive nostalgia; loss of interest in present-day activity

HORNBEAM: Mental exhaustion; feelings of being stuck in a rut, uncreative, or in the wrong line of work; fatigue; dissatisfaction with work and responsibility

IMPATIENS: Impatience; irritability; agitation

LARCH: Feelings of worthlessness or inferiority despite ability; low self-esteem

MIMULUS: Excessive self-consciousness; fear of socializing; fear of known things

MUSTARD: Despair; gloom; depression without cause

OAK: Being overly persistent; refusing to give in; fighting the same fight over and over

OLIVE: Exhaustion; broken spirit; overwork

PINE: Feelings of guilt; self-reproach; apologetic attitude about things not one's fault

RED CHESTNUT: Overanxiety about the welfare of others; fear of impending disaster

ROCK ROSE: Helplessness; panic; feelings of terror

ROCK WATER: Being inflexible; being a perfectionist; being too hard on oneself or feeling victimized

SCLERANTHUS: Excessive indecisiveness

STAR OF BETHLEHEM: Feelings of sorrow; shock; trauma

SWEET CHESTNUT: Hopelessness; profound despair

VERVAIN: Excessive sense of injustice and of fighting for the underdog; perfectionism

VINE: Tyrannical, overbearing behavior; excessive determination in a leader

WALNUT: Inability to sever ties to the past or cope with change, including life transitions or milestones

WATER VIOLET: Aloof, overly reserved or dignified behavior, which may lead to isolation

WHITE CHESTNUT: Hyperactive mind; excessive worry and argument

WILD OAT: Confusion; inability to find one's purpose in life

WILD ROSE: Fatalism; apathy; lack of ambition to make changes in one's life

WILLOW: Feelings of self-pity and gloom; resentment of perceived unfair treatment

Rescue Remedy is a combination of five flower essences: star of Bethlehem, rock rose, impatiens, cherry plum, and clematis. The most frequently used remedy, it treats feelings of panic, mental numbness, shock, terror, fear of flying, response to startling noise—any emotional state of emergency or loss of control, even trauma experienced in the past that is still disturbing. In addition to the tincture, which can be added to any skin wash preparation, douche, or compress, Rescue Remedy is made into a cream that can be applied topically to cuts, bruises, stings, sunburn, and other injuries. Also, Rescue Remedy is used for prevention of panic, such as before a stressful activity or event, and is reported to increase healing and recovery from surgery.

See also AUSTRALIAN FLOWER REMEDIES.

Baily, Philip M.   Medical doctor and author of Homeopathic Psychology: *Personality Profiles of the Major Constitutional Remedies* (Berkeley, Calif.: North Atlantic Books, 1995).

Balch, James, and Balch, Phyllis   Authors of *Prescription for Nutritional Healing*, 2nd ed. (Garden City Park, N.Y.: Avery Publishing, 1997).

Ballentine, Rudolph M.   Medical doctor and homeopathic physician, creator and director of the Center for Holistic Medicine in New York City. A psychiatrist, herbalist, Ayurvedic practitioner, and teacher, Ballentine has written numerous books, including *Diet and Nutrition: A Holistic Approach* (Honesdale, Pa.: Himalayan Publishers, 1978); *Joints and Glands, as Taught by Swami Rama* (Himalayan,1977); *Theory and Practice of Meditation* (Himalayan, 1986); *Radical Healing: Integrating the World's Great Therapeutic Traditions to Create a New Transformative Medicine* (New York: Harmony Books, 1999); *Yoga and Psychotherapy: The Evolution of Consciousness* (with Swami Rama and Swami Ajaya, Ph.D.); (Himalayan, 1976); *Science of Breath* (with Swami Rama and Alan Hymes, M.D.); (Himalayan, 1979); and *Transition to Vegetarianism: An Evolutionary Step* (Himalayan, 1987). Ballentine studied psychology at Duke University and the University of Paris (Sorbonne). He received his M.D. from Duke. He was on the faculty of the Louisiana State University School of Medicine, Department of Psychiatry, and studied the Ayurveda and homeopathy in India. For 12 years he served as president of the Himalayan Institute, and for 18 years as director of its Combined Therapy Program, in which he developed models of holistic medical care that have been adopted throughout the world.

Banerjee, P. N. Author of *Chronic Disease: Its Cause and Cure*, 4th edition (Banerjee & Company, Gidni, India, 1971). This book was originally published in 1931.

Barral visceral manipulation A system of bodywork that is geared to releasing restrictions and tension by manipulating the body's organs and connective tissues, developed by the French osteopathic physician Jean Pierre Barral. This therapy is reported to enhance the entire body's functioning, including organ mobility and activity, circulation, hormonal secretions, immune system activity, and muscle function. In addition, Barral's modality may facilitate the release of internalized emotion. He discovered that the organs have a five- to eight-cycle-per-minute rhythm of movement (relative to its position or referring to its function), and when the cycles are impaired, irritation and disease may develop. The Barral technique involves the use of light, precise mechanical force, which rebalances the organ and helps revive its normal function.

Bates Method for Improving Eyesight A relaxation system geared toward restoring the natural use of the eyes and relearning to see developed by the American ophthalmologist William H. Bates, M.D. (1865–1931). A graduate of Cornell University and of the College of Physicians and Surgeons in New York, Bates practiced at Bellevue, Harlem hospitals, Manhattan Eye and Ear Hospital, and the New York Eye Infirmary and taught ophthalmology at the New York Post-Graduate Medical School and Hospital. In 1920, Bates wrote *The Cure of Imperfect Eyesight by Treatment Without Glasses* (New York: Central Fixation Publishing Co., and London: Arther F. Bird), which presented his theory that sight can be deliberately and naturally improved after being diminished by eyestrain, tension, and misuse of the eyes.

behavioral medicine A physical, psychiatric, and psychologic approach to health care that focuses on how behavior relates to states of both health and illness. In opposition to age-old theories that the mind and body were of a different, and therefore separate, nature, Herbert Benson, M.D., author of several books, wrote in *The Mind/Body Effect* (New York: Simon & Schuster, 1979): "The close interrelation between your mind and body cannot be ignored when modern scientific knowledge is considered. The potential exists for thought processes to lead both to disease and to good health." He cited psychosomatic medicine, which is commonly defined as a discipline that recognizes the power an individual's thinking has over his or her physical condition, as a starting point for the rationale of behavioral medicine. He also pointed out that psychological factors affect the conscious perception of and sensitivity to pain and pain relief, and that symptoms of certain diseases such as asthma, rheumatoid arthritis, and colitis are clearly at risk of being aggravated by psychological stress.

"If you are ill," Benson wrote, "extensive tests and procedures may be required to diagnose and treat your ailment. However, even then the risk versus benefit principle should be applied. You should not allow yourself to become convinced that you are sick or becoming sick. Is it not foolish to spend healthy years worried about disease that is not present and may never occur? Many individuals in previous generations appeared to have faith in their own health. People should strive to adopt this attitude. If you become ill, the medical profession is there to help you. There will be enough time for you to work with your physician and to learn how to adjust to an illness if it occurs. . . . You have a right to expect to be as well as possible for as long as possible."

See also BENSON, HERBERT.

Beinfield, Harriet, and Korngold, Efrem Pioneers in the practice of acupuncture and herbal medicine in the United States and authors of *Between Heaven and Earth: A Guide to Chinese Medicine* (New York: Ballantine Books, 1991). Both are licensed acupuncturists, and Korngold is also a doctor of osteopathic medicine.

Bellavite, Paolo, and Signorini, Andrea Medical doctors and authors of *Homeopathy, a Frontier in*

Medical Science: Experimental Studies and Theoretical Foundations (Berkeley, Calif: North Atlantic Books, 1995).

Benson, Herbert   The founding president of the Mind/Body Medical Institute of Pathway Health Network and a Harvard Medical School graduate. Benson, a medical doctor and chief of the Division of Behavioral Medicine at the Deaconess Hospital, teaches at Andover Newton Theological School and conducts medical research, lectures widely, and has written several books, including *The Relaxation Response* (New York: William Morrow, 1975); *The Mind/Body Effect* (New York: Simon & Schuster, 1979); *Beyond the Relaxation Response* (New York: Times Books, 1984); *Your Maximum Mind* (New York: Times Books, 1987); and *The Wellness Book* (New York: Fireside, 1993) (with Eileen M. Stewart, R.N., C, M.S.). Benson lives in Lexington, Massachusetts.

See also BEHAVIORAL MEDICINE.

Bhakhi enema   See ENEMA.

Bikram yoga   A branch of yoga characterized by performing yoga exercises and asanas in a room heated to about 103 degrees.

See also YOGA.

bioenergetics   Also called core energetics, as a component of energy medicine, a technique geared toward helping one connect with lower chakra energy in the treatment of repressed emotions. Energy medicine techniques include Reiki, reflexology, shiatsu, craniosacral therapy, zone therapy, homeopathy, acupuncture, polarity, Phoenix Rising yoga therapy, and breathwork.

See also CHAKRAS; ENERGY.

bioentrainment   The principle that the brain responds to oscillating light, sound, or magnetic-field energies through "entraining," or "conditioning," itself to the frequency of a particular energy. There exist devices designed to induce relaxation by emitting light (usually red light) or energy waves to the brain at an adjustable frequency. This modality is also used to treat seizure activity and memory and vision problems, among other disorders.

biofeedback   A series of electrodermal responses to changes in heart rate, respirations, temperature, muscle tension, perspiration, brain waves, gastric acidity, blood pressure, and other bodily functions recorded on a machine similar to an electrocardiogram. An individual is connected to sensors that pick up signals of involuntary bodily activities. At a time of stress, these signals are recorded by the machine to inform the person how the body handled that stress. The goal of biofeedback is to help recognize these reactions and learn to alter them through relaxation techniques. Biofeedback is useful in reducing stress as a trigger for physical disorders and disease. Patients of biofeedback are usually taught various breathing techniques as a way to overcome anxiety and other stress responses. This is sometimes referred to as "passive volition," which means developing one's capacity to pay attention to and relax the muscles while doing corresponding breathwork.

biological dentistry   A branch of dentistry that emphasizes the importance of tooth alignment and jaw structure, cavities as a source of other illness, nontoxic restoration materials, the impact of dental toxins, and the conservation of all healthy tooth material. Biological dentistry employs various therapies that may be categorized as bioenergetic medicine, including neural and cold laser therapy, oral acupuncture, homeopathy, mouth balancing, and nutrition.

Neural therapy is based on the concept that the body's electrical charge that is channeled throughout the body; an impediment that blocks or injures this charge may lead to cell breakdown and disease. Effective in healing wounds, reducing inflammation, and fighting bacteria, cold laser therapy draws on traditional acupuncture techniques, but with the use of laser beams instead of needles. Oral acupuncture, which involves the injection of saline solution, weak local anesthetics, or a combination of homeopathic remedies into acupoints in the mucous membrane, is used for relief of pain during dental procedures; for the treatment of neuralgia, sinusitis, allergies, and digestive disorders; and for diagnostic procedures. Mouth balancing is a modality that diagnoses cranial structural problems that may cause illness in other parts of the body, such as headaches, shoulder pain, back problems, blurred vision, and temporo-mandibular joint (TMJ) syndrome. Mouth-balancing treatment includes the use of corrective orthopedic braces to be worn in the mouth.

See also ACUPUNCTURE; HOMEOPATHY.

bitter   One of the six Ayurvedic tastes, a substance from bark, tannin, and resin used in tonics to stimulate appetite.

See also AYURVEDA.

blood cleansing   A one- to two-month diet plan aimed at eliminating toxins from the bloodstream. Among the various plans is one that advocates using fresh, organic produce whenever possible; drinking pau d'arco and other teas, green drinks, and specially prepared juices made from aloe vera, carrot, papaya, and other ingredients; doing weekly colonic irrigation; avoiding meat, dairy and fried foods, saturated fats, salt, sugars, sweeteners, sodas, artificial drinks, and canned, frozen, prepackaged, and refined foods; getting early morning sunlight every day; and taking brisk daily walks. There are also blood tonics, including green drinks that are rich in chlorophyll (similar in molecular composition to human hemoglobin), which is also a source of vitamins, minerals, enzymes, and other nutrients that promote optimal cell response and growth. Green drinks are also effective as energy-boosting, anti-infective blood cleansers.

body map   A technique for the diagnosis of illness or dysfunction. A Chinese tongue map, for example, shows each region of the tongue in correlation with other organs and structures of the body. The area at the back of the tongue relates to the uro-genital organs; the midsection relates to the liver, gallbladder, and other digestive organs; just before the tip of the tongue, the lungs are represented; the tip relates to the heart. Chinese doctors also observe the color and condition of the tongue, very often keys to diagnosing a problem. A dark coating on the tongue, for instance, indicates a toxicity in the body, and a dry, shiny tongue indicates dehydration.

Face maps are popular for diagnosis in Asian medical practice. Divided into horizontal thirds, a face's upper portion (intellect) relates to the nervous system. The middle portion (emotion) corresponds to the circulation, and the lower portion (will) to digestion and reproduction. Specific parts of the face—nostrils, chin, brow, lower lip, cheek, and so on—relate to specific organs that may be dysfunctional or impaired and the meridians (energy channels) of the body. In turn, the physical body conditions relate to emotional and psychological constitution of an individual. Nose, pulse, and hand maps are also used by practitioners to identify disorders.

See also ACUPUNCTURE.

body unit   A system of measurement that corresponds to the body's acupuncture points. One unit is equal to the width of the second joint of the thumb, and three body units is equal to the breadth of the second, third, fourth, and fifth fingers held together. Each major body segment has a certain number of body units. For example, five body units may be measured from the navel to the pubic bone, and 12 body units make up the area from the elbow crease to the wrist crease.

See also ACUPUNCTURE.

bodywork   Modern systems for relaxation, physical therapy, stress reduction, and general musculoskeletal and emotional well-being. These include the following: the Alexander Technique; Feldenkrais Method; Trager Approach; Rolfing; myofascial release; Aston-Patterning; Hellerwork; Barral visceral manipulation; Bowen Therapy; acupressure; acupuncture; massage; (Oriental bodywork: shiatsu, jin shin jyutsu); reflexology; Bonnie Prudden Myotherapy; bioenergetics; Therapeutic Touch; Healing Touch; Reiki; polarity therapy; Reichian therapy; hakomi; the Rosen Method; and the Rubenfeld Synergy Method.

Other bodywork techniques include baths, wraps, hydrotherapy, enemas, compresses, overheating therapy, and any other form of a "laying on of hands" that is meant to facilitate a transfer of energy from one person to another for the purpose of healing.

Boericke, William, and Dewey, W. A.   Homeopathic physicians with M.D. degrees and authors of

The Twelve Tissue Remedies of Schuessler (New York: Aperture, 1911), a classic homeopathic volume on W. H. Schuessler's system of homeopathic practice and the golden age of homeopathy in America. Boericke also wrote a homeopathic book, *Materia Medica with Repertory* (Philadelphia: Boericke and Runyon, 1927).

Bogart, Greg   Doctor of philosophy and author of *Therapeutic Astrology: Using the Birth Chart in Psychotherapy and Spiritual Counseling* (Berkeley, Calif.: Dawn Mountain, 1996).

Bohm, David   Physicist and author of *Wholeness and the Implicate Order* (London: Ark Paperbacks, 1983).

Bond, Mary   Author of *Balancing Your Body: A Self-Help Approach to Rolfing Movement* (Rochester, Vt.: Healing Arts Press, 1993).

Bonnie Prudden Myotherapy   A technique for the relief of pain based on the use of manual pressure on areas of the body known as "trigger points," developed by Bonnie Prudden, a veteran authority on physical fitness and exercise therapy and author of *Pain Erasure and Myotherapy* (New York: Ballantine Books, 1980). Prudden's work contributed to the establishment of the President's Council on Physical Fitness and Sports during the 1950s. Trigger points, or places on the body where painful muscle spasm occurs, may be the result of trauma or injury, repetitive motion, prenatal injury, or child or sexual abuse and may be exacerbated by the presence of disease, substance abuse, and the aging process. Although medication can break the spasm-pain-spasm cycle, Prudden's method aims to eliminate the trigger points completely by applying deep pressure on each point for five to seven seconds. The method also involves performing stretches and trigger-point sessions to prevent recurrence of muscle spasm, strains, sprains, dislocations, tension headaches, migraines, temporomandibular joint (TMJ) syndrome, hemorrhoids, prostate muscle spasms, impotence, incontinence, arthritis, lupus, multiple sclerosis, foot pain, leg cramps, and neck, shoulder, arm, hand, back, chest, and abdominal pain.

botanic physicians   Medical doctors who incorporated the use of herbal remedies, after the 19th-century American herbalist Samuel Thomson started a movement of herbalism with legendary success. When 22-year-old Thomson's young daughter contracted scarlet fever in 1791, and the doctor said he could not help her, Thomson proceeded to use steam and warming drinks that broke her fever and cured her. In 1805, a yellow fever (or some other deadly fever) epidemic broke out, and Thomson's patients survived as many others died. By 1839, there were 100,000 Thomsonian practitioners registered in America, and a decade later the Eclectic Medical Institute emerged when physicians and herbalists decided to join forces. Several schools operated in major cities throughout the country from the late 19th century and into the 20th, but patent medicines rose as competitors that crushed the finances of the Eclectics. In Cincinnati, 1939, the last Eclectic Medical School closed forever.

Bott, Victor   Physician and author of *Anthroposophical Medicine* (Rochester, Vt.: Healing Arts Press, 1984), a summary of the medical system, known as anthroposophical medicine, set forth by Rudolph Steiner.

Bowen Method   A hands-on modality designed to balance and positively affect the autonomic nervous system, developed in the 1950s by the Australian lay healer Thomas Bowen. With the fully clothed patient lying prone on a padded table, Bowen advocated a series of moves such as pulling the skin away from a muscle or tendon, then applying gentle pressure, and eventually allowing the specific structure to spring back into its original position. Bowen developed certain patterns for three sets of moves to treat lower back, upper back, and neck problems. Other moves are also added to accommodate the patient's particular health problem. Treatment sessions vary from 20 to 45 minutes. Bowen therapy is also used to provide benefit to individuals with gastrointestinal disorders, chronic fatigue, fibromyalgia, headaches, respiratory ailments, sports- and work-related injuries, and other conditions. Patients have reported that symptoms subsided, and that anger and depression were reduced, after treatments. A variation of Bowen's therapy, known as the Neurostructural Integration Technique (NST), emerged in 1995. It was developed by Michael Nixon-Livy, who wanted to systematize the Bowen Method in order to train health professionals.

Bower, Peter   A medical doctor practicing in Charlottesville, Virginia, where he and his associates combine Osteopathic Manual Therapy, Pilates-based rehabilitation, and health counseling in the medical management of neurological and musculoskeletal problems. Trained in family and emergency medicine, Bower has been a faculty member at the University of California (Davis) Medical School, the University of San Francisco School of Medicine, and the University of Virginia School of Medicine. His focus is on the diagnosis and treatment of repetitive strain and sports injuries, myofascial pain syndromes, and nerve-entrapment syndromes.

   See also OSTEOPATHY; PILATES.

breathing techniques   Variations of breathing, including deep-breathing exercises, used to induce relaxation, as a component of treatment for a wide spectrum of disorders.

   See also BREATHWORK; BUTEYKO TECHNIQUE; YOGA.

breathwork   A wide variety of energy techniques used to activate the higher chakras.

   See also CHAKRAS; YOGA.

Breema bodywork training   See BODYWORK.

Breiling, Brian Joseph   Author of *Light Years Ahead* (Berkeley, Calif.: Celestial Arts, 1996), a book focused on the futuristic therapy using light and energy healing methods.

Brennan, Barbara Ann   Healer, teacher, and author of *Hands of Light: A Guide to Healing through the Human Energy Field*, and *Light Emerging: The Jour-*

ney of Personal Healing (both published by Bantam Books, New York, 1987 and 1993). Brennan runs a school of healing in New York.

broth, cleansing   Clear broths and hot tonics used during a cleansing fast. Broths of onion, miso, garlic, scallion, apple, carrot, potato, and other ingredients, are geared toward balancing body pH and are alkalizing agents. Hot tonics are not broths or teas, but hot drinks made from vegetables, fruits, and spices that have energizing properties. Tonics are meant to revitalize, clear nasal and sinus passages, provide nutrition, create body heat to ward off aches and chills, and fight a hangover. A cold and flu tonic, for example, may be made by combining garlic, cumin powder, black pepper, hot mustard powder, water, turmeric, sesame salt, fresh cilantro, and cooked split peas.

Buegel, Dale, Lewis, Blair, and Chernin, Dennis   Authors of *Homeopathic Remedies for Health Professionals and Laypeople* (Honesdale, Pa.: Himalayan Publishers, 1991). Buegel and Chernin are medical doctors.

Buhner, Stephen Harrod   Author of *Sacred Plant Medicine* (Boulder, Colo.: Roberts Rinehart, 1996), which discusses Native American healing traditions.

   See also NATIVE AMERICAN HEALING PRACTICES.

Buteyko technique   A system of breathing exercises developed by the organization Instep International (http://www.nqnet.com/buteyko/bristrial1.html) that is reported to be beneficial to individuals with asthma. It is named after a Russian physician who developed the nonhyperventilation breathing/relaxation technique in the 1940s. A study funded by the Australian Association of Asthma Foundations was done on the technique at the Mater Hospital in Brisbane, Australia, with positive results, including that the asthma patients' symptoms and need for steroids were significantly reduced.

   See also YOGA.

calmative A substance used as a tranquilizer or sedative in homeopathic and Ayurvedic medicine.

carminative A substance that relieves griping (severe bowel pains) and intestinal gas.

Casey, the Reverand Solanus A Franciscan priest of the Capuchin Order who has been credited as a healer of hopeless cases. Born Bernard Casey on a Wisconsin farm on November 25, 1870, Father Solanus began working odd jobs at age 17 to supplement the family's income after they experienced financial difficulties attributable to crop failures. At 21, however, he entered St. Francis Seminary High School in Milwaukee, and in 1896 he was called to the Capuchin Order, in which he was given the name Solanus. Once ordained in 1904, Father Solanus worked at Sacred Heart Parish in Yonkers, New York, mainly as doorkeeper and sacristan because he was not highly regarded for his scholarship. But the sick and troubled of the parish began to notice his gift for healing and made a point to ask for his prayers for themselves and their loved ones. He also worked at Our Lady of Sorrows in Manhattan and Our Lady of the Angels in the city's Harlem section; at both parishes, Father Solanus made a lasting impression as a worker of miracles. Appointed to the Capuchin Friary of St. Bonaventure in Detroit, Michigan, in 1924, he became well known and was the inspiration of the Detroit Capuchins to establish their soup kitchen, still in operation today. He continued his ministry to the sick and the poor even after he was sent for retirement to the Friary of St. Felix in Huntington, Indiana, in 1946. When he himself became ill, he returned to Detroit, where he died July 31, 1957. His grave is located at Detroit's St. Bonaventure Monastery.

See also FAITH HEALING; PRAYER.

cathartic A substance used as a laxative.

caustic A substance capable of corroding or burning bodily tissue.

Cayce, Edgar Known as "the sleeping prophet," a psychic (1877–1945) who in 1931 founded the Association for Research and Enlightenment, Inc. (A.R.E.), in Virginia Beach, Virginia. Cayce was a photographer, gardener, Sunday School teacher, and father of two. To date he is the subject of approximately 12 biographies and is discussed in more than 300 other books for his ability to enter a sleeplike state, during which he gave information to individuals throughout the world who had life-threatening illnesses, questions, or problems.

Reports say Cayce would lie down on his couch, fold his hands over his stomach, close his eyes, and, with a person's name and location provided to him, offer answers to that person about his or her situation. Frequently he made a lifesaving diagnosis in cases that stumped the medical community. A stenographer would write as Cayce spoke, and one copy of his "reading" was sent to the person and another was kept in his personal files. The A.R.E. holds more than 14,000 readings, which are made available to the public for research. The readings—considered sources of what is now called holistic, or mind-body, medicine—are being studied by medical professionals, theologians, educators, scientists, and others, including a professor and fellow of the American Physical Society who pointed out a connection between the elementary-particle theory and Cayce's psychic access to information that could not possibly have been available to him in a conventional way.

According to the article "Sleeping prophet's legacy lives on in Virginia Beach," by Victor Zak in the February 23, 1997 issue of the *Asbury Park Press,* "Cayce demonstrated powers of clairvoyance at a young age that seemed to extend beyond the five normal senses. He told his parents that he saw and communicated with 'visions,' some of whom were deceased relatives. He reportedly had a photographic memory that enabled him to absorb, through osmosis, the content of school books while sleeping on them. Cayce's education was brief: he went to work after completing seventh grade. At age 21, he developed a throat malady that paralyzed his vocal cords and made him lose his voice. When medical doctors couldn't find a cause or remedy, he sought help from a hypnotist. While under hypnosis, Cayce reportedly diagnosed his ailment and prescribed a treatment in precise, medical terms, later verified by medical investigators. After following the course of treatment, his voice returned.

"Cayce became a national phenomenon," Zak wrote. "In 1910, the *New York Times* ran a story with the headline 'Illiterate man becomes a doctor when hypnotized–strange power shown by Edgar Cayce puzzles physicians.' As word about his unusual ability spread, people came from near and far, asking Cayce to perform psychic 'readings' and prescribe treatments for their ailments. 'What we think and what we eat, combined together, make what we are physically and mentally,' Cayce said during a 1934 reading. His remedies were holistic, often involving diet and massage."

More information and bibliography on Cayce are available by contacting A.R.E., Inc., 215 67th Street, Virginia Beach, VA 23451, or at (757) 428-3588 or (800) 333-4499, or http://www.edgar-cayce.org/edgar-cayce1.html.

See also FAITH HEALING.

cell salts   The ground material of mineral compounds that are produced naturally by the body, such as *Natrum muriaticum,* or sodium chloride (table salt). In a homeopathic remedy, one part salt must be ground with nine parts lactose, or milk sugar, to make *Natrum mur* 1x (x equals 10). This may be used to treat the symptoms of hay fever, for example. A cell-salt remedy made from calcium fluoride, which is found in fibers throughout the body, is used to treat hemorrhoids, varicose veins, hernias, and other problems. According to homeopaths, the more times cell salts are ground, or triturated, the greater their potency. The cell-salt system, also known as tissue salts, and remedies were first developed by the German physician W. H. Schuessler, M.D., who wrote *An Abridged Therapy Manual for the Biochemical Treatment of Disease* (Calcutta: Haren & Brother, 1st Indian ed., 1960), which was in its 25th edition in 1987. Schuessler believed that as natural medicine, cell salts are not only harmless because they are not substances foreign to the body, but beneficial in the treatment of a range of both acute and chronic problems. He utilized calcium, sodium, iron, magnesium, and potassium salts to develop a 12-salt system (long before the discovery of trace minerals such as zinc and selenium). The 12 salts are calcium fluoride (Calc fluor is the homeopathic designation), calcium phosphate (Calc phos), calcium sulfate (Calc sulph), ferric phosphate (Ferrum phos), potassium chloride (Kali mur), potassium sulfate (Kali sulph), potassium phosphate (Kali phos), magnesium phosphate (Mag phos), sodium chloride (Nat mur), sodium phosphate (Nat phos), sodium sulfate (Nat sulph), and silicic acid/silica (Silicea).

Schuessler also believed that cell-salt remedies catalyze natural biochemical reactions in the body and reorganize or balance them so any malfunctioning tissues can function normally. A homeopath must correctly identify which bodily tissues require specific treatment before prescribing a cell-salt remedy. Each type of salt acts a certain way. For instance, sulfur serves to help the body express, or throw off, an unwanted substance, and sodium attracts water. In combination, they may be used as a remedy for edema, the abnormal retention of water in the ankles, legs, hands, and other parts of the body. Among other ailments that may be treated homeopathically by cell salts are fever, hemorrhage, infections, mucus congestion, inflammation, sinusitis, colds, coughs, bronchitis, backache, colic, irritable bowels, bloating, gynecological problems, muscle spasms and cramps, teething pain, nodules, hernia, anxiety, depression, and insomnia.

See also HOMEOPATHY.

cell therapy   The injection of healthy animal cells or extracts of cells, usually from fetal sheep or pigs, into the human bloodstream in an attempt to fight various diseases, impotence, and aging; promote healing; and generally benefit the immune system and overall well-being. A still-controversial treatment developed during the 1930s by the Swiss physician Paul Niehans, who specialized in gland and organ transplantation, the original cell therapy has been banned in the United States since 1985 because of its potential for allergic reactions, infections, and ineffectiveness. However, cell therapy is practiced in Germany, France, Mexico, the Bahamas, and Switzerland. Studies are under way in the United States, Germany, and England to determine the effectiveness of human-to-human cell transplantation, and the use of shark embryo cells, human stem cells, and dendritic cells for the treatment of certain cancers, acquired immunodeficiency syndrome (AIDS), impotence, Parkinson's disease, Alzheimer's disease, burns, arthritis, spinal injuries, heart disease, and diabetes.

According to the second edition of *Alternative Medicine: The Definitive Guide* (Berkeley, Calif.: Celestial Arts, 2002), "Cell therapy is particularly exciting for conditions that involve cells that do not repair or regenerate well, such as the brain and heart, offering new hope for persons suffering from extensive damage in those organs. . . . The broadest definition of cell therapy includes the use of human blood transfusions and bone marrow transplants as well as injections of cellular materials . . . from organs, fetuses, or embryos of animals, or the transplantation of human stem cells, to stimulate healing and treat a variety of degenerative diseases. . . . Several schools of thought exist as to the ideal practice of cell therapy. The various methods include the use of live cells, freeze-dried cells, cells from specific organs, homeopathic formulations, and embryonic preparations. All these techniques have been used successfully, with different methods targeting different conditions."

A contemporary version of Niehans's therapy involves the use of antibodies or freeze-dried cells and pretesting to determine possible hypersensitivity in a patient. There are four main cell types used in combination for revitalization as well as treatment of a specific disease or malfunction: pituitary, liver, male or female reproductive glands, and connective tissue, plus cells from a particular organ or body structure that corresponds with the patient's needs.

See also CELL SALTS.

centesimal scale, homeopathic   The method of measurement, designated by a *c* for *centesimal,* used in homeopathy to determine the strength of homeopathic remedies. For example, after a mother tincture (which roughly refers to a "batch" or "stock") is made, one drop of it is added to 99 drops of water or alcohol. This yields a remedy of 1c potency, which is further diluted by another 99 drops of water or alcohol to create 2c potency. Usually, the highest dose of a homeopathic remedy equals 200c. Homeopathic practitioners say a remedy becomes more potent the more it is diluted.

See also HOMEOPATHY.

chakras   In Ayurvedic medicine, the seven regions, "focuses," or "circles" of the body that follow the body's midline and represent the specific energy and physical, emotional, and spiritual characteristics of each part. *Chakra* is the Sanskrit word for "wheel." Located along the central axis of the body, from the crown of the head to the root of the spine, the chakras govern not only physical functioning but mental consciousness that promotes awareness, personal evolution, and healing.

The first chakra, or root chakra, is centered on the anus, the base of the spine, the descending colon, and the hamstrings; it represents basic survival instincts, security, groundedness, and fears, including annihilation, abandonment, and other types of primal upheaval. The second chakra, the genital or sexual chakra, consists of the gonads, the urogenital structures, prostate, pelvis, and quadriceps, and represents gender, issues of commitment, sexuality, sensuality, and procreation. The solar plexus, or third chakra, incorporates the abdomen, the entire region around the navel, stomach, duodenum, ileum, pancreas, liver, and adrenal glands; it contains the largest portion of nerve tissue after that of the cranium and spinal cord. Emotionally, the solar plexus represents overall physical vitality and mastery.

The fourth, or heart, chakra, is the area just above the diaphragm in the area of the heart. Its main representations are nurturing, love for others, compassion, connection, and the core or center of one's being. Just above the heart chakra is the throat (including the larynx, pharynx, and thyroid gland), or fifth, chakra, which symbolizes communication, self-expression, and creativity. The sixth chakra, consisting of the eyes, pineal gland, and sinuses, governs intellect, perception, and intuitive qualities and is often referred to as the "third eye." The crown of the head, or seventh chakra, functions as a conduit for spiritual consciousness or the source of one's spiritual aura. Each chakra is also associated with an element such as air, water, ether, fire, or earth and with certain colors.

In the practice of Ayurveda, yoga, homeopathy, Reiki, and other disciplines, manipulating the energies of the chakras plays an important role in the healing process.

See also AYURVEDA; REIKI; YOGA.

channels   The pathways known as meridians along which *ch'i*— the body's life force or energy— flows; when illustrated, the meridians in and on the body resemble a road map that is followed by practitioners of acupuncture and acupressure, reflexologists, and other alternative health care providers.

See also ACUPRESSURE; ACUPUNCTURE.

chelation therapy   Derived from the Greek word *chele*, which means "to bind" or "to claw," a method of detoxifying the body, particularly of unwanted metals such as lead, iron, copper, zinc, aluminum, and manganese. Through a process that includes the removal of calcium in plaque that occludes arteries, chelation therapy is reported to restore blood circulation and therefore counteract gangrene, leg cramps, and other vascular disorders; treat Alzheimer's disease, multiple sclerosis, muscular dystrophy, asthma, macular degeneration, chronic fatigue syndrome, ulcerative colitis, emphysema, thyroid problems, scleroderma, viruses, lupus, and Parkinson's and other diseases; and reduce the adverse effects of chemotherapy and radiation therapy and the need for bypass surgery. The three- to four-hour procedure involves an intravenous (IV) injection of ethylenediaminetetraacetic acid (EDTA) into the hand or a finger. As a treatment for occluded arteries, chelation may be

necessary 20 to 50 times, to as many as 100 infusions of EDTA; as a preventive measure, the typical number of infusions is 10, administered one to three times a week. The IV solution may also contain supplements such as vitamins and minerals, as well as gingko biloba and phosphatidylserine, both of which act as chelators one may take orally as well.

So far, although it is considered safer than aspirin, EDTA has been approved by the Food and Drug Administration only for lead and other heavy metal poisoning and the treatment of hypercalcemia (an excessive amount of calcium in the blood). Chelation therapy remains controversial as an alternative treatment of other disorders, although some physicians prescribe it for individuals with cardiovascular problems and claim that it does in fact improve circulation and relieve the symptoms of arteriosclerosis that can lead to more serious problems. Other physicians argue that EDTA is incapable of permeating the arteries' cell membranes and consequently cannot reach a calcium accumulation effectively enough to clear it out. Furthermore, some say the chelation of iron increases the body's production of free radicals, compound substances that cause oxidation and damage bodily tissues.

A substance originally familiar to plumbers for removing calcium deposits from pipes, EDTA was first used therapeutically by the United States Navy to treat lead poisoning in 1948. Somewhat less effective than intravenous administration, oral chelation involves combining EDTA with other chelators, including garlic, vitamin C, carrageenan, rutin, bromelain, and certain enzymes. The enzyme cysteine, for example, may be prescribed for nickel poisoning and presence of excessive free radicals. Also, the action of the drug penicillamine, used as a conventional treatment of several ailments, including metal poisoning and rheumatoid arthritis, is similar to that of EDTA.

A study was conducted in 1958 in Switzerland to determine the effectiveness of EDTA chelation therapy as a preventive measure against cancer. The 231 adults in the study lived near a heavy-traffic highway that may have been exposing them to lead from vehicle exhaust, to which exposure was attributed high rates of cancer mortality and symptoms including headaches, drug and alcohol abuse, digestive problems, depression, fatigue, and anxiety.

ch'i   See QI.

Chinese herbalism   A segment of ancient Chinese medicine that focuses on plants and natural substances as sources of relief for medical and psychological problems. Because the whole plant contains the active ingredients, and because various herbs and other substances may be blended, side effects are minimized or eliminated and results are often enhanced. Chinese herbs—which include plant, mineral, and animal substances—are also meant to treat the root of one's condition rather than just target symptoms or potentially create additional problems by using one specific drug. Since the mythic sage Shen Nung experimented with and codified medicinal herbs 300 years ago, herbalism has become a highly sophisticated, intricate, and systematized practice that involves more than 6000 substances prescribed by practitioners. Each substance has certain qualities and properties that address the body constituents (*qi* [ch'i], moisture, and blood), organ networks, and what are known as "adverse climates": wind, heat, cold, dryness, and dampness. Herbs are categorized according to their nature (warm, cool, or neutral), taste (sour, bitter, sweet, salty, spicy, or bland), configuration (shape, texture, moisture), color, and properties, that is, their ability to relieve a particular ailment. An herbal substance may tonify, or strengthen; consolidate, or condense, astringe, or help concentrate energy, and so on; disperse, or help circulate; or purge, or eliminate, depending upon the diagnosis. For example, since ginseng is a "broad-spectrum" tonic for any deficiency of *qi*, codonopsis augments the *qi* very specifically in the spleen and lungs to treat ailments such as anemia, dehydration, and fatigue. Another herb, scutellaria, which purges heat from the lungs and liver, is used for the treatment of jaundice and infections.

Chinese herbalism, which now has entered mainstream American alternative and complementary medicine, is often used in conjunction with conventional Western drugs and treatments. Individuals with asthma, for example, may be on a reg-

imen of theophylline and other bronchodilators; rather than extend the intake to steroids when the bronchodilators are not effective enough to relieve symptoms, certain Chinese herbs can help reduce mucus production and strengthen the body's *qi* so the need for other medications may be reduced. A person with an ulcer who takes traditional antacids may be further relieved by Chinese herbs that fight heat and dampness in the stomach, help the liver to relax, and decongest impaired flow of *qi*. In general, Chinese herbalism recognizes remedies for illness but interprets illness as an imbalance of body constituents that may show up as patterns consisting of both physical and emotional symptoms. An important aspect of Chinese herbalism is correct diagnosis of a patient's problem; customized herbal treatment of the problem can conquer an entire spectrum of dysfunction. Common Chinese herbs are astragulus, lotus seed, nutmeg, walnut, ginger, cinnamon, radish seed, angelica root, schizandra, poria cocos, licorice, peony, chrysanthemum, ligusticum, honeysuckle, mulberry, raspberry, mustard seed, dianthus, plantain, motherwort, turmeric, myrrh resin, hawthorn, red and black dates, ephedra root, artemisia leaf, agrimony, magnolia, corn silk, corydalis root, peach seed, salvia root, fennel seed, coptis root, dandelion, sargassum, millettia stem, cordyceps, peppermint leaf, sileris root, gardenia, clove, cardamom seed, and unicaria stem. Chinese herbal substances also have Chinese and botanical names.

See also ACUPUNCTURE; CORDYCEPS; EIGHT GUIDING PRINCIPLES; HOMEOPATHY; JING; QI; WESTERN HERBALISM; YIN-YANG.

chiropractic   A widely acclaimed mainstream alternative discipline, dating back to ancient Egypt and other early civilizations, which is based on hands-on manipulations, or "adjustments," of the spinal cord. Modern chiropractic took root in the theory expressed in 1895 by Daniel David Palmer, of Davenport, Iowa, who advocated the teachings of Hippocrates and believed that all illnesses had their sources in the spine and the nervous system. According to chiropractic, a term derived from the Greek words *cheir* and *praktikos*, meaning "done by hand," when vertebrae are subluxated, or dislocated or misaligned, the person experiences any number of ailments, including allergy, headaches, skin conditions, back pain, sciatica, vision and hearing problems, muscle spasms, asthma and other respiratory disorders, peripheral joint injuries, osteoarthritis, herniated disk, and various other musculoskeletal disorders, bursitis, morning sickness related to pregnancy, menstrual problems, sinusitis, whiplash, otitis media, insomnia, colic, bladder infections, carpal tunnel syndrome and other repetitive stress disorders, scoliosis, depression, addiction, and other dysfunctions.

Chiropractors also work with the concept of the body's innate intelligence and ability to heal. Palmer suggested that innate intelligence flowed throughout the nervous system—which corresponds and communicates with every other part of the body—and could be blocked by a subluxation. When the subluxation is relieved, the body has the opportunity to heal itself. This form of chiropractic, now referred to as "straight," adheres to Palmer's original idea of performing only spinal manipulation. "Mixed" chiropractic refers to spinal manipulation and other forms of treatment, including nutritional and exercise counseling, traction, orthotics, ultrasound, diathermy, cryotherapy, massage, and physiotherapy.

The Canadian-born Dr. Palmer, who eventually founded the Palmer College of Chiropractic in Iowa, first reported that after he had performed spinal manipulation on a patient who had been deaf for 17 years, the man's hearing was restored. Apparently the man had a subluxated vertebra that corresponded to an injury he had suffered to his upper spine just before he lost his hearing. Palmer adjusted that specific area, thereby correcting the blockage in the nerves that caused the deafness. The college's first graduates were medical doctors who were convinced of Palmer's philosophy, and case after case seemed to support chiropractic's success despite the fact that there has long been a dearth of scientific study to prove its fundamental principles to the conventional medical community. The New Zealand Royal Commission of Inquiry into chiropractic in 1979 noted, among many, the case of "Duncan C." Duncan, an active, easygoing boy of 11, from February 1977 complained of stiff knees. The stiffness progressed rapidly to his hips and all joints. His doctor saw no active disease in

Duncan's system or joints and recommended 300 milligrams of aspirin four times daily for symptomatic relief. But the pain progressed until the child cried, was unable to dress himself, and was stooped over as if he was an elderly man.

Further hospital test findings proved negative. Emotional trauma was suggested as the cause of Duncan's pain, but no explanation was found there, either. The boy's desperate parents finally took him to a chiropractor. After the first adjustment, Duncan felt sick. Three hours later, however, Duncan was walking "without my knees flapping together," he said. By the next day, his hands were pain-free. After each adjustment, Duncan made considerable progress until he was totally back to normal. He described as a "numb" feeling the absence of the pain to which he had grown accustomed.

Since chiropractors are trained to advise patients when to seek conventional medical care and because there is overwhelming anecdotal evidence of success of chiropractic as an alternative or complementary modality, the spring 1982 issue of the *International Review of Chiropractic* stated: "The Supreme Court has upheld the right of medical doctors to form partnerships or engage in group practice with alternative health care providers, such as chiropractors." An estimated 30 million people in the United States seek and receive chiropractic treatment, and many leading insurance providers include visits to a chiropractor in their coverage plans. A commonsense and holistic approach with an emphasis on prevention and wellness, chiropractic is considered the second-largest primary-health-care field in the world.

Chiropractic adjustments are given during office visits and are considered safe, painless, and noninvasive. Patients may be lying supine or prone or sitting up, depending upon which type of adjustment is appropriate. One's first visit to a chiropractor often requires acute care (the first level of chiropractic), that is, relief of aggravating symptoms or pain. The second level is the restorative phase, which involves maintenance of the realigned spinal column through individualized, repeated adjustments. The wellness phase, or third level of chiropractic care, entails periodic visits to prevent occurrence of new subluxations. More information is available by contacting the American Chiropractic Association, 1701

Clarendon Boulevard, Arlington, VA 22209, or (800) 986-4636, or www.acatoday.com.

See also Appendix I; OSTEOPATHY.

chologogue A substance that increases the flow of bile into the intestinal tract.

Chopra, Deepak A New England endocrinologist originally from India, former chief of staff of Boston Regional Medical Center, and founding president of the American Association of Ayurvedic Medicine. His highly acclaimed books include *Quantum Healing: Exploring the Frontiers of Mind/Body Medicine* (New York: Bantam Books, 1989); *Creating Health; Return of the Rishi; Perfect Health; Ageless Body, Timeless Mind; Creating Affluence; The Seven Spiritual Laws of Success; Unconditional Life, How to Know God: The Soul's Journey into the Mystery of Mysteries; Overcoming Addictions; Spiritual Laws for Parenting; Grow Younger, Live Longer: 10 Steps to Reverse Aging; The Return of Merlin*; and *The Path to Love*. A fellow of the American College of Physicians and a member of the American Association of Clinical Endocrinologists, Chopra is considered one of the foremost U.S. experts in mind-body medicine, particularly for developing a blend of quantum physics and ancient medicine practices and theories. He is currently director of educational programs, CEO, and founder of the Chopra Center for Well-Being, established in 1995 in La Jolla, California, and now at La Costa Resort and Spa in Carlsbad, California (800-854-5000).

cicatrizant A substance or agent that encourages scar tissue to form during the healing process.

coagulant A substance that promotes the formation of clots, such as blood clots.

Coles, Robert A professor of psychiatry and medical humanities at Harvard Medical School, research psychiatrist for the Harvard University Health Services, and the author of more than 50 books, including *The Spiritual Life of Children* (Boston: Houghton Mifflin, 1990); *The Moral Intelligence of Children* (New York: Random House, 1997); and *The Mind's Fate: Ways of Seeing Psychiatry and Psychoanalysis*. Also the James Agee Professor of Social Ethics at Harvard, he won a Pulitzer Prize for his book *Children of Crisis* and other awards for his books about children. Coles has also worked with parents, undergraduates, teachers, community leaders, and medical students and as a volunteer at schools, hospital wards, and clinics.

colonic irrigation The process of injecting enough water (to which herbs or enzymes may be added) through a tube into the colon to fill and cleanse it, also known as an enema, rectal, or clysis. In certain alternative and complementary medicine practices, colonics are used to detoxify the intestinal tract and treat a wide variety of disorders, including hypertension, heart disease, arthritis, depression, and infections. The method evolved from the days before antibiotics had been developed to fight infection, when emptying the bowels was considered therapeutic for a number of ailments. In ancient Greece and Egypt, as well as in Ayurvedic medicine originating in India, colonics were regarded as rejuvenating. During the 1920s and 1930s, inducing bowel movements became a fad treatment called "high colonics." One of the most prominent colonic therapists was John Harvey Kellogg, who treated thousands of patients with gastrointestinal disorders at the Kellogg Sanitarium in Battle Creek, Michigan. Kellogg later founded the Kellogg cereal company in Battle Creek.

The basic concept of colonic irrigation as therapy is to exacerbate the natural process of eliminating toxins and digestive waste materials from the colon and rectum. Colonic enthusiasts believe a buildup of waste materials impedes normal elimination and therefore impedes the immune system and bloodstream. Irrigation may, however, damage the colon by perforating it or injecting amounts of fluid great enough to stretch the bowel out of normal proportion and thus impair its ability to function. In addition, colonics may deplete the body of enzymes and normal colonic flora that keep the intestines functioning normally, particularly in their ability to fight microbial invasion. Contaminated irrigation equipment may also cause potentially life-threatening infections such as amebic dysentery. Colonic irrigation is not recommended for individuals who have Crohn's disease, diverticulitis, hemorrhoids, rectal or colon tumors, or ulcerative colitis. Also, undiagnosed intestinal disorders that require conventional treatment may be aggravated by irrigation procedures. More information is available by contacting the International Association for Colon Hydrotherapy, P.O. Box 461285, San Antonio, TX 78246-1286, or (210) 366-2888.

See also Appendix I.

color therapy A therapeutic method that originated in ancient Egypt, Greece, Rome, Babylonia, and China after the recognition that sunlight therapy relieved skin disorders. Therapy evolved into the use of colored light (red and infrared) for lesions caused by smallpox and German measles. Dr. Peter Mandel, a German naturopathic physician, developed Colorpuncture, which combines the use of acupoints and meridians of acupuncture with wavelengths of colored light, according to an individual's needs. For example, he believes reds, oranges, and yellows strengthen or stimulate acupoints, and greens, blues, and violets subdue them. Mandel also theorizes that the flow of *qi (ch'i)* throughout the body along the meridians, or channels, works with color and light in the same way a fiberoptic network operates.

In Ayurvedic medicine, each chakra, or energy circle, of the body along the vertical midline has attributed to it a specific color, a concept that embraces the link between the body's electromagnetic vibrations and wavelengths of color. In the practice of feng shui, or the Chinese art of placement, color plays a major role in the way an environment and the people in it are affected by colors. There are various techniques involving the use of color as therapy for both physical and emotional problems.

Because color emanates from daylight, a combination of the eight colors of the spectrum (red, orange, yellow, green, blue, violet, turquoise, and magenta) and the radiation inherent in sunlight, many color therapists believe that certain colors correspond with mental, emotional, and physical problems, such as insomnia, depression, behavioral problems, pain, anxiety, asthma, and stress-related ailments. Each color also has its own vibrational frequency and therefore can affect the body's sense of well-being and balance. A therapist may administer light treatments, during which a patient is given a white robe to wear under a light machine with stained-glass filters for about 20 minutes. This may also include the therapist's use of draping colored materials around the patient or using a quartz crystal torch through which light filters. The colors of one's clothing, foods, and personal environments play important roles in color therapy, and the therapist may suggest variations from current choices. Excessive use of one color is said to affect one's health adversely. Red, for example, is reported to lower resistance to pain, raise blood pressure, and affect embryonic cell structure during pregnancy. When blue light, on the other hand, was focused on the hands of 60 middle-aged women at the San Diego State University School of Nursing in 1982, the women experienced a certain amount of pain relief from their rheumatoid arthritis. Other studies, such as one concerning sufferers of migraines, have also been conducted using colored light.

See also AURA; CHAKRAS; FENG SHUI; LIGHT THERAPY.

combination remedies In homeopathy, a mixture of remedies, often at low potency levels, for the treatment of an ailment, akin to the concept of broad-spectrum antibiotics when a particular microorganism is not identified or readily identifiable.

See also HOMEOPATHY.

complementary medicine Any method or modality intended to enhance or supplement other treatments, including traditional Western medicine. Complementary forms of treatment may also be categorized as alternative or integrative medicine.

compress In various branches of medicine, including home remedies and folk medicine practices, a cloth or pad saturated with either hot or cold agents and applied directly to the skin over an area of the body that is swollen or painful. Compresses may also be used in the form of dry, soft folded cloth that is applied firmly over a wound to promote healing through slight pressure and closure.

constitutional remedies In homeopathy, remedies that correspond to an individual's overall physical and mental state and family medical history.

cordyceps   An ancient Chinese herbal remedy, made from the fungus *Cordyceps sinensis* grown in the Himalayan regions of China and Tibet, that is reported to improve athletic performance and training.

See also CHINESE HERBALISM.

counterirritant   A substance that irritates one part of the body to counteract irritation to another part.

cranial osteopathy   See CRANIOSACRAL THERAPY; OSTEOPATHY.

craniosacral therapy   A system of therapy based on the idea that there is a rhythmic pressure and flow of cerebrospinal fluid between the cranium (skull) and sacrum (the base of the spine) that governs the way the craniosacral structures, including the brain, pituitary and pineal glands, spinal cord, and meninges, or membranes, function and maintain the body's well-being. Gentle hands-on "manipulation" of the skull's sutures, that is, the delineations between the sections of cranial bone, and of the spinal column, rib cage, and limbs is reported to restore the flow and alleviate disorders including headache, sinusitis, brain trauma, transient ischemic attack (called TIA, akin to a ministroke), strabismus (cross-eyes), trigeminal neuralgia (sharp pain in the jaw), asthma, colic, Bell's palsy, posttraumatic stress disorder, rheumatoid arthritis, dizziness, hyperactivity, visual disturbances, seizures, postpartum depression, learning disabilities, ear infections, cerebral palsy, autism, and injury to the head, torso, arms, and legs.

The American osteopathic physician John E. Upledger developed CranioSacral Therapy (CST) after conducting a team of researchers—physiologists, biophysicists, bioengineers, anatomists, and others—at the Michigan State University College of Osteopathic Medicine in the 1970s. Upledger decided that his main approach would involve manipulation of the meninges of the craniosacral system. He theorized that cells and structures of the body have the capacity to "remember" physical or emotional shock, which manifests in certain areas he called "energy cysts." In order for the body to function normally again, these energy cysts representing suppressed painful experiences needed to

be dislodged, released, or broken up both physically and mentally; Upledger described the process as the technique of SomatoEmotional Release (SER). Upledger's disciples often combine CST with SER, depending upon their patients' individual needs. Craniosacral therapy is considered a type of energy medicine that targets the memory of past traumas the body subconsciously harbors.

In addition to Upledger's meningeal approach, the sutural approach—manipulation at the cranial sutures—was developed by Dr. William Garner Sutherland, an early 20th-century osteopathic physician. There is still controversy concerning the ability of the cranial bones, which conventional medicine claims are fused together, to move at all, and also concerning the existence of a craniosacral rhythmic impulse. However, there is some scientific and clinical evidence that supports Sutherland's treatment, originally known as cranial osteopathy. Another type of craniosacral therapy, called the reflex approach, combines the techniques of applied kinesiology with the stimulation of nerve endings located within the cranial sutures and in the scalp. A combination of all three approaches is the Sacro-Occipital Technique (S.O.T.), which was developed by Dr. Major B. DeJarnette, a chiropractor and in the 1920s a student of Sutherland's.

Because craniosacral treatments consist of light palpations, as opposed to chiropractic adjustments or more vigorous forms of bodywork, critics claim it cannot be effective. However effective or harmless the therapy may be, it may not be recommended for young children or anyone with a dysfunction that affects intracranial pressure, such as a brain tumor or an aneurysm.

See also OSTEOPATHY.

crystal and gemstone therapy   Derived from the Greek word *krystallos* and the Latin *crystallum*, meaning a lucid substance that has solidified, crystals and gemstones, which are precious and semi-precious stones, were thought by the ancients to be powerful, healing manifestations of electromagnetic energies of the Earth. During a crystal therapy session, crystals or gemstones may be held by the client or practitioner or placed in the room or on the client's chakras, the energy circles along the midline of the body. Some claim they have been relieved of symptoms of wounds, back pain, and arthritis. There are at least 3000 crystal and gemstone substances that have been identified as having specific properties and characteristics. For example, amethyst may be worn or held during meditation by a person who wishes to develop psychic ability or become more spiritual. To relieve stress caused by being unable to speak up about a problem, one may hold a piece of turquoise or aquamarine against his or her throat and concentrate on relaxing and freeing the mind of resentment. Several crystals and stones have been associated with certain glands in the body. Clear quartz, for instance, may be placed on the forehead, chest, and solar plexus; in the palm of each hand; and on the pubic bone during breathing exercises or meditation to help clear energy blockages from the corresponding organs. Clear tourmaline has been used for benefit to the immune system, for general detoxification, and for eye and nervous system disorders. Silver is said to balance hormone levels, reduce lung and throat irritation, and help resolve sexual dysfunction. Wearing peridot is said to benefit the stomach and digestive tract. As folklore, crystal and gemstone therapy functions daily as part of the customs of our culture; for example, an engagement ring harks back to the days when the ancients believed that wearing or carrying talismans put one in tune with universal forces. Healers through the ages have used substances from the Earth to connect with healing power in conjunction with other relaxation and visualization techniques.

Culpeper's Herbal   The seventeenth-century British reference book by Nicholas Culpeper (also spelled Culpepper), *Culpeper's Complete Herbal,* published by W. Foulsham and Co., lists herbs and herbal remedies.

curanderismo   A form of southwestern folk healing performed by a *curandero,* or most revered healer, considered to have a gift from God. *Curanderos,* males or *curanderas,* females, may be consulted for medical, emotional, social, supernatural, and spiritual problems. The *curandero* or *curandera* uses herbs, rituals, water, candles, countermagic, prayer, potions, hexing agents, Tarot cards, and other methods and symbols of healing, depending upon an individual's problem. *Curanderismo* has evolved throughout history—a practice particularly popular among Hispanics and Mexicans in the Southwest—derived from the ages during which medicine, the church, and belief in the supernatural were virtually interchangeable. *Curanderos* as private consultants offer help to people with problems ranging from love relationships and financial difficulties to illness and the effects of "black magic" or "spells" cast by *brujos* (witches).

cymatics   A type of sound therapy developed by the British physician and osteopath Peter Manners in the 1960s. Dr. (Sir) Manners continues to work in the field of cymatics and biomagnetics for medical diagnosis and treatment. He holds the Dag Hammerskjold Merit of Excellence Award for Benefits to Humanity, and he has lectured at the World Health Organization in Europe. The theory of cymatics, derived from the Greek word kyma, or "a great wave," is based on specific sound frequencies that emanate from the millions of body cells. A healthy body's sound frequency is stable, but in the case of illness, the frequency is increased or upset in some way. Practitioners of cymatics use machines that operate on frequencies that reflect a normal state to stimulate cells whose frequency reflects an abnormality or distress. A cymatics practitioner holds a pencil-sized or larger applicator that is connected to an electromagnetic device about the size of an attaché case. Through electroids attached to the body, similar to electrocardiogram leads, the practitioner then directs the sound frequencies to the distressed area of the body. To treat a painful muscle, for example, the frequency is supposed to correct the impaired frequency causing the pain. Certain practitioners also use "aquasonics," which refers to sound frequencies transmitted through water, or other techniques in combination with cymatics to treat asthma, arthritis, a stubborn virus, and various musculoskeletal injuries and to relieve tension. Treatments are painless and seem to lack any adverse effects. Cymatic clinics are located in the United States, Europe, Canada, Japan, Australia, and other parts of the world.

dance therapy Also called dance movement therapy, methods or techniques involving physical motion, accompanied or unaccompanied by music, to achieve stress reduction, release, creativity, playfulness, and self-expression for individuals with emotional disturbances, depression, or other problems. Dance therapists work with people whose problems are connected with their particular way of moving, who can improve their emotional state and resolve issues (assertiveness, self-image, self-identity, trust, etc.) through specific dance movements.

dan tien In Chinese medicine, the body's three energy centers—upper, middle, and lower—where *qi* (or *ch'i*, the vital force or vital energy) is stored. The upper center is between the eyebrows (also known as the "third eye"); the middle is in the center of the torso, and the lower is the lower abdomen.
See also *QI*.

Davis, Adelle A well-known nutritionist and author of *Let's Eat Right To Keep Fit, Let's Have Healthy Children, Let's Get Well,* and *Let's Cook It Right* (New York: New American Library, Harcourt Brace Jovanovich Inc., 1954–1970). During the 1950s and 1960s until her death in 1971, Davis was one of the pioneers of nutrition as a way to treat illness and dysfunction in the body and promote wellness. Believing that nutrition can determine one's physical, emotional, and spiritual status, she studied at Purdue University and graduated from the University of California at Berkeley, did postgraduate work at Columbia University and the University of California at Los Angeles, and received a master's degree in biochemistry from the University of Southern California Medical School. Davis worked extensively with doctors at Bellevue and Fordham Hospitals and

at the Judson Health Clinic. Later she was a consulting nutritionist for physicians at the Alameda County Health Clinic and the William E. Branch Clinic in Hollywood. Davis was married to Frank Sieglinger and was the mother of two children.

decimal scale, homeopathic Designated by an x in homeopathy, the measure of potency of a remedy in tenths; for example, one drop of mother tincture (stock or "batch" of a remedy) is diluted with nine drops of water or alcohol to yield a remedy that is said to have 2x potency.
See also CENTESIMAL SCALE; HOMEOPATHIC.

decoction From the Latin words *de* and *coquere,* or to boil down, the homeopathic term for a herb or combination of herbs that are boiled in water, which is then reduced to make a concentrate. When a decoction, essentially a liquid medicinal preparation, does not require a precise strength, it may be made by boiling five parts of the herb or vegetable or crumbled pieces of a drug with 100 parts water for 15 minutes. In traditional Western medicine, there are no specific decoctions.

deep-muscle massage See MASSAGE.

demulcent From the Latin word *demulcens,* meaning "to stroke softly," a substance or agent, such as glycerin, honey, lanolin, and olive oil, that soothes, moisturizes, softens, and protects mucous membranes. Demulcents are used in homeopathy.
See also HOMEOPATHY.

depression, effects of In bioenergetic healing and vibrational medicine, a theory that the energy produced by clinically or psychotically depressed individuals had negative effects on plant growth after they had been asked to "treat" or hold onto bottles of saline solution used to water the plants. In studies in the 1960s on the true nature of hands-on healing practices, that is, studies to determine whether results occurred because of psychological factors such as belief or faith or because of an actual transfer of physical energy from the healer to an individual, Dr. Bernard Grad, a gerontologist at McGill University in Montreal, Canada, used plants as the "healees" to eliminate the possibility of faith or personal belief in the healing process. Grad engaged a local healer to treat barley plants watered and grown in the normal fashion and barley plants he had deliberately watered with saline solution to inhibit their growth. The healer was not told which plants had been watered with saline solution; the healer-treated plants were reported to be taller and more robust and to have higher levels of chlorophyll than the control group of normal plants. On days when the healer was not feeling well physically or emotionally, Grad determined that the healing energy was "off."

See also VIBRATIONAL MEDICINE.

depurgative A substance or agent that cleanses the blood, such as echinacea and colostrums.

detoxification Any process, internal and external, geared toward purifying the body, that is, ridding it of foreign or toxic substances and wastes. Detoxificants or detoxifiers include many varieties of herbs as well as vitamin C and other nutrients.

See also *AAMA*; CHELATION THERAPY; COLONICS.

dhatus In Ayurvedic medicine, the body's seven essential components: (1) *rasa*, or plasma; (2) *rakta*, or the blood tissue or red blood cells; (3) *mamsa*, or muscle tissue; (4) *meda*, or adipose tissue; (5) *asthi*, or bone tissue; (6) *majja*, or nerve tissue and bone marrow; and (7) *shukra*, semen and reproductive tissue.

See also AYURVEDA.

diets, specific See MACROBIOTIC DIET; NUTRITION.

digestive Any substance or agent that aids the normal functioning of the gastrointestinal tract and the process of digestion.

dina chariya A regimen geared toward healthful daily living set forth in Ayurvedic medicine.

See also AYURVEDA.

distant healing Any method or technique such as Reiki, prayer, or meditation, that may be performed by an individual despite a physical distance between the healer and the recipient of healing energy.

See also CAYCE, EDGAR; DOSSEY, LARRY; PRAYER; REIKI.

doshas Also known as the *tridoshas*, the three fundamental body types categorized in Ayurvedic medicine—*pitta, vata,* and *kapha*—considered the foundation of all biological, emotional, and physiological aspects of a person. Although the three distinct *doshas* provide the basis for body types, combinations of *doshas* are recognized as more the rule than the exception and demonstrate characteristics in common. Ayurvedic practitioners believe that when the *doshas* are out of balance, illness may occur.

See also AYURVEDA.

Dossey, Larry American medical doctor who has studied the power of prayer as it relates to the practice of medicine. He is the author of several books, including *Healing Words: The Power of Prayer* (HarperSanFrancisco, 1993); *Prayer Is Good Medicine; Meaning of Medicine* (New York: Bantam, 1991); and *Recovering the Soul* (Bantam, 1989). Dossey documents evidence gathered by control-group experimentation on the therapeutic effects of prayer, including prayers of people at great distances from the persons being prayed for and for those with catastrophic illnesses. He also theorizes that healing is linked to a "nonlocal mind" that accesses various phenomena such as remote viewing, distant clairvoyant observations, and other forms of "focused consciousness" different and distinct from faith healing or a placebo effect.

See also NONLOCAL MIND.

douche, herbal A lavage or administration of water on or into a body cavity performed to cleanse and to restore normal functioning and balance. Medicinal or nutritive herbs may be added to the fluid wash for an enhanced effect, particularly to subdue irritation or relieve pain. For example, an herbal douche that may be helpful in cases of vaginitis may contain calendula flowers, pau d'arco, tea tree oil, white oak bark, squaw vine, mild white clay with hazel bark and leaf, and sage or vinegar in one quart of water. Ordinary saline solution is an effective nasal douche for congestion caused by allergies or colds.

See also HERBALISM.

dowser, medical   The term derived from the name given in 1838 to people who used divining (or dowsing) rods to find water or other natural resources, which now refer to individuals who use a dowsing instrument, such as a pendulum, to locate and diagnose a physical malfunction or disease. Also known as medical radiesthesia, medical dowsing corresponds to a certain psychic ability of the dowser, who reportedly receives intensified energy in the form of involuntary muscle tremors or movement in his or her hands as the dowsing device is held.

See also VIBRATIONAL MEDICINE.

drama therapy   Methods or techniques involving role playing, acting out stories, and other activities geared toward helping individuals improve relationships, social skills, and personal issues. Drama therapists guide groups in the creation of drama as a way to address factors including awareness and sensitivity, behavior, imagination, team effort, and general understanding of interpersonal interaction. People with a wide range of physical and emotional problems may benefit from drama therapy.

dreams, diagnostic; healing   The concept of dreaming—constructed in the right brain as opposed to the literal construction of left-brain thinking—as a way to connect with the higher self and as the source of dream-symbol interpretation that may possibly help in the diagnosis and treatment of illness. Some therapists and alternative medicine practitioners recommend keeping a dream diary (dreams can occur during waking or sleeping hours) to determine patterns of symbols or ideas. Some spiritual philosophers and advocates of various types of vibrational medicine maintain that

the dream state provides the opportunity for an aspect of our spirit to leave our physical body and have direct experience with another dimension of existence, which may be referred to as an astral plane. This may offer insights into the true nature of health and illness and add to the entire body of information on mind-body medicine and healing.

Dunbar, Helen Flanders   American psychiatrist (d.1959), who was a founder of the subspecialty called consultation-liaison psychiatry and a proponent of mind-body medicine. Dunbar also believed that mental, social, and environmental factors affect physiological functioning. The daughter of a physicist, Dunbar earned her undergraduate degree at Bryn Mawr in 1923 and her medical degree at Yale Medical School in 1930. She later acquired the degrees B.D., Ph.D., and D.Med.Sci. After spending a year in Europe, she became affiliated with Columbia University and the Presbyterian Hospital, where she was appointed psychiatrist to the medical service. She was a member of the American Psychoanalytic Society and authored more than 80 books and articles. Her work was influenced by ancient physicians and philosophers, the work of Cannon and the flight or fight response, Selye's theory on the general adaptation syndrome, and other 19th- and 20th-century researchers who sought scientific evidence of what Dunbar called, for want of a better term, "psychosomatic" medicine. She studied 600 patients with heart disease, diabetes, and fractures at Presbyterian Hospital, and in 1936 discovered that psychological factors had a significant effect on the causes of the disease and the disease process. This led her to coin the term "accident-prone personality." Dunbar also conducted research by providing personality profiles (later known as "personality constellations") that connected chronic disorders such as asthma, migraine, ulcerative colitis, and peptic ulcer with certain personality types.

At the same time, Chicago psychoanalyst Franz Alexander theorized on a "specificity hypothesis," saying that specific but unresolved emotional problems caused chronic tension, dysfunction, and finally structural changes in certain organs. Dunbar believed that the disorders were not "specific" but complex, and she did not accept Alexander's "specificity hypothesis." She published her book *Emotions and Bodily Changes: A Survey of Literature on Psychosomatic Interrelationships* in 1936, and *Psychosomatic Diagnosis* in 1943. She thought that the research findings would lead to appropriate prevention techniques and treatment. In 1939, Dunbar founded and served as the first editor of the *Journal of Psychosomatic Medicine*, a post she held for eight years. (The journal is now published by the American Psychosomatic Society.) Dunbar's contributions to the study of psychosomatic medicine spurred Rockefeller Foundation grants to general hospitals in 1934 and 1935 with the mission of encouraging the collaboration of psychiatrists and other physicians. The Mount Sinai Hospital in New York and Rochester Medical School pioneered in consultation-liaison services. In the mid-1970s, the National Institute of Mental Health provided grants to 130 consultation-liaison programs.

Dyer, Wayne W.   An American doctor of counseling psychology and popular proponent of mind-body practices who has lectured, conducted workshops, appeared on television, and written several books, including *Real Magic* (New York: HarperCollins, 1992), *Everyday Wisdom, Your Erroneous Zones, Pulling Your Own Strings* (New York: HarperCollins Publishers, 1995), *The Sky's the Limit, Gifts from Eykis, No More Holiday Blues, Your Sacred Self, What Do You Really Want for Your Children?*, and *You'll See It When You Believe It* (New York: Avon Books, 1989).

ear-candling Sometimes also called ear-coning, a home remedy dating back to 2500 B.C. for removing ear wax, fungus, or impurities that supposedly cause a blockage of the ear canal or discomfort in the ears and sinuses. Made from paraffin- or beeswax-soaked natural fibers such as linen or cotton and specifically tapered into cone shapes and allowed to dry and harden, an ear (or auricular) candle is a hollow wax cylinder approximately 10 inches long. (Variations of this include wax-soaked newspaper and pottery cones through which herbal smoke is blown. Also, various herbs, honey, or other substances may be added to the wax.) After being fitted into a hole in a protective plate, it is lit and the smaller (unlit) end placed in the ear canal as the patient lies on his or her side. A collecting plate catches melting wax from the burning end of the candle. The rationale for this procedure is that the burning candle creates a convection or vacuum that sucks out undesirable material from the ear, although there is no evidence that any suction is created. The ear-candling session lasts approximately 45 minutes, and practitioners, also known as "earconologists," claim that two to eight sessions may required before complete relief is experienced. Ear-candlers do not recommend the procedure for individuals who have perforated or artificial eardrums or those who have ear tubes.

Ear candles are not approved by the Federal Drug Administration (FDA) and are banned in Canada. Despite anecdotal reports that ear-candling relieves earache, sinus headache, swimmer's ear, temporomandibular joint (TMJ) pain, auricular herpes zoster, Ménière's disease, vertigo, stress-related problems, allergies, tinnitus, hearing problems, and other ailments, particularly those of horn players and singers, who are said to have a greater earwax buildup, the process is generally considered dangerous—largely because of burns and the potential for puncturing the eardrum—and ineffective. Conventional medicine states that compacted earwax or any other impairment or injury of the ear should be attended to by a physician.

Eastern medicine Various disciplines of medical practice derived from ancient lands including Egypt and countries of the Middle and Near East, continental Asia, China, Japan, and other regions. Ancient Indian medicine, or Ayurveda; traditional Chinese and Japanese medicine; and a wide range of additional practices, such as *qigong*, t'ai ch'i, yoga, and massage, have now been introduced into the United States as alternative/complementary treatment modalities.

effleurage A technique of massage involving slow, rhythmic strokes.

See also MASSAGE.

eight principal patterns Also known as the eight guiding principles, the diagnostic method in traditional Chinese medicine that uses the principles of yin-yang (both of these are composites of a person's illness), cold-hot (either lack of or excess of body heat), interior- exterior (also called internal-external, referring to afflictions of the inner organs, blood vessels, bones, nerves, etc., or skin, muscles, hair, joints, superficial muscles, etc.), and excess-deficiency (either a surplus or lack of the basic body constituents such as blood, *qi (ch'i)*, and moisture). Chinese practitioners believe a person's illness is related to any or a combination of these eight concepts. Treatment is determined by one or more of the principles.

See also EMPTY HEAT; QI; YIN-YANG.

electroacupuncture A technique of acupuncture involving the use of battery-powered devices that stimulate acupoints through needles, rubber electrodes, or a metal probe.

See also ACUPUNCTURE.

electromagnetic force In physics, magnetism generated by an electrical current. Alternative medicine practitioners work to realign, balance, or otherwise manipulate the electromagnetic energy in and around the human body as treatment for illness and as modalities for promoting relaxation and well-being. The electromagnetic field may be accessed with or without the laying on of hands.

See also AYURVEDA; ENERGY; RADIONICS; REIKI; THERAPEUTIC TOUCH; VIBRATIONAL MEDICINE.

emotional freedom technique (EFT) A branch or method of energy psychology.

See also ENERGY.

Empty Heat In traditional Chinese medicine, a yin deficiency also known as internal heat, such as fever, inflammation, redness, swelling, pain, thirst, dryness, constipation, or agitation.

See also EIGHT PRINCIPAL PATTERNS; YIN-YANG.

endorphins Polypeptides, protein chemical substances produced naturally by the brain that, when activated by other substances, exercise, or various emotional states, create a sensation of well-being, analgesia, or euphoria similar to that induced by opiates. The polypeptides bind to opiate receptor sites of the brain related to the perception of pain. When endorphins are released, the threshold for pain increases, and an individual feels more comfortable as a result. The most active of the polypeptides is *B-endorphin*. The word *endorphin*, coined in 1976, is a combination of *endo*genous and mor*phine*. Related are enkephalins, pentapeptides produced naturally in the brain that also have opiate-receptor ability and potent painkilling effects.

enema, therapeutic See COLONICS.

energy From the Greek word *energeia*, or the Latin *energia*, both meaning activity, the power or capacity to work or to empower, that is, to set things in motion (kinetic energy), put things in position (potential or stored energy), and create light, heat, ionizing radiation, or sound. On a metabolic level, for example, when the intake of oxygen combines with the intake of sugar and fat, a chemical reaction occurs in the body that concurrently produces heat, or energy, and cellular waste products, which result in fatigue. Energetics is the science or study of human energy, such as that used in doing work or exercising. The conservation of energy refers to the theory that energy cannot either be created or be destroyed; instead, it is changed into other forms. Bioenergetics is the study of the transfer of energy and the way one living system relates to others; biodynamics refers to the study of the energy, or life force, of living matter. Types of bioenergy include (1) metabolic: the fuel that empowers fundamental cellular processes; (2) bioelectrical: the movement of fluids and substances throughout the body and nervous system activity, including the brain's ability to process information and perceive the world; (3) biophotonic: found in all the body cells' nuclei for cell-to-cell communication; (4) subtle bioenergies: *qi (ch'i)*, or life force, and prana (breath) that flows throughout the body (meridians, chakras, muscles, skin, etc.), particularly for the coordination of bodily functions and defense against illness; (5) etheric: for subtle-energetic growth, development, and repair of the body (this may be similar to subtle bioenergies); (6) astral: thought forms for the processing of emotions and emotional energy; (7) mental: abstract thought forms for creativity and intellectual functioning; and (8) spiritual: soul energy that is said to flow or transfer from lifetime to lifetime and is remembered by the physical cells.

It is generally accepted by all the traditional life sciences that the human being is an energy system. In Ayurvedic medicine, all energy generates from cosmic consciousness, and all five forms of energy—water, fire, air, ether, and earth—are present in all forms of matter, including in each person and representative of the five senses and manifested in the doshas, or body types. Ayurvedic practitioners believe in the goal of balancing one's energy in order to move each individual into harmony with cosmic consciousness.

Practitioners of other forms of alternative medicine, such as Therapeutic Touch and Reiki, believe that human energy may be used as a healing modality and can be directed, modulated, balanced, and interfaced with other modalities. With their techniques, they pursue the concept that the transfer of energy from one human being to another is not only a natural event, but a continuous one, whether it is intended to be or not. Intentionality adds to the healing power of energy transfer.

See also AYURVEDA; ELECTROACUPUNCTURE; ELECTROMAGNETIC FIELD; ENERGY MEDICINE; REIKI; THERAPEUTIC TOUCH; VIBRATIONAL MEDICINE; YIN-YANG.

energy medicine A form of treatment for pain and various illnesses that employs electrical currents. In mainstream medical practice, electroencephalograms (EEGs), electrocardiograms (ECGs), magnetic resonance imaging (MRI), and transcutaneous electrical nerve stimulation (TENS) energy medicine may be thought of as energy medicine. In alternative practice, electroacupuncture, auricular acupuncture, cymatics, light therapy, sound therapy, and microcurrent electrical therapy are some of the available treatments. People who have pacemakers or bleeding disorders or who are pregnant should not consider certain forms of energy medicine.

Microcurrent electrical therapy involves placing electrodes over painful areas of the body (or areas opposite where the pain occurs) and running an electrical current into them in order to relieve the pain. The TENS technique is reported to stimulate the body's natural production of endorphins (chemically similar to morphine) and to prevent the brain from perceiving pain sensations. TENS has been used in the treatment of pain associated with arthritis, sciatica, neuralgia, shingles, chronic back pain, and dental, musculoskeletal, cancer, angina, menstrual, migraine, carpal tunnel, and nerve damage pain.

See also CYMATICS; ELECTROACUPUNCTURE; LIGHT THERAPY; RADIONICS; SOUND THERAPY; VIBRATIONAL MEDICINE.

energy transmutation See ENERGY.

environmental medicine Treatment modalities geared toward disorders, including allergies, ear infection, and sinus headache, that are believed to be caused by environmental factors, such as pollution and toxins. Treatments may involve nutrition and modification of diet, detoxification techniques such as chelation therapy and heat depuration (high-temperature saunas to encourage excretion of toxins through the skin), immunotherapy (any method used to boost the immune system), and desensitization, particularly enzyme potentiated desensitization (EPD), which relies on small doses of the allergen combined with beta glucoronidase, a natural enzyme, administered orally or intravenously to recondition the immune system to fight the allergic reaction. A long time may elapse before the desensitization process becomes effective. Among other (and controversial) environmental treatments are the administration of the solvent dimethyl sulfoxide (DMSO) and the hormone dehydroepiandrosterone (DHEA).

See also CHELATION THERAPY; DETOXIFICATION.

enzyme therapy The administration of supplements, enzymes including Donnazyme, Cotazyme, Creon, zymase, Ultrase, Pancrease, and other conventional substances, for the treatment of enzyme deficiency that results from cystic fibrosis, Gaucher's disease, and celiac disease, among other ailments. Digestive problems such as lactose intolerance and chronic intestinal gas may be helped by certain over-the-counter enzyme products.

Produced by living cells, an enzyme is an organic catalyst that cannot perform independently but is a complex protein that can initiate change in other substances without being changed itself. Enzymes are found throughout the body, such as amylases in saliva and in the intestine; ptyalin, also in the mouth; pepsins and lipase in the gastric juices, trypsin, chymotrypsin, and carboxypeptidase in pancreatic juices; and intestinal juices; including enteropeptidase, maltase, lactase, sucrase, and nucleosidases. Each enzyme has a specific action; rennin is an enzyme that coagulates milk; thrombin, an enzyme that is formed in shed blood and leads to the formation of fibrin for clotting. Other enzymes work to split fats, starches, sugars, amino acid compounds, mucoproteins, and proteins; to join enzymes; and to aid in the process of oxidation, fermentation, and chemical conversions. Cellulase, an enzyme not produced by the body but obtainable only through supplements made from plants and meant to digest fiber, is used for relief of gas and bloating as well as other ailments, including vaginal yeast infections and facial pain or paralysis. A lack of protease, which digests proteins, may cause anxiety, hypoglycemia, appendicitis, cancer, bone problems, and various infections.

Although enzyme depletion occurs with digestive disorders, it may also be caused by root canals, radiation, irradiated foods, pasteurization, heavy metals, mercury amalgam dental fillings, bovine growth hormone, hybridization and genetic engineering, microwaving, geopathic stress zones, chemical additives and pesticides, and excessive unsaturated and hydrogenated fats. In the body are approximately 22 digestive enzymes produced for each stage of digestion.

In alternative medicine, plant enzyme therapy is considered to have beneficial effects for those with chronic digestive disorders, sore throat, hay fever, ulcers, osteoporosis, myasthenia gravis, and candidiasis, and for anyone who wishes to increase nutrient absorption, especially in the case of nutrient deficiency. Pancreatic enzyme therapy is reported to benefit individuals with pancreatic hypertrophy (enlargement); inflammation, such as in sports injuries; viral disorders, including human immunodeficiency virus (HIV); heart disease, multiple sclerosis, cancer, bone fractures, and dental and respiratory infection; and as a preventive measure before surgery. In sum, enzyme therapists rely on a patient history; his or her dietary history; two palpation tests (the therapist's use of touch to identify dysfunctional or painful areas, called palpation points), one after a two-hour fast and another 45 minutes after the patient has eaten a meal; blood profile; and a 24-hour urinalysis to diagnose a person's ailment. Then the therapist is able to prescribe specific enzymes (some preparations contain nine or more enzymes); a healthy diet that contains whole, unprocessed, and raw foods; and any other method geared toward the patient's recovery. Other supplements, such as vitamin and mineral coenzymes, are often prescribed in conjunction with other treatment. Heat-stable, diffusible coenzymes of low molecular weight serve as enzyme activators. Coenzyme A, for example, plays an important role in the biosynthesis of fatty acids and sterols. Coenzyme Q10, an antioxidant nutrient, is said to energize the body and strengthen cardiac health. Other enzymes are also credited with having anti-inflammatory and antiaging properties. For additional information on enzyme therapy, contact the American Dietetic Association, 216 W. Jackson Boulevard., Suite 800, Chicago, IL 60606, or (800) 366-1655; or Dr. Howard Loomis, D.C., 21st Century Nutrition, 6421 Enterprise Lane, Madison, WI 53719, or (800) 662-2630 or (608) 273-8100.

essence Any integral force, part, character, or general energy of a living being or substance. According to traditional Chinese medicine, the essence (or *jing*) represents the body's supply of *qi*, or *ch'i*, meaning "life energy," and is considered the most refined substance of the human body. The Chinese believe one's essence manifests in the skin, tongue, and hair, and in one's fertility, potency, and creativity. These characteristics are said to determine a person's ability to ward off debilitation and promote longevity.

See also BACH'S FLOWER REMEDIES; ESSENTIAL OILS; *JING*.

Eternity Medicine The name given by Dr. Larry Dossey in his book *Reinventing Medicine: Beyond Mind-Body to a New Era of Healing* (HarperSanFrancisco, 1999, pp. 206–216) to a therapy that involves music, presence, and other means of conveying compassion and empathy to a person who is dying. "This provides the support for the revelations and wisdom that usually come to the dying—the regaining of their 'missing half,' which is imperishable. The great task of Eternity Medicine is to facilitate and not to obstruct this process," Dossey wrote.

See also DOSSEY, LARRY; FAITH HEALING; NONLOCAL MIND.

exercise In alternative medicine practices, controlled physical exertion that is directed toward a specific goal, such as relieving stress or rehabilitating one's constitution. In Ayurvedic medicine, for example, aerobic exercise, which includes a variety of sports, is geared to a person's body type, or dosha. Virtually all practitioners of conventional and alternative medicine recommend some form of physical exercise for optimal overall health.

See also AYURVEDA; DANCE MOVEMENT THERAPY; YOGA.

external In traditional Chinese medicine, any outside factor causing an effect upon the body, such as a particular climate, elevation, or other condition.

See also YIN-YANG.

extracts, herbal Ayurvedic, traditional Chinese, Native American, homeopathic, and other preparations from plants used as remedies.

See also ESSENTIAL OILS.

exudative Any substance or agent that causes the expression of fluid or other substance, such as applying heat to an infected wound to help remove pus.

face analysis In Ayurvedic medicine, the assessment of the skin, features, lips, color, and other characteristics of the face in order to diagnose impairment or disease process.

See also AYURVEDA.

faith healing A term coined in 1885, referring to the use of prayer and belief in the power of God to treat disease and other forms of distress. Faith healers may also employ a laying on of hands to enhance the effect. Although certain factions of conventional medical practitioners argue against the effectiveness and premise of faith healing, there have been many well-documented and observed cases in which the ill person was cured of his or her affliction. Miracles are reported to have occurred in the process of faith healing in places such as Lourdes, France, and Machu Picchu, Peru.

Strong belief in a higher power has evolved into mind-body medicine, which is now embraced by the general public and many health professionals, many of whom also advocate treating disease integratively, that is, using both conventional and alternative and complementary methods that are beneficial. Dr. Herbert Benson describes "the faith factor" as "remembered wellness and the elicitation of the relaxation response. . . . People who chose an appropriate focus, that which draws upon their deepest philosophic or religious convictions, were more apt to adhere to the elicitation routine, looking forward to it and enjoying it. . . . Affirmative beliefs of any kind brought forth remembered wellness, receiving top-down, nerve-cell-firing patterns in the brain that were associated with wellness. . . . When present, faith in an eternal or life-transcending force seemed to make the fullest use of remembered wellness because it is a supremely soothing belief, disconnecting unhealthy logic and worries"

(excerpted from *Timeless Healing: The Power and Biology of Belief*, by Herbert Benson, M.D., New York, Scribner 1996). In *Love, Medicine & Miracles* (New York: Harper & Row, Publishers, 1986), Bernie S. Siegel, M.D., wrote: "We had a physician named Herb who came to our group. He said he meditated every night while he walked the dog. One night, while walking down the street, he heard God say to him, 'You are Jesus.' Herb said, 'I'm Jewish.' God said, 'I know that. So was Jesus.' Herb thought, 'I guess God is telling me to heal myself by the laying on of hands.' He started patting himself all over as he stood out there in the street. When he came to the group and told this story, I asked him, 'Did it ever occur to you that God was saying, You need to become loving and spiritual?' Being a physician you reacted in a mechanical way and did something mechanical, like patting yourself all over, but the message is 'Change and be spiritual.' "

In *The Science of Mind* (50th Anniversary Edition, G. P. Putnam's Sons, New York, 1926 and 1988), Ernest Holmes wrote: "It would be difficult to believe in a God who cares more for one person than another. There can be no God who is kindly disposed one day and cruel the next; there can be no God who creates us with tendencies and impulses we can scarcely comprehend, and then eternally punishes us when we make mistakes. . . . Most men who believe in God believe in prayer. . . . But we should bear in mind that the prayers which are effective—no matter whose prayers they may be—*are effective because they embody certain universal principles which, when understood, can be consciously used.*"

Larry Dossey, M.D., author of *Healing Words: The Power of Prayer and the Practice of Medicine* (HarperSanFrancisco, 1993), maintains that it is the intention of the healer or the one who prays that accounts for effectiveness. "Everyone has heard of dramatic examples of healing in which highly specific, directed strategies were used in imagery and prayer," Dossey wrote. "In one well-known example, the person imaged her cancer as a piece of red meat, and her immune cells as a pack of ravenous wolves who attacked the meat and destroyed it. . . . Although stories such as [this] are anecdotes and do not count as hard evidence, we would be foolish to ignore them. In their support there is ample solid scientific evidence that directed, highly specific imagery can bring about changes in the body."

See also BENSON, HERBERT; CAYCE, EDGAR; DOSSEY, LARRY; MEDITATION; PRAYER, POWER OF; RELAXATION RESPONSE; SIEGEL, BERNIE S.

fasting From the Anglo-Saxon word *faestan*, meaning to hold fast, the ingestion of fluids, particularly water, during a period when no solid food is taken. Fasting is largely considered a body-purification or cleansing process in alternative and complementary medicine. In Ayurvedic medicine, effective fasting requires that one take into account his or her *dosha*, or body type. For example, a *vata* body type should not fast for more than three days because a longer fast may cause anxiety (a "vatic crisis"), whereas a *kapha* body type may fast extensively. Also, certain juices, if one is observing a juice fast, are recommended for each *dosha*—grape juice for *vata*, pomegranate for *pitta*, and apple juice for *kapha*. Herbs in the form of tea may be beneficial. Fasting has particular value in the event of fever, cold, arthritis, or constipation. Ayurvedic practitioners believe fasting gives the digestive system a rest as well as a way to neutralize or release toxins that may have built up.

Homeopathic practitioners view fasting as a cleansing technique that must be well managed in order to prevent nutrient deprivation, lack of energy, stress, and starvation. Fruit and vegetable juices, lemon water with honey or salt, and herbal teas taken every two hours may provide a cleansing but not depleting fast. Also, a cleansing diet (low-fat, high-fiber) is often less stressful and as effective as fasting. Other practitioners of alternative medicine tout fasting for a few days as "natural biofeedback" that helps one pay attention to what nutrients the body needs and create a means of ridding the body of waste materials. Most experts suggest beginning a fast by reducing food intake the day before and ending a fast by gradually reintroducing solid foods into the diet.

Conventional medicine regards fasting as drinking only water and taking in no food, a practice that adversely affects normal metabolism that supplies essential nutrients, such as glucose, to body tissues. Problems may include water retention, depletion of normal gastric juices, lessened ability to fight infection, protein or potassium deficiency, gout attacks, gallstones, dry skin, menstrual problems, headache, and impairment of hormone production. In children, who have a smaller glycogen reserve than adults, the lack of food interferes with fat metabolism and may induce ketosis or mild acidosis. Under certain conditions, such as in a temperate climate and with reduced physical activity, an individual may survive on water for approximately two months, but without food or water, death may occur in approximately 10 days. For the purpose of weight loss, conventional practitioners often recommend eliminating a meal per day or fasting for not more than one day. Unsupervised and prolonged fasting may be fatal, and, as a rule, children should not fast.

Naturopathic practitioners frequently recommend brief fasts for individuals with arthritis, rheumatoid arthritis, eczema, asthma, psoriasis, and irritable bowel syndrome (IBS) and for victims of environmental toxins. More information on weight-loss and detoxification fasting is available by contacting the American Association of Naturopathic Physicians, 2366 Eastlake Avenue, Suite 322, Seattle, WA 98102, or (206) 323-7610.

See also DETOXIFICATION THERAPY; *DOSHA*; HOMEOPATHY; NATUROPATHY.

febrifuge In homeopathic medicine, an herbal or mineral or combination remedy that fights fever, such as *Ferrum phos* 6x. Aspirin, acetaminophen, and other conventional drugs, known as antipyretics, also counteract fever. In Ayurvedic medicine, *ghee*, made from boiled, strained, unsalted butter, is administered to relieve chronic fever.

Feldenkrais method A system of rehabilitation developed by the physicist Moshe Feldenkrais, an Israeli born in Russia who, after suffering a severe knee injury, replaced his previous ways of physically moving with more efficient habits that proved healthier and more efficient. Also a martial artist and athlete, Feldenkrais said, "Each one of us speaks, moves, thinks, and feels in a different way, each according to the image of himself that he has built up over the years. In order to change our mode of action, we must change the image of ourselves that we carry within us." He interpreted this self-awareness as a mind-body connection, in that human beings have complex systems of intelligence and emotion that govern physical functioning. He believed that if physical movement (including breathing) became impaired, psychological and even other physical problems would result. Touted as effective for stress-related problems, chronic pain, headaches, temporomandibular joint (TMJ) disorder, multiple sclerosis, cerebral vascular accident (stroke), cerebral palsy, and other ailments, the Feldenkrais method of bodywork consists of two components: Awareness Through Movement and Functional Integration, both terms registered service marks of the Feldenkrais Guild [P.O. Box 489, Albany, OR 97321, or (503) 926-0981 or (800) 775-2118]. Awareness Through Movement involves gentle, nonaerobic motions, such as sitting and standing, along with specific movements in 45-minute to one-hour sessions once a week for four to six weeks. Sessions may be continued for as long as preferred by an individual. Feldenkrais practitioners perform Functional Integration—gentle manipulation of muscles and joints not exceeding one's normal range of motion—on an individual who is standing, sitting, or lying down. There are no reports of adverse effects of this therapy, which also provides supportive conditioning for athletes, dancers, and others who wish to improve their flexibility, balance, and mobility.

Training in the Feldenkrais method, which became popular in America during the 1970s, is available throughout the country and requires 160 training days in the span of four years. Feldenkrais training is popular among physical therapists, but a medical or health background is not necessary to become a practitioner.

feng shui The ancient Eastern art of placement according to subtle Earth energies and their relationship and impact on human life. Considered an environmental science, traditional Chinese feng shui (a combination of the Chinese words for wind and water) is employed in many aspects of life including nutrition, medicine, exercise, the arts, and interior and exterior design. As a philosophical system, feng shui and its variations acclimate to most cultures and societal requirements because of the general acceptance of the idea that the characteristics of our surroundings affect physical and mental health. Harmony, the auspicious flow of *qi* (*ch'i;* life force or energy), and creation of a balance between yin and yang forces (positive and negative, or the universal opposites, such as Sun-Moon and cold-heat) are among the goals of feng shui practices. The Five Elements of wood, fire, earth, metal, and water provide the basis for different energies, personalities, and associations. The position of windows, doors, utilities (particularly water-related, including sinks, toilets, and appliances); furniture, cabinets, architectural details, and materials; and accessories, plants and living creatures, colors, shapes, and textures of objects; lighting; exterior factors such as roads, bodies of water, mountains, and trees; Chinese astrology and numerology; and location are all factors taken into account in feng shui, which attempts to enhance well-being, harness good *ch'i,* or counteract negative conditions or energy. One feng shui approach is based on the Bagua map, an entire floor plan with each area and direction (north, south, east, and west) designated as a symbol of human life—health, family, children, love and marriage, wealth, work, knowledge, helpful people, fame, and reputation. The use of an indoor water fountain, for example, is thought to enhance wealth and beneficial energy and richness of life. Use of the color red is considered stimulating and dominant and representative of warmth, prosperity, anger, and passion; blue may evoke feelings of contemplation, peacefulness, mystery, patience, suspicion, and melancholia. Each feng shui concept is rooted in practicality and the interplay of elements and may be adapted to individual problems and needs. As feng shui practice has entered the mainstream Western art of interior design, it has also found favor among methods for complementarily treating physical and mental illness.

See also *ch'i;* FIVE ELEMENTS; *QI;* YIN-YANG.

fever therapy   See ISSEL'S FEVER THERAPY.

Five Elements   Air (or metal), water, ether, fire, and earth, which represent individual and environmental energy and constitution in various Asian, Native American, and other traditions of medicine. The Five Element concept is based on the belief that all people have a connection to and interpersonal reaction with the physical and spiritual foundation of nature. In the Tantric tradition (one of the Indian schools of thought), for example, air is symbolized by a sphere and represents locomotion, fire is symbolized by a triangle and represents expansion, water is symbolized by a crescent and represents contraction, and a square symbolizes the Earth and cohesion. Ether's symbol is a circle made with dashes, and its tendency is to provide space. These relate to individual processes of healing. In Ayurveda and traditional Chinese medicine, the Five Elements relate to body types and constitutions, chakras (centers of energy down the midline of the body from the crown to the base of the spine), internal organs, and spiritual approaches and experience. Also in Ayurveda the Five Elements involve taste testing, that is, a method to determine how different foods and herbs affect each person. For instance, Ayurvedic practitioners believe that an excessive intake of bitter foods and medicinal herbs may intensify the elements of air and ether and cause one to become disoriented. "Hot" foods are said to intensify the fire element and are not recommended for fiery, hot-tempered, irritable individuals. Sweets represent earth and water elements, and, as a result of water and earth characteristics of leading to growth and the desire for more, lead easily to obesity. Medicinal herbs and foods and therapeutic activities such as yoga correspond to the Five Elements.

The Five Elements also play a role in feng shui, the Chinese art of placement, in terms of fire, metal, wood, water, and earth. In one's environment, as in one's personal biopsychosocial intake, each element must be represented in balance with the others for an optimal sense of well-being.

See also CHAKRAS; DOSHA; FENG SHUI.

flotation therapy   The use of a lightproof, sound-insulated float tank for the purpose of restricted environmental stimulation technique (REST), a deep relaxation modality. The tank holds approximately 10 inches of skin-temperature water mixed with Epsom salts to make it five times denser and more buoyant than seawater. A person gets in the tank to experience a floating sensation. According to an article by Barbara Ritacco in the October 2002 issue of *Options* (West Paterson, N.J.), the central nervous system "experiences a dramatic restriction of external stimuli in the float tank. This triggers relaxation response by inhibiting the release of stress-related chemicals such as cortisol. This, in turn, inhibits the release of neurotransmitters that are associated with distress, with the fight and flight response, and its consequent muscular tension and anxiety. . . . One hour in the float tank is the physical equivalent of six hours of sleep. . . . (Other benefits include) an accelerated learning process (due to the Theta State) and a loosening of muscles. Flotation therapy helps treat asthma, digestive tract conditions, cardiovascular conditions, psychological and emotional conditions, addictions, and chronic pain conditions." Flotation therapy is often combined with guided imagery and music therapy. The article goes on to say there are no adverse effects of flotation therapy, and famous advocates include Carl Lewis (in preparation for the 1988 Seoul Olympics), the Dallas Cowboys since 1981, the Australian Institute of Sport since 1983, and the 2000 USA Olympic Squad. The average length of a float is one hour, which costs approximately $45 to $75 per hour.

See also GUIDED IMAGERY; HYDROTHERAPY; MUSIC THERAPY.

flower remedies   Also known as "soul therapy," the use of flower essences to treat various physical and emotional ailments. Flower essence remedies are made throughout the world, including England, the United States (California), India, Australia, Japan, Africa, and Europe. Among the literature on flower essence remedies are *Flower Essence Repertory*, by Patricia Kaminski and Richard Katz (The Flower Essence Society, Nevada City, Calif., 1994); *Care of the Soul: A Guide for Cultivating Depth and Sacredness in Everyday Life*, by Thomas Moore (New York: HarperCollins, 1992); and *The Encyclopedia of Flower Remedies*, by Clare Harvey and

Amanda Cochrane (London and San Francisco: Thorsons, 1995).

See also AUSTRALIAN FLOWER REMEDIES; BACH FLOWER REMEDIES.

folk medicine   A term coined in 1878 referring to the traditional medicine of a particular culture as practiced by physicians and nonprofessional health providers. Folk medicine most often involves the extensive use of foods and herbs as remedies for a multitude of ailments, many of which have been adopted into the Western mainstream as alternative and complementary medicine options. Treatments may also include spiritual or religious rituals, diagnostic and healing techniques in accordance with a society's specific beliefs and lifestyle, and psychological counseling.

See also *CURANDERISMO*; FAITH HEALING; *KAHUNA*; NATIVE AMERICAN HEALING PRACTICES; *SANGOMA*.

fomentations, herbal   In Ayurvedic medicine warm, moist applications that are infused or treated with herbs.

food therapy   Food nutrients, herbs, and various diets considered to be therapeutic or healing. Healing foods have always been known to humankind. Oranges, for example, were known centuries ago as treatment for respiratory disorders such as allergies and asthma, infections, aging (Arabs of the 17th century applied dried, oil-soaked oranges to discourage graying of hair), and indigestion (the peel was made into a tonic). Grapefruit and its varieties, such as pomelo, are reported to improve circulation and prevent breast cancer. Among common foods considered both nourishment and remedy are papaya (for excess stomach acidity); honey (for inhibition of bacterial infection, ulcers, and acne and promotion of healing); tuna, salmon, and other fatty fish (for rheumatoid arthritis and other inflammation); cranberry (for urinary tract infection); garlic (for high blood pressure, high cholesterol level; cancer, and infection); brazil nuts (for asthma); fava beans (for Parkinson's disease); yogurt (for yeast infections); rice (for diarrhea); broccoli (for colon cancer); watercress (for lung cancer and smoking-related diseases); bran (for constipation); savoy cabbage (for prevention of cancer); apricots (for low libido); and milk (for insomnia and anxiety). Hundreds of foods are believed to help counteract the symptoms and processes of hundreds of ailments. Food therapy also includes a multitude of diets and dietary restrictions or specifications according to individual need. One of the best-known diseases that requires a highly specified diet is diabetes. Food therapy complements herbal therapy, the use of vitamins and mineral supplements, and bodywork.

See also MACROBIOTICS; NATUROPATHY; NUTRITION.

Freud, Sigmund   The Austrian neurologist (1856–1939) long credited as "the father of psychoanalysis." During the years 1892 to 1895, Freud introduced the technique of free association to the practice of psychiatry. He went on to develop theories on dream interpretation, repression, sexual deviation, guilt, the unconscious, psychosomatic pain, and many other groundbreaking psychodynamic methods and concepts that are considered important in contemporary psychiatric practice. Freud's ideas contribute significantly to the foundation of the mind-body philosophy related to various alternative and complementary medicine modalities. In *A Practical Guide to Vibrational Medicine* (New York: Quill/HarperCollins Publishers, 2000, p. 113), Richard Gerber, M.D., wrote: "There is no question that there is often a deeper meaning behind illness, relationships, and the simple events of everyday life. We must learn to walk that fine line between understanding the meaning of our lives on the physical plane while still paying attention to our spiritual roots in the multidimensional worlds that underlie and energize physical energy."

See also ART THERAPY; DRAMA THERAPY; HYPNOSIS.

***fu zheng* therapy**   In traditional Chinese medicine, the fortification of one's constitution, typically administered as a tonic soup made of astragalus root, codonopsis root, tangerine peel, polygonatum rhizome, poria fungus, lycii berries, red dates, black or shiitake mushrooms, seaweed, vegetable or chicken stock, yams, leeks, and scallions.

galactagogue A substance or agent that stimulates the secretion of milk.

Galen, Claudius Greek physician and writer (129–ca. 199) and founder of experimental physiology whose theories on medical practice were acclaimed during the Middle Ages and the Renaissance and are still considered pivotal in medical history. The distinguished Galen served as chief physician to the gladiators in Pergamum, after which he went to Rome to be admitted to the court of Marcus Aurelius and Lucius Aurelius Verus. Later he became physician to Commodus, son of Aurelius. One of Galen's ideas was that light and darkness could affect one's mental state: "The color of the black humor induces fear when its darkness throws a shadow over the area of thought," he wrote. He is also believed to have said, "He cures most in whom most are confident," referring to a mind-body influence on healing and the relationship between healer and patient.

gan In traditional Chinese medicine, the term designating herbs that are sweet-tasting, such as *gan mao ling*, prescribed for the initial symptoms of a cold.

Gandhi, Mohandas K. (Mahatma) Leader of the Indian nationalist, nonviolent movement against the British and known as father of his country (1869–1948) who championed the integration of mind, body, and spirit. For example, he believed exercise was as necessary to the quality of life as air, water, and food and that lack of exercise affected the mind as well. Called the Mahatma, or Great Soul, Gandhi greatly influenced political, literary, ethical, and spiritual thinking throughout the world.

Gattefossé, René-Maurice The French chemist who coined the term *aromatherapy* in 1937 and developed it as a method of healing. After he burned his hand while working in his family's perfume laboratory, he put his injured hand into lavender oil, which reduced the redness and helped stimulate healing of the area. This gave Dr. Gattefossé the idea to explore curative properties of other fragrant substances.

See also AROMATHERAPY; ESSENTIAL OILS.

generals In homeopathic medicine, the counterpart of particulars, or symptoms that are expressed in terms of "I am," which refer to the whole person.

See also HOMEOPATHY.

Gerson therapy The German physician Max Gerson (1881–1959) in the 1930s immigrated to the United States and developed nutritional treatments for diabetes, migraines, tuberculosis, and cancer. Born in Wongrowitz, Germany, and considered a humanitarian physician, Gerson treated Dr. and Mrs. Albert Schweitzer for diabetes and other problems, believed that a low-salt vegan diet; additional fruit and vegetable juices; various supplements such as iodine, niacin, potassium, and pepsin; detoxifying coffee enemas; and enzyme therapy could both prevent and eliminate cancer. His methods proved successful for patients in various stages of melanoma; survival rates studied in 153 of Gerson's cancer patients were higher than those of patients receiving conventional treatment for melanoma. Gerson's daughter, Charlotte, and her staff continue his work at The Gerson Institute, in Tijuana, Mexico. Gerson organizations are the Max Gerson Memorial Cancer Center of CHIPSA, 670 Nubes, Playas de Tijuana, B.C., Mexico; the Gerson Research Organization, 7807 Artesian Road, San

Diego, CA 92127-2117 or (800-759-2966) and the Gerson Institute, P.O. Box 430, Bonita, CA 91908-0430 or (619-585-7600).

See also NUTRITIONAL THERAPY.

glandulars Also called raw glandular extracts, the fluids or soluble gland tissue from animal glands believed to provide an alternative healing method beneficial in the treatment of various disorders. For example, raw adrenal glandular is used to stimulate the adrenal glands and help in the treatment of chronic fatigue syndrome, arthritis, diabetes, infections, and ulcers. Other essential glandulars include raw brain, raw female complex, raw heart, raw kidney, raw lung, raw liver, raw male complex, raw mammary, raw orchic, raw ovary, raw pancreas, raw pituitary, raw spleen, raw thymus, raw thyroid, and raw uterus, each extract corresponding to disorders of each gland. Glandular, or cellular, therapy is often combined with the administration of a specific amino acid and is based on the idea that like cells help like cells.

See also CELL THERAPY.

green superfoods A common way to refer to sources of essential nutrients such as protein, fiber, chlorophyll, vitamins, minerals, and enzymes. Among the "superfoods" are green and blue-green algae, chlorella, spirulina, aloe vera, barley grass, wheat grass, and alfalfa. The algae, or phytoplankton, are a rich source of beta-carotene, vitamin B_{12}, and gamma-linoleic acid (GLA), an essential fatty acid. Chlorella contains the highest known source of chlorophyll, the green coloration of plants that facilitates the process of photosynthesis. Photosynthesis involves the light absorbed by chlorophyll as our primary source of energy—generally, the formation of carbohydrates from carbon dioxide, and from the chlorophyll in plant tissues, the formation of hydrogen as water.

Spirulina, an alga (or seaweed) that thrives in ocean and alkaline water, provides protein containing all 21 amino acids, all the B vitamins, beta-carotene, essential fatty acids, minerals, and trace minerals. Aloe vera juice from the succulent plant is a natural oxygenator, antiseptic, astringent, and topical treatment for burns, ulcerations, and skin disorders. Green and other grasses contain large numbers of enzymes, minerals, vitamins, chlorophyllins, and proteins, and alfalfa, the basis for liquid chlorophyll, is rich in minerals. The green superfoods are popular constituents of nutritional therapy.

See also NUTRITION.

Grinberg Method A type of reflexology called "Footwork" developed by Avi Grinberg that attempts to prevent pain and alleviate chronic pain by teaching practitioners and laypeople to discern the steps along the process of a physical or emotional crisis and use the techniques of Footwork to counteract them.

See also REFLEXOLOGY.

guided imagery Various methods or techniques that draw upon an individual's imagination, thought patterns, emotions, senses, and personal experience as the "theme" of a meditative, relaxation exercise. Considered an adjunctive treatment for illness, guided imagery is used to promote deep relaxation and healing; to aid tolerance and reduce side effects of medical procedures; to decrease pain, stress, anger, and grief; and to increase the therapeutic aspects of self-empowerment and self-control. For example, the radiation oncologist and author O. Carl Simonton successfully employed guided imagery as a technique cancer patients can use to promote their recovery process. He suggested that patients imagine the radiation as "bullets of energy" hitting and shrinking the cancer cells. Imagery is also beneficial for the treatment of chronic headaches, back pain, allergies, hypertension, gastrointestinal spasms and disease, autoimmune diseases, injuries and trauma, irregular heartbeat, and gynecological problems.

See also MEDITATION; SIMONTON, O. CARL.

gunas In Ayurvedic medicine, the three attributes found in nature, that is, in all organic and inorganic matter: *satva* (essence, awakening, light), *rajas* (movement, or dynamic energy), and *tamas* (inertia, darkness, and static or potential energy). The *gunas* are part of the Samkhya philosophy of creation, which includes the beliefs that sound is the *guna* of ether, touch is the *guna* of air, sight is the *guna* of fire, taste is the *guna* of water, and smell is the *guna* of earth. Ether, air, fire, water, and earth represent the five elements of the universe. The practice of Ayurveda, also called the science of daily living, is rooted in the ancient Indian system of knowledge. The Ayurvedic physician Charak established the idea that there are 20 fundamental *gunas*, among which are 10 opposite pairs, such as male and female, slow and fast, and dull and sharp. When one understands the universe in these terms, he or she can recognize characteristics of both health and illness. In addition, food and drugs in Ayurveda are based on the action and reaction of the 20 *gunas*.

See also AYURVEDA.

Hahnemann, Samuel C. F. The German physician (1753–1843) who developed the theory and practice of modern homeopathy, an alternative medical discipline based on the concept *Similia similibus curantur*—"Like cures like."

Hahnemann, who was revered for his work in pharmacology, hygiene, public health, industrial toxicology, and psychiatry, made such an indelible mark on medical history that in Germany all medical students are required to study homeopathy as part of the general curriculum. Born Friedrich Christian Samuel in Meissen, Germany, Hahnemann studied medicine in Leipzig. He married Henriette Kuchler (1764–1830), the adopted daughter of the owners of the Mohren-Apotheke in Dessau, and they had 11 children. Five years after Henriette died, he married again. His second wife, Melanie D'Hervilly (1802–78), accompanied him to Paris in 1842, the year before he died. He is buried in Père Lachaise cemetery in France. A Samuel Hahnemann Memorial, which was a gift of the American Institute of Homeopathy and authorized by Congress in January 1900, stands on Massachusetts Avenue and 16th Street, NW (Scott Circle), in Washington, D.C. There a bronze statue of Hahnemann sits on a pedestal bearing the Latin phrase meaning "Like cures like" in front of a curved wall. Four bronze panels on the wall portray Hahnemann in his days as a medical student, a laboratory chemist, a teacher, and a bedside physician.

After establishing a pharmacopeia of what he called "Simples," the system newly dubbed "homeopathy" in 1808, Hahnemann also published his theories in the works "Essay on a New Principle" (1796) and "Organon of the Rational Art of Healing" (1810). Later, after homeopathy came to be known as the "new medicine," he further developed his method and remedies and published more of his findings in Dr. Hufeland's German pharmacology review, Journal of Practical Pharmacology and Surgery, under the title "Essay on a New Principle for Ascertaining the Curative Powers of Medicines, with a Few Glances at Those Hitherto Employed." It was the fourth edition of Hahnemann's *Organon* (1829) and the first edition of *The Chronic Diseases* (1828) on which the classical practice of homeopathy was based. Both works discuss the single dry dose and the wait-and-watch philosophies characteristic of homeopathy, carried into the 20th century by the prominent homeopath James Tyler Kent. Some of Hahnemann's teachings have been lost, including his views on Hippocratic temperaments, symptomatology, Gestalt, the LM (50 millesimal) potencies (previously addressed in the sixth *Organon* of 1843), diathetic constitutions, and case management strategies.

See also HOMEOPATHY.

hakomi Derived from a word in the Hopi language meaning "Who are you and how do you stand in relation to these many realms?," a type of bodywork that incorporates touch, massage, movement, energy work, bodily realignment, and an individual's mindful and spiritual awareness of his or her own emotions, issues, insights, and coping mechanisms. Through physiological manipulation and the unfolding of personal defenses such as armoring, hakomi teaches one how best to use his or her coping mechanisms. Developed by Ron Kurtz, author of *Body-Centered Psychotherapy: The Hakomi Method* (Mendocino, Calif.: LifeRhythm, 1990), hakomi is intended to promote relaxation, an increased sense of security, and healing. The Hakomi Institute, P.O. Box 1873, Boulder, CO 80306 or (888-421-6699), www.hakomiinstitute.com, offers information, referrals, and training.

hatha yoga See YOGA.

Hay, Louise American metaphysical teacher and author of 18 books, including *You Can Heal Your Life* (Carson, Calif.: Hay House, 1987); *The Power Is Within You* (Hay House, 2003) and *Heal Your Body: The Mental Causes for Physical Illness and the Metaphysical Ways to Overcome Them* (Hay House, 1994). Since beginning her career as a Science of Mind minister in 1981, Hay has developed the reputation of helping people discover and affirm their ability to heal and grow toward daily well-being through meditation and positive thinking. Her affirmation "I deserve love," among her earliest work that drew public acclaim, provided a landmark for the beneficial effects of mind-body philosophy. Hay's works have been translated into 25 different languages in 33 countries around the world, and she operates Hay House, Inc. publishing company in Carson, California, at (800) 654-5126.

See also HOLMES, ERNEST.

heat therapy See HYPERTHERMIA.

Hellerwork Named for the aerospace engineer Joseph Heller, this is a type of bodywork similar to Rolfing involving deep tissue massage and "movement reeducation," geared toward relieving muscular tension; stress, back, neck, and shoulder pain; sports injuries; and respiratory ailments. Heller was born in Poland in 1940, was educated in Europe, and immigrated to Los Angeles, California, at age 16. In 1962 he earned a degree in engineering from Cal Tech. Eventually he left engineering and turned to the field of structural bodywork and bioenergetics, which led him to serve as director of Kairos, the Los Angeles Center for Human Development, and as the first president of the Rolf Institute. Coauthor with William Henkin of *Bodywise* (Berkeley, Calif.: Wingbow Press, 1991), Heller believed that as the body became realigned with the Earth's natural gravitational field, the emotional impact of unconsciously harboring tension and impairing optimal breathing needed also to be addressed. He felt that chronic tension in the muscles caused the body to fall out of

vertical alignment and lose flexibility and energy. By "relearning" to sit, stand, walk, run, and lift more efficiently, one can regain good posture and range of motion. The Hellerwork program consists of eleven 90-minute sessions, each of which focuses on a combination of physical movement and manipulation to reduce stress and foster energy and mind-body awareness to correct imbalances from prolonged stress or trauma. Hellerwork is not recommended for individuals with cancer, rheumatoid arthritis, or other inflammatory conditions. More information is available by contacting The Body of Knowledge/Hellerwork organization, 406 Berry Street, Mount Shasta, CA 96067, or (530) 926-2500. Heller's website is josephheller.com\bio.html.

See also ROLFING.

herbalism The practice of using plants as a source of medicine for a multitude of illnesses. Herbalism spans many cultures, but it began in most of them as traditional remedies and preventive medicines, especially in regions in which physicians and hospitals were not readily available. Many well-known modern pharmaceuticals originate from herbal remedies, among them digoxin, a vital cardiac drug from the common garden flower foxglove (*Digitalis purpurea*). Herbs have always been recognized for their various effects on health. Mint, for example, is perhaps the most common remedy for digestive problems and is often an ingredient in preparations for indigestion and other gastrointestinal disturbances, and echinacea is known to have potent immune-stimulating properties. Although herbal medicine lost much favor for many years in the United States after the 20th-century development of antibiotics, it is a thriving business today, with hundreds of herbal preparations available over the counter in health food stores, pharmacies, and supermarkets. Although the federal Food and Drug Administration (FDA) does not regulate the production of herbal remedies and at one time threatened to remove all supplements from public access, Congress responded to the public's clamoring for herbals by passing the Dietary Supplement Health and Education Act (DSHEA) of 1994, which limits what herbal-preparation manufacturers can claim about their products' scope and efficacy. Herbalism is a major component of traditional Chinese (and other Asian) medicine and Ayurveda, traditional Hindu and Indian medicine.

See also AYURVEDA; NATIVE AMERICAN MEDICINE; TRADITIONAL CHINESE MEDICINE.

herbal wraps Cloth or another substance such as seaweed saturated with herbal preparations and applied to the body for therapeutic and cosmetic purposes. Herbal wraps may be used to counteract excess body fluid or fat (e.g., cellulite), aching muscles, and dry or distressed skin and to provide concurrent relaxation and aromatherapy.

herbs, Ayurvedic See AYURVEDA.

Hering's Law of Cure A homeopathic theory developed by Dr. Constantine Hering (in some sources spelled Herring), one of the founders of the American homeopathic movement, that "the curative process moves from within outward, from the more important to the less important organs, in the reverse order of the onset of the symptoms, and from above downward." Rudolph M. Ballentine, M.D., writes in *Radical Healing* (Harmony Books, New York, 1996): "A patient with asthma may find that as his lungs clear, his skin breaks out. Physicians of the old school like to call asthma 'eczema on the inside . . . .' The reason it's a move in the direction of cure is that the lungs are more vital than the skin. As we get stronger, we tend to push the disorder out toward the surface. This is the opposite of suppression. . . . We express the disorder the way dirty water is expressed from a sponge. . . . Herring's Law of Cure, as it is called, also stipulates that as you move toward better health, old symptoms will return in reverse order of their original appearance. When the asthma goes away, the eczema returns."

See also HAHNEMANN, SAMUEL C. F.; HOMEOPATHY.

Hippocrates Greek physician of the fifth century (ca. 460–ca. 377 B.C.), considered "the father of modern medicine." In harmony with traditional medical practices throughout the world as well as with contemporary alternative and complementary medical practices, Hippocrates' major tenets are that physicians should observe all, evaluate honestly, assist nature, work for the good of the patient, treat the whole person and not simply the illness, and, above all, do no harm. In addition, modern chiropractic employs Hippocrates' idea that all illness stems from anomalies of the spine. In Hippocrates' writings, he described the symptoms of many illnesses and embraced the idea that certain foods could cause what has now long been established as allergic reaction.

Hippocrates, the son of a physician, traveled and practiced medicine extensively in Greece and Asia Minor; taught at the medical school in Cos, Greece, the island on which he was born; and wrote and/or collected material (some scholars believe that some of the writings in the collection were by his disciples, or Hippocratists, and possibly other authors) for works known as *Corpus Hippocraticum* (the Hippocratic collection). The collection consists of anatomy, physiology, medical ethics, general pathology and descriptions of clinical subjects, gynecology and obstetrics, diseases of children, mental illness, prognosis, treatment by diet and drugs, and surgery. The collection—approximately 72 books and 59 treatises—was assembled in the fourth century B.C. at the great Library in Alexandria, Egypt, which was intended by the ruling Ptolemies to be the site of the entire scope of human knowledge.

The Hippocratic oath, widely associated with and credited to the teachings of Hippocrates but not necessarily his exact concept, is an ethical code and a pledge taken by nurses, physicians, and other health professionals at graduation, marking the beginning of their professional careers. The oath serves as a guide to appropriate behavior and intent, particularly that health care professionals help or at least do no harm to the patient or family, honor confidentiality, and act with purity and discretion.

holistic medicine A discipline of Western medicine that incorporates some theories of Eastern and other medicines and the recognition of the patient as both a physiological and a psychological being. Holistic practitioners believe that psychological factors affect well-being and disease processes. They employ various techniques, including relaxation, guided imagery and visualization, and hypnosis, along with conventional methods of treatment appropriate to the ailment, and they advocate the patient's participation in his or her own healing. Most types of alternative and complementary medicine, also known as integrative medicine, embrace the concept of the patient as a biological, psychological, sociological whole (often documented as a biopsychosocial profile), and treatments that also include conventional medicine are geared to suit the individual's needs. Moreover, holistic medicine seeks to prevent physical and emotional illness as well as proactively maintain well-being. Organizations such as the American Holistic Nurses Association, based in Flagstaff, Arizona, and the American Holistic Medical Association, based in McLean, Virginia, have been founded in order to encourage health professionals to practice mind-body medicine.

See also Appendix I.

holistic nursing   See Appendix I; HOLISTIC MEDICINE.

Holmes, Ernest   Author of *The Science of Mind* (New York: G. P. Putnam's Sons, 1988), a definitive textbook and motivational reference on how one's attitude and emotions affect health and well-being.

homeopathy   An alternative treatment system based on the theory that "like cures like," that if, is a substance causes a symptom, it can conversely cure it when taken in a highly diluted form or in minute quantity. Remedies are made from plant, animal, and mineral sources and are available at health food stores and pharmacies. Recognized as a scientific method of medicine, homeopathy was developed in the late 18th century by the German physician Samuel Hahnemann (1755–1843), who decided to focus on symptoms rather than on the seemingly futile quest for causes. He observed that symptoms of a disease could be induced in a healthy individual by certain substances. The malaria remedy cinchona, for example, could produce malaria-like symptoms, Hahnemann observed, and he experimented with numerous plant, mineral, and animal substances on himself and other volunteers. This "proving" procedure, as he called it, gave credence to the ancient idea that a substance could both cause and cure symptoms, depending upon the dosage and the patient's overall condition. He

went on to develop potentized remedies: each substance was diluted many times until the preparation contained only the essence of the original substance, thus making the remedy more powerful.

Hahnemann believed in the laws of nature and incorporated them into his theories. Four basic principles created the foundation of homeopathy as a healing art and science: (1) similars cure similars; (2) a single remedy is used (one medication at a time); (3) the minimal dose is used, and (4) the potentized remedy is employed.

According to *The People's Repertory* (Santa Fe, N.M.: Full of Life Publishing, 1998) by Luc De Schepper, M.D., Ph.D., C.Hom., D.I.Hom, L.Ac., "A homeopathic remedy is an almost infinitesimally small dose of a medication which—if given in a bigger dose to a healthy individual—would provoke symptoms similar to those presented by the patient. Western medical doctors often practice 'unconscious' homeopathy when they give vaccinations and allergy shots. In general, Western medical treatment is successful when it follows this important Law of Similars (to create a similar [*not the same*] artificial 'disease' picture, not the disease itself, but information about the disease which helps the body to organize its defenses). As the body's vital energy pushes back like a rebound effect against the 'shadow disease' created by the remedy, it also pushes the actual disease from the inside to the outside." Vaccines and immunizations to prevent various diseases and allergies engage the Law of Similars by administering trace amounts of a disease component, such as a virus, to promote an antibody-producing immune response in the body.

The basic concept of homeopathy, named from the Greek words *homoios*, meaning "similar," and *pathos*, "suffering," may be found in ancient medical practices and now has a history of more than 200 years. In addition to the Law of Similars (like cures like), Hahnemann, who was appalled by certain conventional methods of the time such as bloodletting, the use of leeches, and purging with high doses of mercury, lead, and other toxic substances, proposed the Law of the Infinitesimal Dose, that the more a remedy is diluted, the greater its potency, and that illness is specific to an individual—in sum, holistic medicine.

Described universally as a humane, low-cost, nontoxic, noninvasive system of medicine that especially offers benefits to individuals suffering from diseases that fail to respond to conventional treatment modalities, homeopathy is an alternative and complementary option chosen by more than 500 million people in the world, says the World Health Organization (WHO), which should be integrated into conventional medicine. Also, the federal Food and Drug Administration (FDA) recognizes homeopathic remedies as official drugs, listed in the *Homeopathic Pharmacopoeia of the United States* (HPUS), first published in 1897 (published by the American Institute of Homeopathy, 1980). The FDA regulates the manufacturing, labeling, and dispensing of homeopathic remedies, many of which are available over the counter in health food stores and pharmacies throughout the world.

Although conventional medicine practitioners claim there is no benefit offered by homeopathy or its thousands of remedies, proponents continue to believe in its efficacy for relief from a multitude of illnesses and conditions. Despite some disdain for the premise of a remedy's "energy imprint," "essence," or "memory" of symptoms that calls forth the body's "vital forces" to elicit relief of those symptoms, homeopathic treatment gained favor during the 1849 cholera epidemic in Cincinnati, Ohio: only 3 percent of the victims treated with homeopathic remedies died, while 40 to 70 percent of the victims treated with conventional methods died of the disease. In New Orleans, homeopaths treated 1945 victims of the 1879 yellow fever epidemic, with a 5.6 percent death rate, while conventional treatment resulted in a 16 percent death rate.

Believed to be compatible with other medical interventions and disciplines, homeopathic treatments are "of tremendous value in reversing diseases such as diabetes, arthritis, asthma, epilepsy, skin eruptions, allergic conditions, mental or emotional disorders, especially if applied at the onset of the disease," according to George Vithoulkas, director of the Athenian School of Homeopathic Medicine in Athens, Greece. "The long-term benefit of homeopathy to the patient is that it not only alleviates the symptoms but it reestablishes internal order at the deepest levels and thereby provides a lasting cure" (excerpted from *Alternative Medicine:*

The Definitive Guide, Celestial Arts, Berkeley, Calif., 2002, p. 273).

Homeopathy is practiced in the United States, Europe, India, Mexico, Argentina, Brazil, and elsewhere, and annual sales in the United States of homeopathic remedies now exceed $150 million, indicating a yearly increase in their use of 20 to 30 percent in the last 20 years.

home remedies   Also called folk remedies and usually based on family history and methods handed down from one generation to another, actions that individuals can take on their own to help combat illness and augment treatments prescribed by a physician or other health professional. For example, one home remedy for aching feet is to massage them with olive or sesame oil. Another example is the use of honey, which has antiseptic and calming properties, for sore throat, diarrhea, hay fever, asthma, and topical wounds. It is said that the ancient Greek physician Hippocrates touted a combination of honey, water, and certain herbs as an antipyretic. Eating sprigs of parsley dispels bad breath, and mint has long been known as a remedy for indigestion. Home remedies may also be based on ethnic traditions and beliefs.

See also FOLK MEDICINE; HIPPOCRATES.

Hoxsey therapy   A combination of herbs—red clover, buckthorn bark, burdock root, stillingia root, barberry bark, chaparral, licorice root, cascara amarga, and prickly ash bark—in a potassium iodide solution, plus a regimen of nutrition, supplements, and counseling developed as a holistic treatment for cancer by the coal miner–turned–herbal folk healer Harry Hoxsey (1901–74). According to reports, the cancer medicines were handed down to the Illinois-born Hoxsey from his great-grandfather. Hoxsey's personal charisma and his belief in the herbal solutions led him to fight accusations of quackery from several powerful organizations, including the American Medical Association (AMA) and the Food and Drug Administration (FDA). Two federal courts ruled in favor of Hoxsey's tonics as "therapeutic," however, and Hoxsey operated the Hoxsey Cancer Clinic in Dallas, Texas, which had branches in 17 states. In a 1953 federal report to Congress, the AMA, FDA, and National Cancer

Institute (NCI) joined forces to hinder Hoxsey's method, and the Dallas clinic, which at the time had 12,000 patients, shut down in 1960. The FDA banned the sale of all Hoxsey tonics, and all Hoxsey's alleged requests for scientific investigation of his formulas went unanswered. In 1963 it reopened as the Bio-Medical Center in Tijuana, Mexico, under the auspices of Hoxsey's longtime clinical nurse, Mildred Nelson, R.N. Hoxsey chose to stay in Dallas and work in the oil business.

The solutions were made for both internal and external use (the topical version was a paste that contained zinc chloride, antimony sulfide, and bloodroot, a wildflower herb popular as a skin cancer remedy among Lake Superior Native Americans). Since laboratory studies of its effectiveness were conducted, the Hoxsey formula has been reported to reduce tumors, inhibit tumor growth, and provide antioxidant and antiestrogen activities that are known to have a deleterious effect on cancerous cells. The botanist James Duke, Ph.D., of the U.S. Department of Agriculture, found all the herbs used by Hoxsey to have anticancer properties; they are cited in *Plants Used Against Cancer* (Lawrence, Mass.: Quarterman Publications, 1981), a compendium of medicinal plants used in folk remedies compiled by the NCI chemist Jonathan Hartwell. Lymphoma, melanoma, and skin cancer patients have responded particularly favorably to the Hoxsey therapy. Hoxsey believed that his herbal preparations balanced the chemical process in the body; his idea was that cancer is a systemic disease that "occurs only in the presence of a profound physiological change in the constituents of body fluids and a consequent chemical imbalance in the organism." Hoxsey also wrote the book *You Don't Have to Die* (New York: Milestone Books, 1956), which is now out of print.

Information about this treatment is available at the Bio-Medical Center, P.O. Box 727, 615 General Ferreira, Colonia Juarez, Tijuana, B.C., Mexico 22000, or 011-52-66-84-9011, 011-52-66-84-9081, or 011-52-66-84-9376.

humectant   A substance used as a moisturizer.

humors, the four   The ancient theory that human temperament and propensity for disease are based on the proportion of the major bodily fluids—blood, phlegm, black bile, and yellow bile—in one's system. When all the humors were balanced, an individual maintained health, and the body needed to expel any excesses in order to keep the humors in balance. Hydrotherapy, largely based on the use of water internally and externally, along with a diet and exercise regimen, became popular in the 19th century as a means to affect the humors. Blood represented a warm, moist state; phlegm represented cold and moist. Yellow bile was considered warm and dry; black bile was thought of as cold and dry. Certain diseases or conditions were associated with a certain humor. If the level of one of these humors became excessive or deficient, illness occurred in three stages: first, the humoral change; second, fever or what was called "boiling"; third, the discharge of one of the humors in the form of urine, feces, phlegm, bleeding, sweating, vomiting, and so on. Hippocrates is said to have espoused this theory, for which he was later criticized.

See also HIPPOCRATES; HYDROTHERAPY.

humor, use of   The practice inspired by Proverbs 17:22, "A merry heart doeth good like a medicine," of employing laughter and enjoyment as ways to assuage pain, stress, and anger, all of which may lead to illness. It has also been shown that laughter stimulates the body's natural production of endorphins, chemicals almost identical to the painkiller morphine. In mind-body medicine, laughter, optimism, and other qualities associated with pleasure are believed to have a positive impact in the treatment of disease.

See also COUSINS, NORMAN; SIEGEL, BERNIE S.

hydrotherapy   Any therapeutic method that involves the internal or external use of water for the treatment of disease, injury, or dysfunction. Hydrotheraphy and hydrothermal therapy are known to many cultures, including those of ancient Rome, Greece, China, and Japan. Hydrothermal therapy involves varying temperature of the water according to need, as in hot baths, saunas, wraps, and packs. Therapeutic water treatments have been known and used for centuries as an all-purpose therapy based on the ancient concept of the four bodily humors and the need to diminish or expel excessive humors such as phlegm and bile. Water is also a significant component in the traditional Chinese and Native American healing systems. A major proponent of hydrotherapy was Vincenz Priessnitz (1799–1851), whose system of administering water therapeutically in numerous ways along with an appropriate nutrition and exercise regimen sparked the establishment of hydropathic institutions in the United States and Europe. Enthusiasts in Priessnitz's day were called "hydropaths." Since the time of St. Bernadette Soubirous, the waters of Lourdes, France, have been a destination for thousands of people seeking faith healing or a water cure.

The 19th-century Bavarian monk Father Sebastian Kneipp helped repopularize the therapeutic use of water, which has healing properties based on both mechanical and thermal effects. Hydrotherapy stimulates the body's reaction to hot and cold, to the protracted application of heat, to pressure exerted by the water, and to the sensation of the water or being in the water. The nerves of the skin carry impulses into the body, where they can encourage the immune system to produce stress hormones, increase circulatory and digestive processes, and reduce pain. Generally heat soothes and relaxes the body, slowing the activity of internal organs, and cold invigorates and intensifies internal activity. For example, muscle tension and stress anxiety may warrant a hot bath or shower. Fatigue may respond well to a warm bath or shower followed by a brief cold shower. Baths, pools, hot tubs, or any body of water in which one can be submerged offer relief from the pull of gravity, and water's natural movement gives the body a gentle massage that helps relieve muscle spasm and poor circulation. Hydrotherapy and hydrothermal therapy are chiefly used to tone up the body; to stimulate digestion, blood flow, and the immune system; to reduce or alleviate pain; and to reduce stress. Besides soothing tired, tense muscles, hydrotherapy quiets the lungs, heart, stomach, and endocrine system by stimulating nerve reflexes on the spinal cord. Various case reports and observational studies and a number of controlled studies indicate successful use of hydrotherapy. In a 40-person study at the University of Minnesota, 85 percent of the participants preferred a whirlpool bath to a still bath because whirlpools had a more direct impact on the ravages of stress and anxiety than a still bath.

A number of hydrotherapy techniques are available: baths and showers, neutral baths, sitz baths, contrast sitz baths, foot baths, cold-mitten friction rub, steam inhalation, hot compresses, cold compresses, alternating hot and cold compresses, heating compresses, body wrap, wet sheet pack, and others. For most douches, the water stream should always be directed from the outer parts of the body toward the heart. After douching, dry off excess water, dress, and exercise. Among various douches are the following (1) In a knee douche, water streams from the right small toe, along the outside of the lower leg to the hollow of the knee, then along the inside of the leg and over the sole of the foot. Repeat the process on the other leg. This may help treat headache, migraine, hypotension, insomnia, contusions, and varicose veins and other vascular injury. It is not recommended for urinary tract infections, irritable bladder, sciatica, or during menstruation. (2) A thigh douche uses the same method as the knee douche but includes the upper thigh to promote better circulation. This may help treat rheumatism, varicose veins, arthritis, and certain forms of paralysis. (3) A lower trunk douche, essentially the same procedure as a thigh douche but including the lower torso, is used to help treat diabetes mellitus, meteorism (distention caused by gas in the abdomen or intestine), enlargement of the liver, enlargement of the gallbladder, and stone formation. (4) For an arm douche, direct the water stream from the outside of the right hand to the shoulder, then back on the inside of the arm. Repeat the process for the left arm. It is useful for cold hands, nervous disorders, neuralgia and paralysis, rheumatism of the arms, heart problems, vertigo, headaches, and catarrh in the nose and throat. (5) For a chest douche, direct water to the arms first. This is useful for chronic bronchitis and bronchial asthma, and angina pectoris *Caution:* Moderate the temperature if there is risk of angiospasm. (6) An upper trunk douche is used for the upper torso and arms. It can improve blood flow to the lungs, heart, and pleura. It is useful for the treatment of bronchitis, bronchial asthma, disease of the larynx and vocal cords, headaches, nervous excitability, varicose veins of the legs, toning, and stimulating cardiac and respiratory activity. Do not use if there is blood stasis in the pulmonary circulation. (7) Back douches are useful for the treatment of weakened back muscles, back pain, spinal disease, multiple sclerosis, bronchial asthma, and nearly all diseases of the lung. *Warning:* Do not use for debilitated patients or those with neurasthenia. Neck douches help alleviate headaches, migraines, tension in the shoulder and neck, hypersensitivity to changes in the weather, mild depression, tinnitus, vertigo, and arthrosis of the hand and finger joints. *Warning:* It is not to be used by persons with high blood pressure, enlargement of the thyroid, or raised intraocular pressure. (8) A facial douche should proceed from the right temple downward to the chin, upward to the left temple, from right to left over the forehead, and repeatedly from the forehead to the chin, then in circles over the face. This helps relieve headaches and migraines, trigeminal neuralgia, and toothaches and relaxes tired eyes. *Caution:* Keep the eyes closed.

Saunas and steam baths are similar. Sauna heat acts more quickly to eliminate toxins through the skin, though some consider the moist air of a steam bath to have a more satisfying effect on the respiratory system. A sauna promotes deep relaxation while it stimulates circulation, increases heart rate, has an immune-modulating effect, promotes hormone production, encourages mucosal secretions in the respiratory system, opens the airways, reduces resistance to respiration, regulates the vegetative system, and induces a sense of well-being. Children may take saunas from age two to three years. Saunas are used to relieve pulled muscles in the back, chronic rheumatoid arthritis, bronchial asthma, unstable hypertension (stages I and 11), and impaired peripheral blood circulation. However, saunas should not be taken by individuals who have acute rheumatoid arthritis, acute infection, active tuberculosis, sexually transmitted diseases, acute mental disorder, inflammation of an inner organ or blood vessels, significant vascular changes in the brain or heart, circulatory problems, or acute cancer. To prevent ill effects of excessive heat, wipe your face often with a cold cloth and stay in the sauna no longer than 15 to 20 minutes. Saunas are not recommended for pregnant women.

Baths may be warm and rising-temperature baths or may employ herbs and other substances added to the water. The rising-temperature hip bath, for example, is taken in a tub filled with tepid water. Hot water is then gradually added until the level reaches the navel. The final temperature should be 103–104° Fahrenheit. Afterward, the patient is wrapped for warmth. This form of bath should last 15 to 30 minutes, not more than three times per week, and is not recommended for individuals who have cardiac or circulation disorders, hemorrhoids, or varicose veins. A cold foot bath, in which the feet are placed into calf-high cold water, may help relieve varicose veins, susceptibility to edemas, headaches, low blood pressure, circulatory problems, sleeplessness, susceptibility to the common cold, sweaty feet, or a contused ankle. However, it is not recommended for individuals who have chronically cold feet, hypertension, irritable bladder, urinary tract infection, diabetes, or vascular occlusion. A rising-temperature warm foot bath may work well for individuals experiencing the onset of a common cold or cold feet or for treatment of tension but is not effective for those with varicose veins, edema, or lymphostasis. Other therapeutic baths include herbal baths (using valerian, lavender, linden, chamomile, hops, burdock root, sage, lemongrass, and many other herbs), the cold arm bath, the rising-temperature arm bath, and the sitz bath.

The sitz bath is generally taken in a hip bath as a cold, rising-temperature, or warm sitz bath. Before a sitz bath, warm the feet in a warm foot bath. Parts of the body not immersed in water should be covered. A cold sitz bath may help hemorrhoids or inflammation of the anus; a warm or rising-temperature sitz bath may relieve difficulty in voiding the bladder, an irritable bladder, and inflammation or infection of the prostate or enhance preparation for pregnancy. Do not use warm or rising-temperature sitz baths for hemorrhoids.

In another form of bath, the wrap is largely a supportive measure for treating fever and local inflammation. The person receiving treatment should be in a relaxed position while a linen cloth moistened with cold water (warm water for respiratory diseases), well wrung out, is wrapped tightly, but not restricting circulation, around the appropriate part of the body. The moist linen cloth is in turn wrapped with a dry cotton or linen cloth. The patient is then usually wrapped in a blanket or another cloth and rests for 45 to 60 minutes or, if the intention is to induce sweating, for up to three hours. If the wrap does not feel warm after 15 minutes, a hot water bottle or hot tea may be offered. If the patient feels ill or uncomfortable, the wrap should be removed immediately. Various wraps include neck (for sore throat), chest (for neuralgia and upper respiratory disease), body from the costal arch to the pubic bone (for inflammatory diseases, ulcers, fever, cramps), trunk (for high fever), hip (for prostatitis, vaginitis, hemorrhoids, anal eczema, inflammation in the pelvic cavity), calf (for lymphostasis, edema, withdrawal of heat in fever and phlebitis; in varicose veins the effect can sometimes be amplified by applying earth or loam poulstices), and joint wrap (for rheumatoid arthritis and arthrosis).

Wraps also employ water as a healing method. A wrapping cloth is soaked in a hot infusion or decoction of herbs, wrung out, and applied to the patient's body. Alternatively, the wrap may receive a coating of hot mud mustard flour, or fango. As a further alternative, hayseed may be placed in a sack and steamed. This wrap may aid the treatment of painful chronic diseases such as arthrosis, renal disease, or cystitis and may stimulate blood flow. Always make certain that the temperature of the wrap is tolerable before applying it. For a cool wrap, cooled cataplasm is spread onto the wrapping cloth and placed on the affected body area. Crushed ice in a plastic bag may also be repeatedly applied for one minute, then removed for four. This may be therapeutic for various inflammatory arthropathies, sprains and strains, and pleurisy. Ice packs can also be used for headaches. When using ice packs, place a thin cloth between the pack and the skin to prevent frostbite. In addition, any application of cold is not indicated for individuals who have Raynaud's disease.

General hydration of the entire body—a response to thirst and loss of water through elimination and perspiration—is extremely important. Experts suggest drinking eight glasses of water per day.

See also HUMORS, THE FOUR.

hyperthermia Various types of heat treatment geared toward increasing blood circulation and extensibility of soft tissues, extracting toxins from cells, increasing tissue-cell function, and inducing muscle relaxation and pain relief. The two main types of heat treatments are superficial and deep. Superficial heat treatments involve applying heat topically—to the outside of the body. Deep heat treatments through ultrasound or electric current direct heat toward specific inner tissues and structures. Heat treatments are beneficial before exercise, when warming the soft tissues makes muscles more flexible and prevents the possibility of injury to "cold" muscles. Different ways to convey heat include conduction—the transfer of heat from one object to another, with objects in direct contact with each other; conversion—turning another form of energy into heat; radiation—the transmission and absorption of electromagnetic waves to produce heat; and convection—creating heat when a liquid or gas moves past a body part.

Hot packs, a popular form of heat treatment, use conduction as the medium of heat transfer. Moist heat packs are readily available in hospitals, walk-in medical care centers, physical therapy centers, sports training facilities, and elsewhere. With a therapeutic temperature not exceeding 131°F (55°C), the hot pack is placed over several layers of towels or pads for not more than 20 or 30 minutes to produce comfortable warmth for the patient. Some commercially prepared hot packs may be warmed in a microwave before being applied to the patient.

Hot-water bottles have long provided superficial heat treatment. A vinyl or rubber bag with a stopper at the opening forms the "bottle," which is half-filled with hot water ranging between 115°F and 125°F (46.1–52°C). Covered by a towel or other protective cloth or pad, the hot-water bottle is placed on the treatment area until the water has cooled. Electric heating pads may also be used, although safety issues are to be considered.

Melted paraffin wax containing mineral oil conducts superficial heat and is often the topical heat treatment of choice for uneven surfaces such as the hands. Paraffin placed in a small bath unit solidifies at room temperature and is used as a liquid heat treatment when heated at 126–127.4°F (52–53°C). In what is commonly known as the "dip and wax method," the patient dips a hand or other body part eight to 12 times into the paraffin. The hand is then covered with a plastic bag and a towel for insulation for approximately 20 minutes.

Hydrotherapy, a heat treatment involving submersion in water, is prescribed for many musculoskeletal disorders. Hydrotherapy tanks and pools are generally set at warm temperatures up to 150°F (65.6°C). Because the patient may perform resistance exercises while in the water, higher temperatures may place undue strain on the heart, lungs, and circulation as the treatment becomes more physically demanding. Because of this, many hydrotherapy baths are now being set at 95–110°F (35–43.3°C). There are also units available with movable turbine jets, which provide a light massage. Some people find that a brief dip in a hot tub or spa before exercise is beneficial as a warmup.

Fluidotherapy was developed in the 1970s as a dry-heat modality consisting of cellulose particles suspended in air. Units are manufactured in different sizes, and some are restricted to treating only a hand or foot. The turbulence of the gas-solid mixture provides heat to objects immersed in the medium. Temperatures of this treatment range from 110°F to 123°F (43.3–50.5°C). While massaging and increasing the flow of blood to the limb, fluidotherapy allows the patient to exercise the limb during the treatment.

A deep-heat treatment, ultrasound waves administered by way of an ultrasound transmitting device, penetrates the body to provide relief to inner tissue. Also a diagnostic tool, ultrasound energy occurs in the acoustic or sound spectrum and is undetectable to the human ear. By using conducting agents such as gel or mineral oil, the ultrasound transducer warms areas of the musculoskeletal system. Certain areas of the musculoskeletal system absorb ultrasound better than others. Muscle tissue and other connective tissue such as ligaments and tendons absorb this form of energy very well; fat absorbs it to a much lesser degree. Ultrasound has a relatively long-lasting effect, continuing up to one hour.

Diathermy, another deep-heat treatment, which enjoyed much popularity between the 1940s and 1960s before the use of ultrasound, employs an electrode drum used to apply heat to an affected area. The drum has a wire coil surrounded by dead space and other insulators such as a plastic housing. Several layers of towels are placed between the unit and the patient. This device works on the premise of a magnetic field's effect on connective tissues. One advantage of diathermy over various other heat treatments is that although fat resists an electrical field, it does not resist a magnetic field. Diathermy is reported to be helpful to individuals with chronic low back pain and muscle spasms.

Any kind of heat treatment should be supervised. The patient's heat sensitivity should be assessed to prevent burns and other injury, and the skin over the affected area should be clean. After heat treatment, symptoms of dizziness and nausea, local irritation, or discoloration should be charted. Treatments should be administered at least one hour apart, if more than one is necessary. Any heat treatment may cause damage if there are excessive temperatures or improper insulation or treatment duration. Overexposure to heat may cause redness, blisters, burns, or reduced blood circulation, and in ultrasound therapy, excessive heat over bony areas with little soft tissue (such as hands, feet, and elbows) may cause pain and possible tissue damage. Exposure to the electrode drum during diathermy may produce hot spots.

Heat treatments are not recommended for individuals with circulation problems, heat intolerance, or lack of sensation in the affected area. Sluggish or impaired blood circulation may contribute to heat-related injuries. Heat treatments also should not be used for pregnant women or individuals afflicted with heart, lung, or kidney diseases, or on areas above the eye or heart, or over areas where there are metal surgical implants.

See also HYDROTHERAPY.

hypnotherapy   Also referred to as hypnosis, varied techniques used by psychiatrists, psychologists, and other psychotherapists to guide the patient into a state of altered awareness, deep relaxation, or trance in order to help treat anxiety, panic attacks, addictions, and numerous other psychological and somatic problems. Hypnosis has also been used successfully as a substitute for pharmaceutical anesthesia. The system is founded on the idea of the power of suggestion—that one's emotional status has a significant effect on one's physical status, a concept dating back to ancient Greece, India, and Persia.

Franz Anton Mesmer (1734–1815), a German physician, introduced hypnosis—what he called Mesmerism—to the medical community in the late 18th century. Mesmer's theory was that when magnetic forces existing in all matter became unbalanced, disease occurred, and he believed he could transfer his body's "animal magnetism" to another through the use of magnets, iron rods, and "mesmerizing," or highly soothing, verbal suggestions that induced a trancelike state. Despite the fact that the healing potential of mind over matter and deep relaxation states including trance emerged, Mesmer's theories could not be scientifically proved by a committee of investigators in the French medical community, among whom were the American statesman Benjamin Franklin and the French physician Josef de Guillotin. Mesmer was branded a quack and banned from practicing in France.

It was later that the British ophthalmologist James Braid explored Mesmer's ideas with his patients and renamed the technique hypnosis, after Hypnos, the Greek god of sleep. Dr. Sigmund Freud, known as the father of modern psychiatry, used hypnosis in his practice in the 19th century, but not until 1955 was hypnotherapy recognized by the British Medical Association as a bona fide medical treatment. In 1958 the American Medical Association also officially recognized hypnosis; that recognition eventually led to the establishment of several professional associations, including the American Society of Clinical Hypnosis and the American Institute of Hypnotherapy, whose members are physicians, psychologists, dentists, and other health professionals.

Contemporary hypnosis has been shown to help the body release endorphins and enkephalins (morphine-like chemicals naturally produced by the body to assuage pain and promote a sense of well-being), improve circulation, lower blood pressure and heart rate, and generally elicit deep relaxation that is beneficial in fighting stress, anxiety, depression, chronic pain, and disease of many kinds. Many hypnotherapists say that the patient benefits most if he or she is willing to participate in the process of hypnosis, and that people who are not willing cannot be hypnotized.

See also Appendix I; MESMERISM; WEISS, BRIAN.

Imaginal Therapy   See ISLAMIC SUFI HEALING PRACTICES.

infusion   A liquid injected into a vein, or a substance steeped in hot or cold water and ingested for therapeutic purposes. A tea is considered an infusion, for example. In Western medicine, an intravenous infusion may be a solution containing electrolytes, nutrients, and pharmaceutical agents. An infusodecoction is an infusion followed by a decoction, that is, a medicine stock that contains a crude drug that is first steeped in cold water and then placed in boiling water.

insulin potentiation therapy   Also known as IPT, an alternative method for the treatment of certain cancers, involving the administration of a small dose of insulin to cancer patients with the intention of inducing hypoglycemia, or low blood sugar level. It is believed that once low blood sugar level is achieved, low doses of intravenous conventional chemotherapy may be more effective, because insulin potentiates the cells' ability to be permeated by the cancer medications. Cancer cells have more insulin receptors than normal cells, and therefore insulin provides a boost to the anticancer drugs. In addition insulin can stimulate proliferation of certain cancer cells, to create a larger, more receptive target for the chemotherapeutic agents.

Interior Realignment   A feng shui approach devised by Denise Linn, of Seattle, Washington, author of *Past Lives, Present Dreams; Sacred Space: Clearing and Enhancing the Energy of Your Home; The Hidden Power of Dreams*, and *The Secret Language of Signs: How to Interpret the Coincidences* and *Symbols in Your Life*.

See also FENG SHUI.

intuitive touch   Since the beginning of time people have used various styles of touch to try to soothe and heal family and friends. While scholars feel that massage originated in China it is certain that each country throughout the world had developed and passed down their methods for treating the body with the hands. Ancient writings of Egypt, Persia, Greece, Rome, and Asian countries mention the positive effects from the use of massage.

We instinctively rub, press, pat, or in some way touch when we ache, feel pain, or just don't feel right. Intuitively we are applying self-treatment to try to create a more balanced state. Everyone is qualified to help themselves and with a little effort, are able to help others too. The simple understanding that humans are equipped to heal themselves, and that we can also help others, is the underlying foundation of shiatsu. If we live according to natural laws we really shouldn't have many troubles. Unfortunately we don't consistently live that way and humankind has had to devise ways to deal with the suffering that we experience. Ultimately to regain wholeness we must change our way of living. There are many tools that we can use in this process. Shiatsu is one of them.

Shiatsu practitioners have long been considered authorities on treating minor diseases in Japan. In general, the Japanese public favors shiatsu treatment and, for many years, these practitioners have played a major role in health maintenance. The previously mentioned forms of massage and shiatsu are wonderful tools for the betterment of health. With life forever changing, even these techniques must continue to evolve.

See also SHIATSU.

iridology   A preventive, diagnostic method developed more than a century ago by the Hungarian homeopathic physician Ignatz von Peczeley, which was based on the concept that examining the iris, or the colored part of the eye, could reveal hidden disease in the body before the appearance of the symptoms. When he was a child, von Peczeley observed that an owl with a broken leg also had a black mark in his iris. Later the doctor observed the same eye mark in a human patient with a broken leg; that discovery led him to investigate marking in the iris as a sign of dysfunction or impairment somewhere else in the body.

The ancient Greeks, Egyptians, and Chinese maintained that a person's eyes held information about his or her health. Hippocrates said, "Behold the eyes, behold the body." On the premise that eyes are not only the mirrors of the soul, but also of the body, iridology practitioners claim it is possible to make a diagnostic reading of the iris to discover the weakened parts of the organism, the latent tendencies, the patient's vitality, the condition of the organs, and the disease processes.

Iridology is reportedly a safe, painless, quick, and economical diagnostic method without radiation that helps discover any constitutional weakness before a clinical outbreak occurs. It is considered a unique preventive method used to determine the body's tendency toward certain ailments (for example, certain characteristics of the iris may show a sluggish digestive system or detect hereditary predispositions to cardiac or arthritic diseases) and its present degree of stress, with the advantage of requiring only observation with a light and a magnifying glass. Iridologists may make a videotape or photographic slide of the iris using a special camera, which they can then project onto a larger screen for examination. Color, texture, fibers of the iris, and markings and their positions in the eye are the indicators of problems or potential problems. The left iris corresponds to the left side of the body, and the right iris corresponds to the right. An eye chart has been developed—an illustration similar to the "body map" on the soles of the feet in reflexology—to designate parts of the eye as they relate to other parts of the body; for example, the area immediately surrounding the pupil relates to the stomach. Iridologists believe that blue-eyed people may have tendencies toward excessive acidity that may cause ulcers and arthritis, brown-eyed

individuals may tend to experience gallbladder dysfunction and other problems caused by impaired ability to metabolize fats, and green, gray, or mixed-color irises (called "biliary irises") may indicate gastrointestinal difficulties. Although iridologists take an extensive personal and medical history of each patient and may be qualified to offer nutritional advice or prescribe certain treatment, iridology cannot replace other diagnostic methods in conventional and alternative medicine. It is reported on some websites pertaining to iridology that some Russian scientists are developing irischromotherapy, which involves curing disease through the iris. More information is available by contacting the Hellenic Medical Association of Iridology, Lidias 2, Thessaloniki, Greece 544 53, or info@iridology.gr, or telephone 0113 0310 906086.

Islamic Sufi healing practices   An ancient Islamic religion-based system of meditation, chanting, prayer, herbs, special diet, use of essential oils, and other practices that are believed to bring about healing. Sufis are Muslim mystics. According to Web information on Sufi healing, Sufis revere the healing of the sick as the most important of all services to humanity, and a book has been written on the 800-year tradition of this "divine science" of the Christi Order (one of the Sufi healing orders). "Among the many topics covered are dietary recommendations of the Prophet, the preparation of herbal formulas, healing with essential oils, illnesses arising at various stages of the soul's evolution, fasting and prayer, talismans, and the 'infallible remedy.' Hakim Chishti is a naturopathic physician and one of the only recognized Tibb practitioners in the United States. As a Fulbright Research Scholar, he studied Tibb medicine in Afghanistan and has participated in international health symposia in Afghanistan, India, and Pakistan. Working from original material, he has translated the handbooks of Avicenna and the standard text on Tibb medicine, *Mizan-ul-Tibb*. He is the author of *The Traditional Healer's Handbook* (Rochester, Vt.: Healing Arts Press, 1991)."

Another healing order is an international network of people called the Sufi Healing Order. Its website states: "Initiation into the Healing Order strengthens one's inner connection with illuminated

Beings of Healing, through our link with Pir-o-Murshid Inayat Khan, founder of this order. Members work with healing practices on a daily basis to increase their capacity for the Divine Healing Power to come through. A commitment to healing includes one's own personal healing and involves ongoing purification and clarity of intention. The Healing Order aims to make the Sufi Teachings about healing available through seminars and workshops. Special training courses are provided for conductors as well as for members who are involved in professional healing work. The Healing Ritual is a group activity of the Healing Order, in which members pray for the healing of those who have asked for their names to be on the Healing List. Healing circles are facilitated by healing conductors and serve those who have asked for healing. Healing conductors may also provide classes in healing. Candidates for the Healing Order are encouraged to contact their local conductor. In addition members are encouraged to visit hospitals, and to help their friends when they are not well.

"The purpose of the Sufi Healing Order is to awaken humanity to a greater realization of the power of the Divine Spirit to heal, thus to bring about a better state of physical, mental and spiritual health, and so to fulfill the law of God. The basic principle of the Healing Order is that the soul is the Divine Beneath; it purifies, revivifies and heals the instrument through which it functions," said Hazrat Inayat Khan. "The secret of healing is to rise by the power of belief above the limitations of this world of variety, that one may touch by the power of intelligence the oneness of the whole Being. It is there that one becomes charged with the almighty power, and it is by the power of that attainment that one is able to help oneself and others in their pain and suffering. Verily, spirit has all the power there is."

"The beauty of the group work is that it illuminates the personal satisfaction of being endowed with special powers. Healing is looked upon as a gracious act of solidarity with human suffering, inspired by attunement with the Holy Spirit and allowing oneself to become a pure channel for the divine power. We therefore beckon upon your cooperation and goodwill in helping us to fulfill this great task, if indeed it finds a resonance in your being," said Pir Vilayat Khan.

According to the practitioner Ismael Mazzara, "Sufi healing practices cover a number of therapies, including traditional Eastern aromatherapy (based on fragrances called 'attars'), and traditional cupping, which is practiced in both traditional Chinese and Islamic medicine. I find it particularly effective with dancers and athletes who need fast relief from muscular aches and pains. (See www.chishti.com.) Other aspects of Sufi healing work are best discussed in personal consultation. Imaginal Therapy, a system of therapeutic visualization (http:www.farancenter.org) is effective in helping you change how you see yourself in your present situation, and change toward a direction you want. It's particularly effective in pain relief and in helping to cope with the fear and anxiety that often accompanies serious illness. In combination with auricular acupuncture, the benefits are enhanced. We periodically offer workshops in London for health professionals and for the general public." (See ismael@mazzara.demon.co.uk. The U.S. website is Sufi Healing Order. The contact in Germany is Kabir, email CaduceusFindeisen@ T-Online.de; telephone 011 05821-477129.)

See also FAITH HEALING; PRAYER, POWER OF.

Issels's fever therapy   An alternative cancer treatment, a method of raising body temperature to as high as 105° Fahrenheit in order to stimulate the immune system, one of several whole-body therapeutic methods developed by the German physician Josef Issels. Part of Issels's "whole-body therapy," as it was known, active fever, was induced on a monthly basis by administering the drug Pyrifer, which was made from treated *Escherichia coli* bacteria. Passive fever was produced by placing the patient in a cylinder containing electrodes that administered ultrashort waves.

Issels also advocated a diet of raw organic foods, very low-dose chemotherapy, surgery, radiation, ozone therapy, administration of organ extracts and organic ribonucleic acid (RNA) and deoxyribonucleic acid (DNA) (proteolytic enzymes to destroy the protein coating around tumors), vitamins and minerals, and psychotherapy. In addition, he recommended the removal of infected teeth and tonsils and of metallic dental fillings (particularly mercury amalgam), since they could have a deleterious effect on immune system functioning. Issels wished to motivate cancer patients to participate fully in their care and healing and encouraged them to go mountain-climbing, jog, and do other daily exercise. Studies conducted at King's College Hospital in London and at the University of Leyden in Holland indicated that approximately 17 percent of Issels's patients, considered to be in terminal stages of illness, led cancer-free lives for at least five years after being diagnosed with less than one year to survive. During the 1950s and 1960s, however, the German medical community charged Issels with fraud and manslaughter. In 1960 he was incarcerated. Eventually he was acquitted of all charges, and he now has retired to Florida. Ahmed Elkadi, M.D., and his colleagues at the Panama City Clinic in Panama City, Florida, are offering a "multimodality immunotherapy program" based on Issels's methods. Additional information on fever therapy is available from the foundation for Advancement in Cancer Therapy (FACT), P.O. Box 1242, Old Chelsea Station, New York, NY 10113, or (212) 741-2790, or P.O. Box 215, 200 East Lancaster Avenue, Wynnwood, PA 19096, or (215) 642-4810.

Iyengar yoga   See YOGA.

J

James, William The American philosopher and psychologist (1842–1910), who led the movement called pragmatism or the pragmatic method and wrote several works, including *The Principles of Psychology* (1890. Reprint, New York: Dover Books, 1950), *The Varieties of Religious Experience* (1902. Reprint, New York: Penguin, 1982), and *Essays in Radical Empiricism* (New York: Longman, Green, 1912). A graduate of Harvard University in 1869 with a medical degree, James suffered a panic disorder that fostered his interest in physiological psychology. In his lecture "Pragmatism" in 1907, he said: "The philosophy which is important in each of us is not a technical matter; it is more or less our dumb sense of what life honestly and deeply means. It is only partly got from books; it is our individual way of just seeing and feeling the total push and pressure of the cosmos." In 1884 James theorized: "Our feelings of [bodily] changes as they occur is the emotion. We feel sorry because we cry . . . not that we cry because we are sorry." In other words, the accelerated heart rate, sweaty palms, butterflies in the stomach, and other visceral changes translate the impression or perception of the changes into an actual emotional reaction. James and the Danish physician Carl Lange, who believed that emotions are a result of stimulation of the vasomotor system, together established the idea that fundamentally emotions of all kinds produce similar physical responses. In the James/Lange theory, as it was called, is evidence of the link between mind and body and the way each can produce effects in the other.

jing In traditional Chinese medicine the term for the fundamental energy that is the essence of all life.

jingluo The Chinese word for the body's invisible but well-documented meridians, channels, or pathways along which flows *qi* (or *ch'i*), the vital force or basic life energy.

See also ACUPUNCTURE.

jin ye In traditional Chinese medicine, the term referring to body fluids.

juices and juice therapy A nutritional regimen based on the idea that the juice of fruits and vegetables offers many important vitamins, minerals, and enzymes to help the body detoxify and function at its best, in that many diseases and disorders are related to poor diet. In the book *Juicing for Life: A Guide to the Health Benefits of Fresh Fruit and Vegetable Juicing*, by Cherie Calbom and Maureen Keane (Garden City Park, N.Y.: Avery Publishing Group, 1992), *juice* is defined as "water, flavors, pigments, enzymes, vitamins, minerals, and anutrients (flavonoids, etc.). Juice is all these substances working synergistically to give your body the materials that promote healing, energy, and protection from disease. . . . And juices should be part of a comprehensive approach to wellness." The authors also wrote that the late Dr. Max Bircher-Benner, of the Bircher-Benner clinic in Europe, believed cooking and processing food destroy its living energy, and that the most nutritive energy is obtained from plants because they undergo the process of photosynthesis. Among the most popular are the juices of carrot, apple, kale, spinach, ginger root, celery, beet, cabbage, garlic, broccoli, parsley, potato, turnip greens, pineapple, cantaloupe, pomegranate, green pepper, collard greens, sprouts, red Swiss chard, pears, berries, grapes, and tomatoes. Juice enthusiasts maintain that juices of all kinds are beneficial to health and complement treatment of ailments ranging from anxiety to varicose veins. Juices are used also as components in weight loss, cleansing and detoxification diets, and fasting.

See also DETOXIFICATION THERAPY; FASTING; GERSON, MAX; HOXSEY THERAPY.

Jung, Carl The Swiss psychologist and psychiatrist (1875–1961), who founded analytic psychology and described the concepts of introverted and extroverted personality types, archetypal personalities, and the collective unconscious and universal synchronicity of thoughts and events. Educated at the universities of Basel and Zurich (where he earned an M.D. in 1902), Jung worked in the psychiatric clinic in Zurich and was on the staff of the Berholzli Asylum of Zurich headed by the prominent Swiss psychologist Eugen Bleuler. Jung also collaborated with Sigmund Freud and wrote articles and books including *The Psychology of the Unconscious* (1921. Reprint, Mineola, N.Y.: Dover, 2002). In addition, Jung taught at the Federal Polytechnical University in Zurich and was a professor of medical psychology at the University of Basel.

Jung's works greatly influence modern psychological concepts including those embraced in various disciplines of mind-body medicine.

kahuna A Hawaiian witch doctor. The term was coined in 1886; its basic philosophy involves "the three selves"—high, or superconscious *(aumaka)*; middle; conscious *(uhane)*; and low; subconscious *(unihipili)*—and "the three invisible subtle bodies" *(kino-aka)* of each self. The high self is the least dense; its center is above the crown chakra; and it is rooted in the heart chakra. The middle self is more dense and is centered in the brow chakra. The low self is the most dense; its center lies within the solar plexus chakra. In addition, *kahunas* believe in the harmonious interaction of "the three voltages" (levels of life energy or psychic energy) *(mana/prana)*: the Low self controls the supply and use of *mana* and converts it to a higher voltage *(mana-mana)* for use by the middle self. The low self uses *mana* to maintain the physical body. The middle self uses *mana* to think and feel. The two together must supply *mana* to high self. The high self converts *mana* to *mana-loa*, which in turn becomes a potent healing, or "miracle-making" force.

See also FAITH HEALING; SANGOMA; VOODOO.

kapha One of the *doshas*, or three main body types, in Ayurvedic medicine. *Kapha* also refers to the moon force, the opposite of the sun force, both of which are considered to be basic life forces or elements.

See also AYURVEDA.

ki The Japanese equivalent of QI, or *ch'i*.

kinesiology Commonly known as applied kinesiology (AK), a noninvasive system centered on testing the muscular range of motion, strength, and capacity of individuals with muscle injury or disease. Muscle testing helps the practitioner evaluate neuromuscular function as it relates to the structural, chemical, and mental physiologic regulatory mechanisms. From the Greek *kinesis*, meaning "motion," kinesiology is the study of movement and a blend of Western technology and the theories of energy flow throughout the body along the meridians, or invisible energy pathways mapped out by practitioners of acupuncture and traditional Chinese and Asian medicine. Focused on determining "subclinical" problems (predisposition to disease, or subtle indications of potential problems), kinesiologists offer diagnosis and treatment of aches and pains, joint stiffness, headaches, food sensitivities, digestive problems, and phobias.

Members of the International College of Applied Kinesiology, founded and developed by the chiropractor Dr. George Goodheart, Jr., have made considerable advances in the field. AK is used as a diagnostic tool to determine what is wrong and what to do for a patient. An applied kinesiology examination depends upon knowledge of functional neurology, anatomy, physiology, biomechanics, and biochemistry and is combined with standard physical examination procedures, laboratory findings, X rays, and the patient's personal and medical history. The various procedures developed by Goodheart and others in the International College of Applied Kinesiology are derived from many disciplines, including chiropractic, osteopathy, medicine, dentistry, acupuncture, and biochemistry, and are currently being used by doctors of chiropractic, osteopathy, homeopathy, dentistry, and medicine.

Applied kinesiology has two major components: one is an aid to diagnosis. Muscle testing helps diagnose what is functioning abnormally—the nervous system, lymphatic drainage, vascular supply to a muscle or organ, a nutritional excess or deficiency, a problem with the cranial-sacral-temporo-mandibular joint (TMJ) mechanism, or an imbalance in the meridian system. By testing individual muscles the examiner can determine what affects the relative strength of the muscle on the basis of his or her knowledge of the basic mechanics and physiological functioning of the body.

The second part of applied kinesiology involves treatment. Balancing the malfunction may be accomplished with nutrition, chiropractic, osteopathic cranial techniques, acupuncture, myofascial techniques, nervous system coordination procedures, and other modalities. More information is available at www.icak.com.

Kirlian photography   A photographic technique to produce images of the human electrical energy field for diagnostic purposes. Developed in 1939 by the Russian electrician Semyon Kirlian and his wife, Valentina, Kirlian photography with either a single-plate or two-plate process reveals the quality of one's energy by indicating one's capacity to resonate with the electrical frequency that passes through the plate. Unbalanced yin and yang may be determined, as well as effects of long-term medication, the stage of cancer one may be in, and the optimal fertile period during the menstrual cycle of women who are having difficulty conceiving. Safe for everyone except babies and individuals with any metal implant, such as a pacemaker, in their bodies, the technique is said to be helpful also for people who have suffered emotional trauma, such as divorce, or serious problems with children or career.

Either Kirlian procedure simply requires pictures of one's hands and feet, or fingertips and toes. The images that show up correspond to the patient's energy level on that particular day; if one is in a total state of exhaustion, for example, no image may appear. If a person is experiencing intense feelings, the images may have "splines," referring to the fuzziness around the outlines of the prints. A body logic counselor "reads" the Kirlian images in terms of one's amount of tension or imbalance. Acupuncturists sometimes use Kirlian photographs to enhance their diagnostic ability.

Krieger, Dolores   A registered nurse and Ph.D. who developed Therapeutic Touch, a healing technique employing the body's electromagnetic field and innate ability to heal. The author of books including *Accepting Your Power to Heal* (Santa Fe, N.M.: Bear & Company Publishing, 1993), she and the natural healer Dora Van Gelden Kunz interpreted several ancient healing practices and established Therapeutic Touch as an extension of professional skills for persons in the health field. It is now taught in more than 80 colleges and universities in the United States and in 67 other countries. Krieger is professor emerita at New York University. Therapeutic Touch, which most often induces deep relaxation, has been beneficial to patients with headaches, burns, bone fractures, asthma, reproductive ailments, cancer, acquired immunodeficiency syndrome (AIDS), and other illnesses. Other books by Dolores Krieger are *The Therapeutic Touch: How to Use Your Hands to Help or to Heal* (Englewood Cliffs, N.J.: Prentice Hall, 1979) and *Living the Therapeutic Touch: Healing as a Lifestyle.*

See also BIOENERGETICS; THERAPEUTIC TOUCH.

kripalu   A form of yoga.
See also YOGA.

Krishnamurti, Jiddu   An Indian teacher and spiritual leader (born in Madanapalle, India), 1895–1986, and former head of the Order of the Star of the East, an organization founded by Annie Besant (president of the Society, a group of clairvoyants) and Charles Webster Leadbeater (one of the chief lecturers in the Society). After dissolving the order in 1929, Krishnamurti went on to travel and lecture on topics including meditation, enlightenment, energy, passion, and other mind-body concepts in the interest of promoting world peace.

kriya   See YOGA.

ku   The term in traditional Chinese medicine referring to the bitter taste of herbs.

Kübler-Ross, Elisabeth   A medical doctor, psychiatrist, proponent of mind-body medicine, internationally known thanatologist, and author of several books, including *On Death and Dying* (New York: Macmillan, 1969), *Questions and Answers on Death and Dying* (New York: Macmillan, 1974), *To Live Until We Say Good-Bye* (Englewood Cliffs, N.J.: Prentice Hall, 1978), *Living with Death and Dying* (Macmillan, 1981), *Remember the Secret* (Milltree, Calif.: Celestial Artist, 1978), *Death: The Final Stage of Growth* (Prentice Hall, 1971), *Working It Through* (Macmillan, 1982), *AIDS: The Ultimate Challenge*, and *On Children and Death* (New York: Macmillan, 1983).

kundalini A type of energy or force thought to move up through the body's chakras to promote spirituality.

See also CHAKRAS; YOGA.

Kunz, Dora Van Gelder A healer and collaborator with Dolores Krieger in developing Therapeutic Touch.

See also BIOENERGETICS; KRIEGER, DOLORES; THERAPEUTIC TOUCH.

Law of Contraries The allopathic principle of counteracting an ailment, for example, fighting a fever by administering an antipyretic such as aspirin and giving a cool bath. Ayurvedic medicine suggests two treatment options: one based on the principles of contraries—the cool bath to combat the temperature—or the other based on the homeopathic principle of similars (the Law of Similars), which entails bundling up in blankets and drinking a hot beverage until the fever breaks. Each approach is valid, but the choice of one or the other depends upon other factors in the patient's situation.

See also HOMEOPATHY; LAW OF SIMILARS.

Law of Similars The homeopathic principle of treating ailments with like properties, such as treating frostbite initially with cold applications that gradually become warmer. The idea is to trigger the body's innate adaptive response rather than shock it with an opposite stimulus. Immunizations and vaccinations are considered to follow the Law of Similars because the injection of minute amounts of the allergen or pathogen creates an immune response in the body.

See also HOMEOPATHY; LAW OF CONTRARIES.

laying on of hands A healer's use of touch for the purpose of transmitting or transferring healing energy to an individual. Many alternative and complementary treatments include the laying on of hands, such as chiropractic and Reiki.

See also BIOENERGETICS; FAITH HEALING; VIBRATIONAL MEDICINE.

light therapy The use of full-spectrum, ultraviolet laser light and color as treatment for depression, chronic pain, and other problems, particularly those caused by malillumination, which is now linked with suppressed immune functioning, substance abuse, Alzheimer's disease, cancer, stroke, alopecia, fatigue, skin damage, dental caries, anger, and seasonal affective disorder (SAD).

Tibetan, Chinese, Ayurvedic, and other medical practitioners throughout history have recognized that each color—a product of light—has its own transformational and healing characteristics and may be directed toward physical, emotional, mental, and spiritual healing. For example, green, associated with the liver and gallbladder, is thought to be a healing color that also evokes comfort, nurturing, stability, and balance and counters anger, judgment, and criticism. Moods and performance are influenced by the circadian rhythm, that is, our work-sleep cycle in the course of the 24-hour day. Superimposed on the daily cycle are other biological cycles, such as estrus and, in animals, and diurnal or nocturnal lifestyle. winter hibernation. Also, the substance melatonin, which is produced by the body during hours of darkness, requires daylight to keep it in synchronization with the real world. Without daylight, the body adjusts naturally to a 25-hour rhythm, that requires light to reach the eyes, which actually transmit not only images, but fundamental environmental information that helps regulate hormone levels. Although humans do not respond to light as plants do, the need for sunlight is crucial.

"Light therapy has now become an accepted form of therapy, and a new ingredient of daily routine for those who find relief from the symptoms," writes Michael A. Ferenczi in an essay online at www.nimr.mrc.ac.uk/MillHillEssays/1997/sad.htm. "Treatment is safe. There have been a few reports of patients temporarily developing a mild form of manic behaviour as a result of light therapy, and some incidence of headaches, but these have disappeared after readjustment of the therapy schedule. No deleterious effects on the eyes have been reported. Some do not find relief, and in their case, SAD may be superimposed on other psychological problems, or the diagnosis of SAD may not be appropriate. Attention should be given to the quality of the light used in light therapy. The illuminated area should be large so as to avoid uncomfortable glare, and the presence of ultraviolet rays should be minimized by careful choice of the light source and by the use of filters. Some alternative forms of light therapy have been developed. For example, a dawn simulator used at wake-up time which slowly reduces darkness over a forty-five minute period to a low light level of 100 lux is apparently also effective in alleviating SAD symptoms. A light visor producing constant low light illumination has had mixed results, and was not readily accepted by patients. Of course exposure to natural daylight is highly recommended whenever possible and not surprisingly winter holidays in the sun invariably relieve SAD symptoms. Exercise is also found to be beneficial, but the effects of outdoor exercise may in part result from the accompanying exposure to daylight.

"Light therapy is used regularly to treat various forms of sleep disorders and is used also to overcome the effects of jet lag and changes in shift-work schedules. Here, the timing of the light therapy is all-important as it is used to accelerate the establishment of the appropriate pattern of melatonin secretion. Light therapy is used in the morning or before the work shift. In these applications, oral ingestion of melatonin before going to sleep also helps to reset the circadian rhythm, and is found to be effective in promoting sleep. Disruption of sleep patterns is often observed in the very old and in patients suffering from dementia, with poor links between night-time and sleeping time. It has been suggested that light therapy is effective in restoring the circadian rhythms and the sleep pattern in such patients. One possible explanation for the effect of light therapy in this case may be a result of the increased opacity of the cornea in the elderly. Above the age of sixty, the cornea transmits to the retina less than two thirds of the light which it transmits in young people. This means that the light cues are not as marked in the elderly as they are in the younger popula-

tion, resulting in the possible de-phasing of the circadian rhythms. It is reported that some forms of blindness are also accompanied by loss of circadian rhythms."

liniment   From the Latin *linimentum*, or "smearing substance," a liquid such as tincture of green soap or camphor, mixed with oil, alcohol, or water and applied topically by rubbing sore or injured parts of the body.

liver flush   Herbal remedies designed to rid the liver of excessive toxins, sludge, and stones caused by fats, proteins, and consumption of large quantities of food over a period of years. One liver flush consists of drinking lemon juice (or cider vinegar) in water with a teaspoon of honey and a teaspoon of royal jelly; another treatment is an olive oil liver flush along with a coffee enema. Liver detoxification also may involve fasting with vegetable and fruit juices and taking various supplements, such as milk thistle, beta-carotene, vitamin C, vitamin E, herbal teas, and chlorella.

See also COLONICS; DETOXIFICATION; JUICING.

longevity medicine   An alternative discipline now considered a subspecialty of conventional medicine, focused on early diagnosis of predisposition to and prevention of age-related diseases and on the enhancement of cardiovascular, immune, and endocrine systems in order to prolong life. The objectives of longevity medicine include slowing the aging process for individuals, thereby in turn increasing life expectancy in the population; extending the number of years individuals may be free of age-related diseases; and increasing physical, mental, and emotional vitality. Factors that intensify the aging process include genetic characteristics, excessive free-radical production, stress, hormonal imbalance, poor nutrition, toxic overload, impairment of the immune system, occluded arteries and lymph vessels, and sluggish brain cell functioning. Two organizations are centered on the many longevity-medicine preventive measures and treatments: the American Academy of Anti-Aging Medicine (www.worldhealth.net) and the International College of Advanced Longevity Medicine (www.healthy.net/icalm).

lymphasizing   The process of removing waste materials from the extracellular space by increasing the flow of lymphatic fluid in the body, described by C. Samuel West, N.D., in *The Golden Seven Plus One, Conquer Disease with Eight Keys to Health, Beauty, and Peace* (Orein, Utah: Samuel Publications, 1981).

A related theory and technique may be found in the *Textbook of Dr. Vodder's Manual Lymph Drainage* (Heidelberg, Germany: Haug Publishers, 1990) by H. and G. Wittlinger, which describes a massage technique designed to increase lymph drainage from diseased or dysfunctioning parts of the body.

macrobiotics A whole-food, nondairy, vegetarian diet geared to restoring and maintaining health by considering the energetic qualities of food and one's total lifestyle. Macrobiotics defines the world in terms of expansive energy (yin) and contractive energy (yang). Macrobiotic diet theory suggests eliminating all food that is processed, fragmented (including vitamins), toxic (e.g., the nightshade family) or either expansive such as alcohol, or contractive, such as meat. The following are the basic concepts of a macrobiotic diet (1) Consume organically and locally grown foods in season as they become available, or foods that may be stored without artificial preservation or refrigeration. Alternatively, eat foods grown in the same latitude where you live. (2) Consume cooked whole grains and recipes made from whole grains and cooked vegetables, adjusting proportions and preparation methods according to activity, climate, and seasonal fluctuations of temperature and humidity. (3) Use solar-evaporated seawater salts in preparation of foods, as well as traditionally aged miso and shoyu, umeboshi, and seaweeds. Drink undyed, three-year-old roasted twig tea (kukicha) as preferred beverage. (4) Use unrefined, cold-pressed seed oils, made from organically grown seeds including sesame, corn, safflower, sunflower, and flaxseed sparingly. (5) Use roasted seeds and nuts, fruit, salads, and fish occasionally as desired, in small quantities, as provided in season. (6) Use beans and bean products as primary sources of protein, along with whole grain and vegetable dishes. (7) Avoid all foods and beverages that contain refined sweeteners, chemical dyes, synthetic flavorings or seasonings, refined oils, and chemical preservatives or that are made from foods grown with chemical insecticides, herbicides, fungicides, or chemical fertilizers or are produced by bioengi-

neering or grown under hothouse conditions. (8) Avoid foods grown in and shipped from warmer latitudes. (9) Avoid "soft" (carbonated, sweetened) beverages, canned goods, alcoholic beverages, artificial sweeteners, and products containing these ingredients. (10) Chew each mouthful of food thoroughly before swallowing.

Organizations for macrobiotic study and practice include the Kushi Institute, P.O. Box 7, Becket, MA 01223, or (413) 623-5741, and the International Macrobiotic Shiatsu Society (IMSS), 2807 Wright Avenue, Winter Park, FL 32789, a forum on a combination of macrobiotics and shiatsu based on the teaching of Shizuko Yamamoto. Macrobiotics is a natural approach to living that includes a whole-foods diet. Shiatsu ("finger pressure" or acupressure) is a touch technique based on traditional Asian medicine. It is similar to acupuncture but does not employ needles. The Yamamoto macrobiotic style is also known as "Barefoot Shiatsu." Founded in 1986 after nearly 50 years of experience by the shiatsu master Shizuko Yamamoto, the IMSS promotes a natural approach to living. Macrobiotic shiatsu combines the power of natural foods in the macrobiotic diet with the traditional Asian healing techniques of shiatsu. As all things belong to nature, it is natural to be healthy and happy. When imbalances arise, simple techniques can help to correct them. In a down-to-earth practical manner, macrobiotic shiatsu unifies body, mind, and spirit.

The practice of eating large amounts of animal food has created bodies that are rigid. To deal effectively with this hard, stiff condition an appropriate shiatsu technique naturally evolved. The macrobiotic shiatsu developed as a response to the Western condition. The aim of treatment is to create balance within the individual.

The most important underlying principle of macrobiotic shiatsu is that everyone has the power to heal him- or herself. Additionally, beyond the formal training and martial arts exposure, intuition and common sense blend into the technique to make it what it is today. Practitioners claim its principal beauty is that it has a large sense of caring for others in a very practical way.

Principles of macrobiotic shiatsu

- Health is the natural condition of human beings.
- Illness and unhappiness are unnatural conditions.
- Health or sickness is not an accident or something without explanation.
- Sickness arises from how we live because of our own actions and thoughts.
- Food is one of the more important factors in determining health or sickness.
- We should eat foods that grow in our environment.
- The strong will naturally help the weak.
- People will naturally help themselves.
- Through interaction with others, you naturally develop beyond your limitations of body, mind, and spirit.
- Purpose of treatment is to stimulate people to go beyond their previous limitations.

Source: http://www.itppeople.com/macrobio.htm

Macrobiotic shiatsu as a holistic treatment, or "whole health shiatsu," is not limited to acupressure, massage, or bodywork. It has been developed from attempting to understand the underlying reasons for ill health, such as the patient's breathing patterns, emotional changes, exercise and dietary preferences, and lifestyle.

See also MASSAGE; SHIATSU; YIN-YANG.

magnetic field therapy A type of alternative medicine practice based on the idea that magnetic fields have healing powers, named after the legendary Greek shepherd Magnes, who noticed that the iron nails of his sandals were pulled by an invisible force to a large rock (now known as the Magnes stone, or lodestone). After he disengaged from the rock, Magnes also noticed that he could walk longer if he placed fragments of the rock in his sandals. Other ancient cultures, including the those of Chinese, Eastern Indians, Arabs, Hebrews, and early Egyptians, used magnets as healing devices. The 16th-century physician Paracelsus believed the entire Earth is a huge magnet, and he advocated use of magnets as healing devices for certain disorders. Other proponents of magnetism as therapy were the French Royal Society of Medicine in 1777; Franz Anton Mesmer, who catalyzed the use of hypnosis and "animal magnetism" in mind-body medicine; the French chemist Louis Pasteur, who claimed that magnets accelerated the fermentation process; and Dr. C.J. Thacher, of the Chicago Magnet Company, who thought that using magnets on the body and in clothing and shoes helped ease disease-related pain in the extremities. Samuel Hahnemann, the father of modern homeopathy, also experimented with and advocated the use of therapeutic magnets.

Contemporary theory says magnetic fields can influence the function of the human body. In his book *A Practical Guide to Vibrational Medicine* (New York: Quill, 2000, p. 266), Richard Gerber, M.D., wrote: "There are a variety of different types and characters of magnetism that exist in the spectrum of natural and man-made magnetic fields. Each of these types of magnetic fields has the potential to overtly or silently influence human biology. It seems that north-versus south-pole fields, static versus pulsed magnetic fields, weak versus strong magnetic fields, and slow versus fast magnetic fields all produce different biological effects upon individual cells as well as upon whole living organisms."

Both internal and external fields of magnetic energy are necessary for human survival. In *Magnet Therapy: An Alternative Medicine Definitive Guide* (AlternativeMedicine.com Books, 2000), coauthored by Dwight K. Kalita, Ph.D., and Burton Goldberg William H. Philpott, M.D., wrote that negative magnetic fields normalize pH; oxygenate cells; resolve cellular edema; usually reduce symptoms; inhibit microorganism replication and slow down infection; reduce pain and inflammation; govern rest, relaxation, and sleep; evoke anabolic hormone production (melatonin and growth hormone); clear metabolically produced toxins from the body; eliminate free radicals; and slow down electrical brain activity. Whereas negative fields have a tranquilizing effect, positive magnetic fields have a stressful effect and disrupt metabolic function, produce acidity, inhibit oxygen flow to the cells, and encourage the growth of microorganisms.

Magnetic field therapy is reported to have beneficial effects on such conditions as toothache, periodontal disease, fungal infections such as candidiasis, kidney stones, calcium deposits in inflamed tissues, edema, stress, heart disease, sleep problems (particularly chronic insomnia), and central nervous system disorders, cancer, injuries, and other conditions. Enthusiasts also claim magnets used in beds, clothing, and chair pads and applied to the body affect the body's ability to combat fatigue and regulate body temperature even in extreme atmospheric conditions. According to studies, the body's electromagnetic fields are affected by the weakest magnetism and harmed if the magnetism is altered in even subtle ways. Some patients may experience pain or symptomatic reactions to certain medications or have more severe reactions to toxins that may be released into the body. Also, magnets are not recommended for use on the abdomen during pregnancy or for prolonged periods. Although magnetic field diagnostic procedures such as magnetic resonance imaging (MRI) have been widely accepted by conventional practitioners, the application of the positive magnetic pole is known to be capable of stimulating tumor growth, promoting addictive behavior, and inducing seizures, hallucinations, insomnia, and hyperactivity. Medical supervision of magnetic therapy is advised.

Gerber also cites an illness called "magnetic-field deficiency syndrome (MFDS)" reported by Japanese researchers, led by Dr. Kyoichi Nakagawa, in the 1950s. Some people in Japanese cities experienced symptoms including chronic fatigue and insomnia that were eventually related to the fact that iron and steel girders in large modern buildings restricted the flow of the Earth's magnetic energy. People who spent significant time in those buildings, it was concluded, did not receive as much magnetic energy as did those who spent time in buildings made of wood or other organic materials. In other experiments, blocking the flow of magnetism by covering the heads and adrenal regions of master dowsers with magnetically shielded material affected their ability to sense weak magnetic fields.

Magnetic belts, braces, pads, and a host of products are now popular with individuals who suffer from arthritis; headaches; chronic back, leg, and foot pain, and many other ailments.

According to Robert Todd Carroll, author of *The Skeptic's Dictionary* (Hoboken, N.J.: John Wiley & Sons, 1994–2003), "Some claim that magnets can help broken bones heal faster, but most of the advocacy comes from those who claim that magnets relieve pain. Most of the support for these notions is in the form of testimonials and anecdotes, and can be attributed to "placebo effects and other effects accompanying their use" (Livingston 1998). There is almost no scientific evidence supporting magnet therapy. One highly publicized exception is a double-blind study done at Baylor College of Medicine that compared the effects of magnets and sham magnets on the knee pain of 50 post-polio patients. The experimental group reported a significantly greater reduction in pain than the control group. No replication of the study has yet been done.

Additional information is available by contacting Bio-Electro-Magnetics Institute, 2490 West Moana Lane, Reno, NV 89509-3936, or (702) 827-9099, and Enviro-Tech Products, 17171 Southeast 29th Street, Choctaw, OK 73020, or (405) 390-3499 or (800) 445-1962.

See also BIOENERGETICS; DOWSING; FENG SHUI; HAHNEMANN, SAMUEL C. F.; MESMERISM; PARACELSUS; YIN-YANG.

malas In Ayurvedic medicine, the body's three waste products: urine, feces, and sweat.

mantra Sanskrit words or phrases (the singular form is *mantram*) that carry energy and vibrations useful in meditation practices. According to Ayurvedic medicine, chanting a mantram or mantra has healing benefits, particularly to achieve balance in body, mind, and consciousness and to nourish spiritual growth.

See also TRANSCENDENTAL MEDITATION; YOGA.

marma In Ayurvedic medicine, the energy points where two or more physical functions meet.

See also *MARMA* PUNCTURE.

marma puncture In Ayurvedic medicine, the insertion of a needle into the body's *marma*, or energy points, at the junction of two or more significant body functions.

massage The scientific method of manipulating the soft tissues of the body for several different purposes: to restore basic functions of all systems of the body as a whole (hence the term *holistic*), release tension by giving the body a chance to heal naturally, boost the immune system, release endorphins, increase circulation, improve muscle tone, and rid the body of toxins.

The healing properties of touch and massage have been used for the past 5,000 years or more. The use of one's hands for the purpose of calming another person has made massage one of the most accessible modalities of healing known to humankind. In ancient times, people of India used massage to strengthen and heal the body. The Bible mentions "laying the hand on the body" and anointing the body with oil as a means of healing. In 460 B.C. Hippocrates, known as the father of medicine, recommended that his patients receive such treatment for overall health and said that all physicians should learn massage techniques. From that point forward, hundreds of variations on the theme have been created and explored by many different cultures. Thai medical history documents that Thai massage was introduced to the world by Jibaka Kumaru Bacha, an Indian doctor, more than 2,500 years ago. He incorporated the use of herbs and minerals, as well as the spiritual aspect of the art. Since then, therapeutic massage has become a respected profession, despite its unfortunate link to prostitution and "massage parlors." In the 1800s, the Royal Central Institute, where massage techniques were looked upon as a science, was established in Stockholm, Sweden. Swedish massage, the basis of all Western forms of massage treatment, is a full-body massage using a variety of oils to nourish the skin—sesame, almond, coconut, and grape seed, to name a few. Of the approximately 400 or so branches of massage, there are several that are widely recognized as Swedish. Deep Tissue, for example, is often incorporated into Swedish massage if the client has problem areas that need specific attention. Although it can be somewhat painful, it can be quite healing if done properly and with caution.

Therapists may borrow techniques from a variety of different kinds of massage and use them according to the client's needs. Among the most common types of massage are the following (1) shiatsu, a Japanese style of massage, is performed on the floor, on a mat, rather than on a massage table, (2) acupressure, similar to shiatsu, mainly uses thumb pressure to stimulate pressure points, (3) neuromuscular, also known as trigger point therapy, uses finger pressure to address painful areas in the muscles, (4) sports massage uses techniques for athletes and other physically active people who have sore muscles or injuries that require special care, such as sprains, strains and tendinitis; before and after physical activity, it can enhance training and prevent injury, (5) craniosacral work aims to locate and correct cerebral and spinal imbalances or blockages that cause sensory, motor, or intellectual dysfunction, (6) connective tissue massage concentrates on the superficial and middle layers of connective tissue (called fascia) to relax, revitalize, and heal the body, (7) manual lymph drainage is a rhythmic pumping form of massage designed to stimulate the movement of lymph fluid through the lymph vessels. It is especially useful in the treatment of lymphedema, a side effect of any surgery in which the lymph nodes are removed or of irradiation administered in the area of the lymph nodes, (8) chair massage often occurs in public settings, such as corporate offices, where time is of the essence and clothes may not be removed. A special chair, rather than a massage table, is used to make the recipient as comfortable as possible while making the back, neck, and arms accessible to the therapist, (9) Reflexology is making use of the hands and feet as maps for the entire body. This is especially useful in cases when massage of certain areas of the body is restricted, (10) The Feldenkrais Method is considered useful for many types of chronic pain, including headaches, temporomandibular joint (TMJ) syndrome, and other joint disorders. Commonly used for athletes, dancers, and other performers, the method is said to improve balance, coordination, and mobility. A session, which may be performed while the person is sitting or lying on the floor, standing, or sitting in a chair, consists of being verbally guided through a sequence of movements designed to relax the body and help abandon destructive patterns, (11) Therapeutic Touch (also known as T-Touch or TT) uses the principle of the universal life force energy that flows in and out of the body. Where there are disease, illness, and pain, they indicate a block of such energy. Practitioners are taught to detect such blockages by passing their hands above the patient's body. Energy imbalances can be equalized, therefore enabling the body to heal. As of 1988, the method was taught in 80 colleges and universities in the United States and in 65 foreign countries, (12) Reiki, similar to Therapeutic Touch, is a gentle technique meant for stress reduction and relaxation. The practitioner may position his or her hands either above or on the body in order to tap into the life force energy and to locate and clear blockages to improve health and enhance their quality of life. Treatments can be performed when the patient is sitting up or lying down and do not require the removal of clothing, (13) Lomi-Lomi massage, a Hawaiian tradition, uses kneading techniques as well as bone adjustment, baths, and religious practices. Hot and cold stone massage uses rock formed by volcanic and sedimentary action to manipulate the muscles and induce relaxation and healing.

Aromatherapy, the use of aromatic essential oils, is often coupled with massage to enhance treatment. These oils are used to affect the way you feel, such as to deepen relaxation, rid the mind of worry, or energize. Aromatherapy adds the air of luxury and pampering to a massage session. Before accepting such treatment, the client should be sure the oils are pure and of good quality. Although massage is considered safe treatment for many diseases and conditions, there are some instances in which it should not be used. Check with a physician before having a massage treatment after recent surgery or when there is acute inflammation or redness, swelling, difficulty breathing, fever, skin rash, varicose veins and other circulatory ailments, cancer, or any other serious illness or infectious disease.

Before booking a massage appointment with a therapist, ask about his or her credentials. It is not uncommon for people with little or no formal education to pass themselves off as certified. A therapist should have completed 500 hours of training at an accredited school and be affiliated with an organization such as the American Massage Therapy Association (AMTA) (see Appendix I). It is preferable to choose someone who is either state or nationally certified. This means the therapist has been taught and tested in the areas of anatomy and physiology, pathology, massage technique, massage-related medical treatment, and ethics. Licensing of massage therapists is now required in 25 states, and an increasing number of states are adopting the National Certification Examination. A national list of trained massage therapists is available from the AMTA. To locate a therapist, contact a local school of massage for the names of qualified local therapists.

See also AROMATHERAPY; ESSENTIAL OILS; FELDENKRAIS METHOD; HELLERWORK; MACROBIOTICS; REFLEXOLOGY; REIKI; THERAPEUTIC TOUCH; TRAGER INTEGRATION.

Mayr intestinal therapy A modified fast using mild laxatives combined with a specified diet and exercise. The Mayr therapy, popular in Europe, is concerned also with an individual's posture and the condition of his or her intestinal tract. More information is available in the book *Health through Inner Body Cleansing*, by Erich Rauch, M.D. (Haug Publishers, Heidelberg, Germany, 1986).

See also COLONIC IRRIGATION.

meditation The art and science of quieting and centering the mind and coordinating breathing for the purpose of achieving deep relaxation and clarity of thinking.

See also TRANSCENDENTAL MEDITATION.

mentals In homeopathic medicine, symptoms related to one's emotional or mental condition and moods.

See also HOMEOPATHY.

meridians In traditional Chinese medicine and other Asian medicine practices, the pathways—also known as *jing-luo*—along which vital energy points carry the body's *ch'i*, or life force. Fourteen pathways go to and from the hands and feet to the torso and head. Twelve main bilateral meridians correspond to the 12 major organs—liver, spleen, heart, stomach, kidneys, lungs, etc. Six meridians pertain to the bladder, gallbladder, stomach, small intestine, and large intestine, and the Triple Burner (which regulates overall body temperature) is related to the transportation of food and fluids throughout the body. Other meridians travel up the front midline of the body and up the spinal column. Chinese practitioners believe imbalances, blockages, or disharmonies along points of any of the meridians cause symptoms of illness.

See also ACUPRESSURE; ACUPUNCTURE; .

mesmerism The technique of "animal magnetism," named for its developer, Franz Anton Mesmer, which was a precursor to hypnosis.

See also HYPNOSIS.

Metamorphic Technique An approach to self-healing and personal development through eliminating limited beliefs about one's potential and patterns both physical and emotional that cause these beliefs. Underlying the symptoms are corresponding patterns of energy, and the metamorphic technique acts as a catalyst to this energy (also known as the life force), gently helping to transform the negative patterns into positive ones.

The Metamorphic Technique originated in the work of Robert St. John, a British naturopath and reflexologist. During the 1960s St. John discovered he could create significant effects by applying a light touch to particular points on the feet that reflexologists call the spinal reflexes. He then developed the spinal reflexes approach in combination with the concept of innate self-healing ability and eventually called the entire process Metamporphosis, particularly because the changes experienced by clients appeared to be enduring. Gaston Saint-Pierre, who studied extensively with Robert St. John during the 1970s, further developed St. John's work and called it the Metamorphic Technique. In 1979 he set up the Metamorphic Association, which was then registered as a charity in 1984, to promote the technique worldwide.

The basis for the Metamorphic Technique, like that of other alternative techniques, is that human beings possess a life force or energy beyond the physical constitution, and that energy may become blocked or unbalanced in some way, causing illness or injury or dysfunction. Moreover, the blockage may be either physical or emotional, current or historical, in origin. The Metamorphic Technique practitioner seeks to repair illness-generating energy patterns.

Acting as a catalyst for the client, the metamorphic practitioner uses a light touch on points known as the spinal reflexes in the feet, hands, and head while remaining unattached to any specific outcome. The Metamorphic Technique is not a therapy or a treatment, since it is not concerned with addressing specific symptoms or problems. Practitioners do not require a personal or medical history to perform this gentle, noninvasive, safe technique. It can be used alone or complement conventional or alternative medicine therapies. No special training, abilities, or background are needed in order to become a practitioner. Clients who wish to transform their behavioral and emotional patterns often seek the Metamorphic Technique as a treatment.

A session usually lasts about an hour. The recipient removes shoes and socks and may either sit or lie down. The practitioner uses a light touch on the spinal reflex points in the feet, hands, and head. Metamorphic Technique practitioners work in a detached way: nonjudgmental, nonmanipulative, relaxing, and energizing.

The Metamorphic Technique has been used a great deal in work with physical and mental disabilities, as well as in schools for children with learning difficulties, in hospitals, in prisons, and in practices that help people overcome addictions, eating disorders, and stress-related conditions. It is also used by pregnant women and midwives, to help bring about an easier pregnancy and birth.

The Metamorphic Association offers these guidelines on the technique:

- A unique tool for personal transformation.
- Not a therapy or a treatment, but a technique that helps trigger your own inner life force, enabling you to better realize your potential.

- Based on a new way of looking at energy patterns. While other approaches often focus on removing energy blockages, the Metamorphic Technique looks at transforming energy patterns. It does not consider people to be "blocked" or "broken" and in need of being "fixed." Instead, it simply notices that you may have patterns that no longer serve you and that you wish to transform. The energy that was involved in creating the old patterns is released and can be used to create new patterns.

- Empowering. Any changes that occur originate entirely from within the recipient. That person's own life force has an innate intelligence of its own. The practitioner simply acts as a catalyst in the process.

- Noninvasive. There is no physical manipulation, nor diagnosis, nor any need to discuss personal problems or medical history.

- Gentle and completely safe.

- Accessible to everyone, and easy to learn and integrate into everyday life.

The Metamorphic Association is a United Kingdom–based registered charity (Charity No. 326525) with an international presence. It functions as a network of people who support each other in learning, sharing, exploring, practicing, promoting and teaching the Metamorphic Technique. As members of the association, they have a common goal: "to promote good health and well-being through awareness, understanding and use of the Metamorphic Technique in the UK and internationally and to uphold standards in practicing and teaching the technique." The Metamorphic Association address is P.O. Box 32368, London SW17 8YB.

miasm   In homeopathic medicine, an underlying pattern of dysfunction that creates and maintains chronic disease processes and their recurrences. The three miasms formulated by Samuel Hahnemann are psora, sycosis, and syphilis. A psoric miasmic pattern refers to itching (e.g., psoriasis), especially skin disorders. A sycotic miasm refers to gonorrhea and other disorders involving mucous membranes. A syphilitic miasm is associated with vital organs and structures of the body, exemplified particularly by syphilis, a venereal disease that eventually destroys all the bodily systems.

See also HAHNEMANN, SAMUEL C.F.; HOMEOPATHY.

mind-body connection   The relationship between the physiological and psychological aspects of the human being, for example, how stress, depression, fatigue, exposure to environmental factors, and other general emotional conditions are manifested in dysfunction and disease. The former section chief at the National Institute of Mental Health, Candace Pert, Ph.D., of Rutgers University, who discovered the neurochemical substances known as neuropeptides, encouraged research on neuropeptides. A common example is endorphins, the body's naturally produced form of morphine, which are both pain-relieving and euphoria-inducing. Alternative and integrative medicine modalities have embraced the mind-body concept as the most significant premise for wide-ranging holistic treatments, including acupuncture, numerous forms of bodywork, bioenergetic therapy, and other methods.

See also ACUPUNCTURE; AYURVEDA; BIOENERGETICS; ENDORPHINS; ENVIRONMENTAL MEDICINE; HOLISM; HOMEOPATHY; VIBRATIONAL MEDICINE; YIN-YANG; YOGA.

molecular nutrition   The application of biochemical and physiological approaches to the understanding of nutrient function and metabolism in systems ranging from the whole animal to the molecular level. Nutrition is a natural science that has a fundamental biological basis. Nutrition-related intracellular processes and pathways have far-reaching implications for human nutrition, nutrient-regulated cell processes, and gene-nutrient interactions, all believed to be vital for human health and longevity. To study such processes and pathways requires a critical knowledge of biochemistry and physiology combined with a fundamental background in basic sciences. The headquarters of The International Society for Molecular Nutrition and Therapy (ISMNT) is the Molecular Cardiology Laboratory Department of Internal Medicine and Cardiology, Philipps University of Marburg, Karl-von-Frisch-Str. 1 35033 Marburg, Germany, or Tel 011 49 6421 286 5032; Fax 011 49 6421 286 8964;

E-mail: ISMNT@mailer.uni-marburg.de; World Wide Web: http://cardiorepair.uni-marburg.de/ismnt.html. Objectives of ISMNT include promoting nutritional research at the molecular level with respect to health and disease and organizing scientific meetings in the area of molecular nutrition, including nutrition related to cancer, cardiovascular diseases, immune disorders, neurosciences, nutritional abnormalities, and vitamins and trace elements.

Source: http://nutrition.tufts.edu/programs/cmn/

Moody, Raymond An American physician and author, born in Georgia in 1944, who documented the near-death experience and is a proponent of the concept of an afterlife, particularly as it pertains to catastrophic trauma or illness. His best-selling book, *Life after Life,* first focused public attention in 1975 on the near-death experience and what it is telling the medical profession Dr. Moody recorded and compared the experiences of 150 persons who died, or almost died, and then recovered. His research describes the results of decades of inquiry into the near-death experience. He outlines nine elements that generally occur during the near-death experience:

A strange sound. A buzzing, or ringing noise, while having a sense of being dead.

Peace and painlessness. While people are dying, they may be in intense pain, but as soon as they leave the body the pain vanishes and they experience peace.

Out-of-body experience. The dying often have the sensation of rising up and floating above their own body while it is surrounded by a medical team, and watching it down below, while feeling comfortable. They experience the feeling of being in a spiritual body that appears to be a sort of living energy field.

The tunnel experience. The next experience is that of being drawn into darkness through a tunnel, at an extremely high speed, until reaching a realm of radiant golden-white light. Also, although they sometimes report feeling scared, they do not sense that they were on the way to hell or that they fell into it.

Rising rapidly into the heavens. Instead of a tunnel, some people report rising suddenly into the heavens and seeing the Earth and the celestial sphere as they would be seen by astronauts in space.

People of light. Once on the other side of the tunnel, or after they have risen into the heavens, the dying meet people who glow with an inner light. Often they find that friends and relatives who have already died are there to greet them.

The being of light. After meeting the people of light, the dying often meet a powerful spiritual being whom some have called God, Jesus, or some religious figure.

The life review. The being of light presents the dying with a panoramic review of everything they have ever done. That is, they relive every act they have ever done to other people and come away feeling that love is the most important thing in life.

Reluctance to return. The being of light sometimes tells the dying that they must return to life. Other times, they are given a choice of staying or returning. In either case, they are reluctant to return. The people who choose to return do so only because of loved ones they do not wish to leave behind.

Moore, Thomas An American psychotherapist, writer, and lecturer who lives in New England with his wife and two children. He has published many articles in the areas of archetypal and Jungian psychology, mythology, and the arts. His books include *Soul Mates* (New York: HarperCollins, 1994). He also edited *A Blue Fire* (Harper-Collins), an anthology of the writings of James Hillman. Moore lived as a monk in a Catholic religious order for 12 years. He has a Ph.D. in religious studies from Syracuse University, an M.A. in theology from the University of Windsor, an M.A. in musicology from the University of Michigan, and a B.A. in music and philosophy from DePaul University. He is a leading lecturer and writer in North America and in Europe in the areas of archetypal psychology, mythology, and the arts.

MORA Concept A therapy that combines acupuncture's meridian therapy, high technology, and homeopathic medicine, described in the book

The MORA Concept, by Franz Morell, M.D., published Karl F. Haug (Heidelberg, Germany, 1990).

See also ACUPUNTURE; HOMEOPATHY.

mother tincture The base stock from which homeopathic remedies are taken.

See also HAHNEMANN, SAMUEL C. F.; HOMEOPATHY; INFUSION.

moxibustion An acupuncture technique involving the use of dried mugwort, an herb that is burned on the ends of acupuncture needles or rolled to form a stick, heated, and applied to the body in order to warm the area, thus increasing the flow of the life force, or *qi* (also *ch'i*).

See also ACUPUNCTURE; QI.

music therapy The application of music by a qualified practitioner to effect positive changes in psychological, physical, mental, or social functioning in the client. Music therapists have been successfully using the effects of sound and music to improve health in clients for years. The substantial research they have produced is helpful in illustrating the potential healthful effects of sound therapy, yet their approach has been so process-oriented that it has not been able to determine exactly how or why it works.

See also SOUND THERAPY.

myotherapy A method of treatment that focuses on the relaxation and restoration of muscles. Massage, Rolfing, Feldenkrais method, and many other techniques are forms of bodywork or myotherapy.

Myss, Caroline An American intuitive healer and author. Myss, a graduate of St. Mary of the Woods College in Indiana, worked as a freelance journalist when she attended a seminar of Elisabeth Kübler-Ross and experienced a "crisis of meaning." Inspired, she attended Mundelein College and received a master's degree in theology. She thereafter started the Stillpoint Publishing Company. During this time in New Hampshire Myss acknowledged and began to demonstrate what she referred to as medical intuitive abilities. As Myss said, "I had all the ambition in the world to be a publisher and all the talent to be a medical intuitive." She started working with holistic doctors, began creating audiotapes, and lectured around the world. She returned to Chicago and wrote *Anatomy of the Spirit* (New York: Harmony Books, 1996), a *New York Times* best-seller, and a year later, *Why People Don't Heal and How They Can* (New York: Harmony Books, 1997), which also became a best-seller. Myss currently gives lectures, seminars, workshops, and educational programs.

nasya In Ayurvedic medicine, the therapeutic inhaling of oils.

National Center for Complementary and Alternative Medicine (NCCAM)
An organization dedicated to the study and promotion of alternative and complementary medicines in the United States. The following are its mission statement and pertinent information. The statement below has been edited. Footnotes in the original document have not been reproduced. For the full text see the NCCAM website at http://www.nccam.nih.gov/.

Decisions about your health care are important—including decisions about whether to use complementary and alternative medicine (CAM). The National Center for Complementary and Alternative Medicine (NCCAM) has developed this fact sheet to assist you in your decisionmaking about CAM. It includes frequently asked questions, issues to consider, and a list of sources for further information.

- Take charge of your health by being an informed consumer. Find out what scientific studies have been done on the safety and effectiveness of the CAM treatment in which you are interested.

- Decisions about medical care and treatment should be made in consultation with a health care provider and based on the condition and needs of each person. Discuss information on CAM with your health care provider before making any decisions about treatment or care.

- If you use any CAM therapy, inform your primary health care provider. This is for your safety and so your health care provider can develop a comprehensive treatment plan.

- If you use a CAM therapy provided by a practitioner, such as acupuncture, choose the practitioner with care. Check with your insurer to see if the services will be covered. (To learn more about selecting a CAM practitioner, see our fact sheet, "Selecting a Complementary and Alternative Medicine Practitioner.")

Questions and Answers

1. What is complementary and alternative medicine?
2. How can I get reliable information about a CAM therapy?
3. Are CAM therapies safe?
4. How can I determine whether statements made about the effectiveness of a CAM therapy are true?
5. Are there any risks to using CAM treatments?
6. Are CAM therapies tested to see if they work?
7. I am interested in a CAM therapy that involves treatment from a practitioner. How do I go about selecting a practitioner?
8. Can I receive treatment or a referral to a practitioner from NCCAM?
9. Can I participate in CAM research through a clinical trial?

1. What is complementary and alternative medicine?

Complementary and alternative medicine (CAM) is a group of diverse medical and health care systems, practices, and products that are not presently considered to be a part of conventional medicine. [1]People use CAM therapies in a variety of ways. CAM therapies used alone are often referred to as "alternative." When used in addition to conventional medicine, they are often referred to as "complementary." The list of what is considered to be CAM changes continually, as those therapies that are proven to be safe and effective become adopted into conventional health care and as new approaches to health care emerge. For more about these terms, see the

NCCAM fact sheet "What Is Complementary and Alternative Medicine?"

2. How can I get reliable information about a CAM therapy?

It is important to learn what scientific studies have discovered about the therapy in which you are interested. It is not a good idea to use a CAM therapy simply because of something you have seen in an advertisement or on a Web site or because someone has told you that it worked for them. Understanding a treatment's risks, potential benefits, and scientific evidence is critical to your health and safety. Scientific research on many CAM therapies is relatively new, so this kind of information may not be available for every therapy. However, many studies on CAM treatments are under way, including those that NCCAM supports, and our knowledge and understanding of CAM is increasing all the time. Here are some ways to find scientifically based information:

- Talk to your health care practitioner(s). Tell them about the therapy you are considering and ask any questions you may have about safety, effectiveness, or interactions with medications (prescription or non-prescription). They may know about the therapy and be able to advise you on its safety and use. If your practitioner cannot answer your questions, he may be able to refer you to someone who can. Your practitioner may also be able to help you interpret the results of scientific articles you have found.

- Use the Internet to search medical libraries and databases for information. One database called CAM on PubMed (see "For More Information"), developed by NCCAM and the National Library of Medicine (NLM), gives citations or abstracts (brief summaries) of the results of scientific studies on CAM. In some cases, it provides links to publishers' Web sites where you may be able to view or obtain the full articles. The articles cited in CAM on PubMed are peer-reviewed— that is, other scientists in the same field have reviewed the article, the data, and the conclusions, and judged them to be accurate and important to the field. Another database, International Bibliographic Information on Dietary Supplements, is useful for searching the scientific literature on dietary supplements (see "For More Information").

- If you do not have access to the Internet, contact the NCCAM Clearinghouse (see "For More Information"). The staff is available to discuss your needs with you and assist you in searching the peer-reviewed medical and scientific literature.

- Visit your local library or a medical library to see if there are books or publications that contain scientific articles discussing CAM in general or the treatment in which you are interested. Thousands of articles on health issues and CAM are published in books and scientific journals every year. A reference librarian can help you search for those on the therapy that interests you.

3. Are CAM therapies safe?

Each treatment needs to be considered on its own. However, here are some issues to think about when considering a CAM therapy.

- Many consumers believe that "natural" means the same thing as "safe." This is not necessarily true. For example, think of mushrooms that grow in the wild: some are safe to eat, while others are poisonous.

- Individuals respond differently to treatments. How a person might respond to a CAM treatment depends on many things, including the person's state of health, how the treatment is used, or the person's belief in the treatment.

- For a CAM **product** that is sold over the counter (without a prescription), such as a dietary supplement, safety can also depend on a number of things:
  - The components or ingredients that make up the product
  - Where the components or ingredients come from
  - The quality of the manufacturing process (for example, how well the manufacturer is able to avoid contamination).

The manufacturer of a dietary supplement is responsible for ensuring the safety and effectiveness of the product before it is sold. The U.S. Food and Drug Administration (FDA) cannot require testing of dietary supplements prior to marketing. However, while manufacturers are prohibited from selling dangerous products, the FDA can remove a product from the marketplace if the product is dangerous to the health of Americans. Furthermore, if in the labeling or marketing of a dietary supplement a claim is made that the product can diagnose, treat, cure, or prevent disease, such as "cures cancer," the product is said to be an unapproved new drug and is, therefore, being sold illegally. Such claims must have scientific proof.

- For CAM therapies that are administered by a practitioner, the training, skill, and experience of the practitioner affect safety. However, in spite of careful and skilled practice, all treatments—whether CAM or conventional—can have risks.

4. How can I determine whether statements made about the effectiveness of a CAM therapy are true?

Statements that manufacturers and providers of CAM therapies may make about the effectiveness of a therapy and its other benefits can sound reasonable and promising. However, they may or may not be backed up by scientific evidence. Before you begin using a CAM treatment, it is a good idea to ask the following questions:

- Is there scientific evidence (not just personal stories) to back up the statements? Ask the manufacturer or the practitioner for scientific articles or the results of studies. They should be willing to share this information, if it exists.
- Does the Federal Government have anything to report about the therapy?
  - ○ Visit the FDA online at www.fda.gov to see if there is any information available about the product or practice. Information specifically about dietary supplements can be found on FDA's Center for Food Safety and Applied Nutrition Web site at www.cfsan.fda.gov. Or visit the FDA's Web page on recalls and safety alerts at www.fda.gov/opacom/7alerts.html.
  - ○ Check with the Federal Trade Commission (FTC) at www.ftc.gov to see if there are any fraudulent claims or consumer alerts regarding the therapy. Visit the Diet, Health, and Fitness Consumer Information Web site at www.ftc.gov/bcp/menu-health.htm.
  - ○ Visit the NCCAM Web site, nccam.nih.gov, or call the NCCAM Clearinghouse to see if

NCCAM has any information or scientific findings to report about the therapy.

- How does the provider or manufacturer describe the treatment? The FDA advises that certain types of language may sound impressive but actually disguise a lack of science. Be wary of terminology such as "innovation," "quick cure," "miracle cure," "exclusive product," "new discovery," or "magical discovery." Watch out for claims of a "secret formula." If a therapy were a cure for a disease, it would be widely reported and prescribed or recommended. Legitimate scientists want to share their knowledge so that their peers can review their data. Be suspicious of phrases like "suppressed by government" or claims that the medical profession or research scientists have conspired to prevent a therapy from reaching the public. Finally, be wary of claims that something cures a wide range of unrelated diseases (for example, cancer, diabetes, and AIDS). No product can treat every disease and condition.

5. Are there any risks to using CAM treatments?

Yes, there can be risks, as with any medical therapy. These risks depend upon the specific CAM treatment. The following are general suggestions to help you learn about or minimize the risks.

- Discuss with your health care practitioner any CAM treatment that you are considering or are using; it is important for your safety and for a comprehensive treatment plan. For example, herbal or botanical products and other dietary supplements may interact with medications (prescription or non-prescription). They may also have negative, even dangerous, effects on their own. Research has shown that the herb St. John's wort, which is used by some people to treat depression, may cause certain drugs to become less effective. And kava, an herb that has been used for insomnia, stress, and anxiety, has been linked to liver damage.
- If you have more than one health care provider, let all of them know about CAM and conventional therapies you are using. This will help each provider make sure that all aspects of your health care work together.
- Take charge of your health by being an informed consumer. Find out what the scien-

tific evidence is about any treatment's safety and whether it works.

- If you decide to use a CAM treatment that would be given by a practitioner, choose the practitioner carefully to help minimize any possible risks.

6. Are CAM therapies tested to see if they work?

While some scientific evidence exists regarding the effectiveness of some CAM therapies, for most there are key questions that are yet to be answered through well-designed scientific studies—questions such as whether they are safe, how they work, and whether they work for the diseases or medical conditions for which they are used.

NCCAM is the Federal Government's lead agency on scientific research of CAM. NCCAM supports research on CAM therapies to determine if they work, how they work, whether they are effective, and who might benefit most from the use of specific therapies.

7. I am interested in a CAM therapy that involves treatment from a practitioner. How do I go about selecting a practitioner?

Here are a few things to consider when selecting a practitioner. If you need more information, see our fact sheet, "Selecting a Complementary and Alternative Medicine Practitioner."

- Ask your physician, other health professionals, or someone you believe to be knowledgeable regarding CAM whether they have recommendations.
- Contact a nearby hospital or a medical school and ask if they maintain a list of area CAM practitioners or could make a recommendation. Some regional medical centers may have a CAM center or CAM practitioners on staff.
- Contact a professional organization for the type of practitioner you are seeking. Often, professional organizations have standards of practice, provide referrals to practitioners, have publications explaining the therapy (or therapies) that their members provide, and may offer information on the type of training needed and whether practitioners of a therapy must be licensed or certified in your state. Professional organizations can be located by searching the Internet or directories in libraries (ask the librarian). One directory is the Directory of

Information Resources Online (DIRLINE) compiled by the National Library of Medicine (dirline.nlm.nih.gov). It contains locations and descriptive information about a variety of health organizations, including CAM associations and organizations.

- Many states have regulatory agencies or licensing boards for certain types of practitioners. They may be able to provide you with information regarding practitioners in your area. Your state, county, or city health department may be able to refer you to such agencies or boards. Licensing, accreditation, and regulatory laws for CAM practices are becoming more common to help ensure that practitioners are competent and provide quality services.

8. Can I receive treatment or a referral to a practitioner from NCCAM?

NCCAM is the Federal Government's lead agency dedicated to supporting research on CAM therapies. NCCAM does not provide CAM therapies or referrals to practitioners.

9. Can I participate in CAM research through a clinical trial?

NCCAM supports clinical trials (research studies in people) of CAM therapies. Clinical trials of CAM are taking place in many locations worldwide, and study participants are needed. To find out more about clinical trials in CAM, see the NCCAM fact sheet "About Clinical Trials and Complementary and Alternative Medicine." To find trials that are recruiting participants, go to the Web site nccam.nih.gov/clinicaltrials. You can search this site by the type of therapy being studied or by disease or condition.

For More Information
NCCAM Clearinghouse

Toll-free: 1-888-644-6226
International: 301-519-3153
TTY (for deaf or hard-of-hearing callers):
1-866-464-3615

E-mail: info@nccam.nih.gov
Web site: nccam.nih.gov
Address: NCCAM Clearinghouse, P.O. Box 7923, Gaithersburg, MD 20898-7923

Fax: 1-866-464-3616
Fax-on-Demand Service: 1-888-644-6226

NCCAM is dedicated to exploring complementary and alternative medical practices in the context of rigorous science, training CAM researchers, and disseminating authoritative information to the public and professionals.

NCCAM has provided this material for your information. It is not intended to substitute for the medical expertise and advice of your primary health care provider. We encourage you to discuss any decisions about treatment or care with your health care provider. The mention of any product, service, or therapy in this information is not an endorsement by NCCAM

NCCAM Publication No. D167
August 2002

Mechanisms of CAM interventions

When the National Center for Complementary and Alternative Medicine (NCCAM) was established in Fiscal Year (FY) 1999, experts were recruited to build an infrastructure capable of supporting a new research enterprise and the Center's future growth. NCCAM also established a program of Specialized Research Centers to build essential research capacity in the complementary and alternative medicine (CAM) community. We launched a program of clinical trials, including the largest and most rigorous Phase III studies ever designed for a range of CAM modalities. We also initiated a portfolio of investigator-initiated research.

During the past year, and with the recruitment of our first Director, we have rapidly expanded our grants portfolio. It now addresses a wide range of conditions and CAM modalities. Based on the input from the communities we serve, our statutory authorities, and the funding NCCAM has received thus far, we developed a strategic plan to wisely guide our future growth and direction.

Our new strategic plan, *Expanding Horizons of Healthcare*, together with our *Strategic Plan to Address Racial and Ethnic Health Disparities* outline a clear, yet flexible research agenda through FY 2005. Consistent with these plans, we have identified priority areas that warrant immediate investments due to pressing public health needs and a dearth of valid scientific information or sufficient maturation of the science. NCCAM's areas of focus include:

1. mechanisms of CAM interventions;
2. cancer;
3. botanicals;
4. health disparities; and
5. integrative medicine and research training.

Cancer Progress Report

One of every four Americans dies of cancer, making it the second leading cause of death. During the year 2000, an estimated 552,200 Americans died of cancer, averaging more than 1,500 deaths per day. Cancer costs this nation an estimated $107 billion annually, including health care expenditures and lost productivity from illness and death.

Many cancer patients use CAM as a primary treatment or, more often, to alleviate the discomfort of conventional cancer therapy; however, the subject goes largely unexplored in dialogues between oncologists and their patients. A recent survey of cancer patients elucidated the extent to which CAM modalities are incorporated in cancer treatment. In total, nearly 85 percent of the patients surveyed used at least one CAM therapy while undergoing conventional oncology treatment. Among the most popular modalities are spirituality, vitamins and herbs, and movement/physical therapies. This survey illustrates not only the need for frank oncologist-patient discussions, but also the need to carefully examine combinations of cancer and CAM therapies. It is possible that some modalities are beneficial, while others are ineffective or otherwise diminish the effectiveness of conventional treatments.

NCCAM's rapidly growing cancer portfolio is directed at CAM therapies appropriate to the treatment of the disease itself, as well as its complications, encompassing both the study of cancer interventions and palliative care. In FY 2000, NCCAM spent more than $4 million in support of cancer research studies—a three-fold increase over FY 1999. Through FY 2001 and FY 2002 we will further expand our support for meritorious research.

Specialty Research Centers. In FY 2000 NCCAM funded two new Specialty Research Centers dedicated to studying the safety and effectiveness of several popular CAM cancer therapies. Awards totaling $8 million each over five years were made to Johns Hopkins University and the University of Pennsylvania. The Johns Hopkins Center is studying the anti-oxidant effects of herbs in cancer cells and the safety and efficacy of PC-SPES (a popular mixture of Chinese herbal medications) in men with prostate cancer. The University of Pennsylvania Center is examining the mechanisms of action, safety, and clinical efficacy of hyperbaric oxygen (oxygen at greater than atmospheric pressures) for the treatment of head and neck cancers.

Gonzalez Therapy.   Certain CAM approaches are controversial, particularly those used instead of conventional regimens for treating cancer. Nonetheless, NCCAM is committed to pursuing rigorous investigations of such therapies for which there is sufficient preliminary data, compelling public health need, and ethical justifications to do so. This is illustrated by our support of a study of an approach advocated by Dr. Nicholas Gonzalez. Dr. Gonzalez treats cancer patients with dietary supplements, including pancreatic enzymes, magnesium citrate, papaya extracts, vitamins, minerals, trace elements, and animal glandular products, as well as with coffee enemas. Very preliminary data suggests the therapy may be effective in prolonging life expectancy for those suffering from pancreatic cancer. Given that conventional regimens for this type of cancer only moderately prolong life, there is sufficient argument from a public health standpoint to evaluate the regimen in a more rigorous fashion. Accordingly, to assess Dr. Gonzalez's protocol, NCCAM and NCI are funding and overseeing a substantive pilot trial of 90 patients with pancreatic cancer at the Columbia-Presbyterian Cancer Center.

Shark Cartilage.   Our cancer research portfolio includes studies of shark cartilage that are also funded in collaboration with the NCI. These studies include an ongoing phase III clinical trial involving over 700 lung cancer patients in the United States and Canada. A second trial will examine safety and efficacy of shark cartilage in patients with a variety of advanced cancers.

Quick Trials.   In conjunction with NCI, NCCAM has embarked upon a creative, new research grant mechanism to simplify the grant application process and to provide rapid turnaround from application to funding. Initially announced for a pilot program in prostate cancer, the Quick Trial mechanism has been used for pilot, phase I, and phase II cancer clinical trials testing new agents, as well as patient monitoring and laboratory studies to ensure timely development of new treatments. We intend to support well-designed studies in such areas as complex CAM systems (i.e., Revici or Ger-

son therapy), high dose anti-oxidants, herbal mixtures, and whole plant extracts.

Future Directions

Supplements to NCI Cancer Centers.   NCI's Cancer Centers possess the infrastructure, organization, leadership, and integrated multidisciplinary objectives enabling them to build and incorporate new programs in emerging areas of cancer research. Rather than attempting to duplicate the success of this program, NCCAM plans to solicit and fund competitive, supplemental awards to existing NCI-funded Cancer Centers. This will permit us to develop innovative pilot projects in areas of cancer CAM research. Emphasis will be placed, where possible, on studies involving minority and underserved populations. Preliminary data from this research will serve as the basis for more definitive clinical trials.

CAM at the End-of-Life.   Cancer patients for whom a cure is not an option face not only death, but also the diminution of quality of life and intractable pain. Perhaps as many as 70 percent of these cancer patients are seeking complementary and alternative therapies to expand their end-of-life care options. NCCAM plans to solicit phase I and II clinical trials of CAM modalities for the prevention and management of symptoms associated with the end-of-life, including secondary side effects of chemotherapy and radiotherapy, and the enhancement of the well-being of persons facing a life-limiting illness. In parallel, we are interested in supporting similar studies for people with HIV/AIDS.

While people have used complementary and alternative remedies for centuries, little is known about how they work. By understanding the underlying mechanisms of CAM modalities, we could better monitor their actions and develop biomarkers that correlate with beneficial clinical outcomes. Thus, we would be better positioned to prove which CAM modalities work and which do not, and to inform the public accordingly.

Phase III Clinical Trials.   One of NCCAM's highest priorities is to conduct Phase III clinical trials of CAM modalities. NCCAM's phase III clinical trials are built upon a substantial body of scientific evidence concerning a given modality. While sufficiently complex in design and ambitious in scope to address the critical scientific issues and patient safety concerns, they are well poised to definitively address the most obvious premise, "Does this modality work?" In collaboration with other NIH Institutes and Centers (ICs), NCCAM currently supports five multiyear, multicenter phase III clinical trials:

1. Hypericum for depression—the National Institute of Mental Health (NIMH);
2. Shark cartilage for lung cancer—the National Cancer Institute (NCI);
3. Ginkgo biloba for dementia—the National Institute on Aging (NIA), the National Heart, Lung and Blood Institute (NHLBI), and the National Institute of Neurological Disorders and Stroke (NINDS);
4. Acupuncture for osteoarthritis pain—the National Institute of Arthritis and Musculoskeletal and Skin Diseases (NIAMS); and
5. Glucosamine/chondroitin sulfate for osteoarthritis—NIAMS.

Specialty Research Centers. In addition to supporting multicenter clinical trials, NCCAM now funds *15 specialty research centers* that form a research infrastructure on which to investigate the mechanisms underlying CAM treatments and their health effects. NCCAM-funded centers cover CAM approaches for many areas of major public health need, including drug addictions, aging and women's health, arthritis, craniofacial disorders, cardiovascular diseases, neurological disorders, pediatrics, and chiropractic research. These centers constitute a major investment of NCCAM's resources and serve as the focal point for initiating and maintaining state-of-the-art multidisciplinary CAM research, developing core research resources, training new CAM investigators, providing community outreach and education, and expanding the research base through collaborative research and outreach to scientists and clinicians.

Efficacy of Acupuncture. More than one million people in the U.S. receive acupuncture, resulting in approximately 10 million treatment visits annually. Acupuncture is administered by a variety of health care providers ranging from conventional physicians to Traditional Chinese Medicine practitioners. In response to this great public interest, NCCAM has funded multiple studies to examine the effectiveness of acupuncture for a variety of conditions. Currently, there is considerable use of acupuncture for the management of both chronic and acute pain. NCCAM supports studies to evaluate acupuncture for dental pain,

back and neck pain, and carpal tunnel syndrome. NCCAM also supports studies of "lesser known" applications of acupuncture, including the treatment of hypertension, cocaine abuse, and pre- and postnatal depression. Investigations of the many different applications of acupuncture should provide us with greater insight into the beneficial use of acupuncture.

Spinal Manipulation. New to NCCAM's research portfolio are studies to examine the efficacy and mechanisms of action of specific types of spinal manipulation, including those employed in chiropractic. Studies include examination of the efficacy of spinal manipulation on chronic neck pain and range of motion, as well as the impact of lumbar spinal manipulation on posture.

Future Directions

Chelation Therapy. Coronary artery disease (CAD) is the leading cause of mortality for both men and women in the United States, with more than 500,000 Americans dying of heart attacks each year. Despite decades of use, studies of ethylenediaminetetraacetate (EDTA) chelation therapy on CAD have been extremely few, very small in size, and of flawed design, offering few conclusions concerning its true safety and effectiveness. To address this important public health issue, NCCAM plans, in collaboration with NHLBI, to solicit applications to conduct the first substantive, multisite, clinical trial, using rigorous trial design and validated outcomes measures, to investigate the *efficacy and safety of EDTA chelation therapy* in individuals suffering from CAD.

Biology of Acupuncture. Despite the growing body of literature that addresses the clinical effects of acupuncture, there are critical scientific gaps. In particular, NCCAM plans to invite seasoned investigators to join us in exploring how acupuncture works. Potential areas of research include the basic biology and biochemistry of acupuncture, its effects at the cellular level, its effects upon body systems (such as the immune and nervous systems), and genetic factors that correlate with responses to acupuncture therapy.

Investigations of the Placebo Effect. The placebo has received an increasing amount of attention recently due to its effect on pain management. In November 2000, NCCAM and the National Institute of Diabetes and Digestive and Kidney Diseases

(NIDDK) cosponsored a major international conference to examine social, psychological, and neurobiological contributions to the placebo effect, and how to ethically employ and evaluate placebo actions in clinical trials. The ultimate outcome of the meeting is the development of a multidisciplinary research agenda in which NCCAM and other ICs may sponsor basic and clinical investigations of placebo mechanisms and use.

Osteoarthritis. The pain and limitation of motion caused by osteoarthritis (OA) are significant contributors to disability and dependence to millions of older Americans. Because current medications for OA are not sufficiently effective for all individuals and may yield dose-limiting side effects, the public is seeking alternative methods of treatment. In conjunction with NIAMS and NIA, NCCAM plans to support innovative research projects that explore the entire repertoire of CAM strategies used by the public in the prevention or treatment of OA. Relevant CAM modalities worthy of further investigation include various forms of manual manipulation, magnet therapy, and s-adenosylmethionine (SAM-e).

. . . Botanicals are among the most popular CAM therapies and Americans rely upon them for treatment and prevention of a number of conditions. These include St. John's wort for depression, Ginkgo biloba for improved memory, and saw palmetto for prostate enlargement. Still, we have much to learn about these products, most notably their relative safety and efficacy, side effects, and interactions with medications. For instance, recent studies suggest that St. John's wort is more effective than placebo in treating depression. While awaiting results of the NCCAM-funded multicenter trial of St. John's wort for depression, we are investigating other properties of St. John's wort. For example, when used with some life-saving drugs, like the AIDS drug indinavir, St. John's wort increases the rate at which the drug is eliminated from the bloodstream, rendering the drug ineffective sooner. This phenomenon has also been observed with certain oral contraceptives and drugs that prevent rejection of transplanted organs. These findings illustrate vividly both the promise and challenges presented by botanicals and other CAM therapies. Through rigorous research, NCCAM helps identify the extent to which individual therapies are safe and effective, as well as under what circumstances an effective CAM modality may interfere with other treatments.

Centers for Dietary Supplement Research. In collaboration with the NIH Office of Dietary Supplements (ODS), NCCAM now funds four Centers for Dietary Supplement Research with an emphasis on botanicals; each totaling approximately $1.5 million per year for five years. The Centers serve to identify and characterize botanicals, assess bioavailability and activity, explore mechanisms of action, conduct preclinical and clinical evaluations, establish training and career development, and help select the products to be tested in randomized controlled clinical trials. The two new Centers NCCAM added in FY 2000 include the Purdue University Center, which focuses on the health effects of antioxidants in botanicals, and the University of Arizona, which studies the use of botanicals for disease prevention and treatment.

Future Directions

Botanical-Drug Interactions. As illustrated by the effects of St. John's wort on the AIDS drug indinavir, botanical products interact with a number of important drugs. This is of concern because 18 percent of individuals taking prescription drugs also use botanicals, high dose vitamin products, or both. However, little reliable research-based data is available to guide consumers and practitioners about the use of botanicals simultaneously with over-the-counter and prescription drugs. NCCAM is now soliciting applications to investigate botanical-drug interactions in vitro, in animal models, and in phase I and II clinical studies, as well as to increase our knowledge of the mechanisms of action of botanicals. One special emphasis will be an examination of interactions between CAM botanicals and HIV/AIDS therapies.

Soy Supplements for Women with Breast Cancer. Some menopausal and postmenopausal women find symptom relief through conventional estrogen replacement therapy (ERT). Moreover, ERT has been associated with benefits such as preservation of cardiovascular, skeletal, genitourinary, and cognitive health. Unfortunately, this therapy is associated with an increased risk of breast cancer, dissuading some women from using it and excluding its application for breast cancer survivors. Not surprisingly, despite its benefits, less than 20 percent of women in the United States use ERT. Many women explore alternative approaches to estrogen replacement to eliminate the risks of conventional ERT, with the hope of reaping the benefits. Soybeans are known to be rich in naturally occurring compounds with estrogen-like activity. Several studies of these popular soy-derived phytoestrogens (PEs) yielded unclear and contradictory results, leaving open the question of whether soy may protect against breast cancer or, like conventional ERT, cause its emergence. NCCAM intends to study these issues and assess the impact in a phase II clinical trial of PE supplementation on the health of women after a breast cancer diagnosis.

Natural Products Development. NCCAM recognizes the great need to study botanicals and has encountered some limitations in doing so. Perhaps the most significant limitation is the lack of standardized products worthy of in-depth study. Consequently, NCCAM plans to solicit applications for the development of standardized botanical products. The availability of sufficient quantities of a given botanical will ensure a reliable supply for clinical and basic research, allowing investigators to make comparisons across studies, between known products, and permit large randomized controlled clinical trials.

Cranberry for Urinary Tract Infections. Cranberries have been used widely for decades for the prevention and treatment of recurring urinary tract infections (UTI), particularly in women. However, no conclusive studies have been conducted in humans. Consequently, NCCAM intends to assess the effectiveness and potential mechanisms of action of cranberry juice and other cranberry products in preventing UTIs in susceptible populations, and to determine the appropriate dosage and duration of therapy.

The NCCAM recently recruited a director for the Office of Special Populations. This office will focus on identifying the extent and nature of CAM use among special populations; studying the application of CAM therapies to the reduction of disparities; increasing participation of underrepresented populations in NCCAM-supported clinical trials; and enhancing the ability of minority institutions to conduct CAM research. In conjunction with the trans-NIH effort to address the health disparities of U.S. racial and ethnic minorities, we have developed our own multi-faceted research plan. This plan will serve as a guide for the development of new research initiatives to address minority health and health disparities through FY 2005.

Magnesium Therapy for Asthma. In the last several years there has been a significant increase in the number of Americans suffering from asthma. Although the prevalence of asthma does not vary substantially by racial/ethnic group, minority groups experience more severe disability and more frequent hospitalization from asthma than Caucasians. Basic and preliminary clinical studies summarized at a recent joint NCCAM/NHLBI workshop suggest that the mineral magnesium sulfate may be an effective new treatment for people with asthma. In collaboration with NHLBI, NCCAM plans to support a definitive study to assess the safety and efficacy of intravenous magnesium supplementation as a treatment for acute asthma. This study would determine the safety and efficacy of magnesium in different subpopulation groups, including different age and racial/ethnic groups.

Epidemiology of CAM Use in Minority Populations. Although the demographics, prevalence, and patterns of use of CAM in the United States have been described for the general population, its use by racial and ethnic minorities is currently not known. NCCAM, in conjunction with the Centers for Disease Control and Prevention (CDC), has begun epidemiological investigations of the use of CAM within minority and underserved populations, emphasizing the use of traditional and folk medicine among immigrant populations and the rural poor. Information gained from these surveys will help to prioritize NCCAM research agendas for individual populations.

Institutional Research Training Awards for Minority Researchers. To improve NCCAM's ability to obtain accurate and effective information that is relevant to the diverse cultures that comprise the United States, we seek to achieve greater diversity among our research communities. We will use the National Research Training Award (T32) mechanism to support pre- and post-doctoral trainees at minority and minority-serving institutions having the potential to develop meritorious training programs in CAM research. Through this effort, we hope to ensure that highly trained minority scientists will be available in adequate numbers and in appropriate research areas and fields so as to meet the nation's CAM research needs.

Future Directions

As part of fulfilling our overall scientific mission, NCCAM will continue to address health disparities. We will continue to focus on diseases that contribute to health disparities and increase our outreach to minority populations. We will also continue to create opportunities for minority scientists and students to pursue research training.

During 2001, the draft version of the Strategic Plan to Address Racial and Ethnic Health Disparities will be posted on the NCCAM Web site for public comment.

Integrative Medicine. Medicine is an ever-evolving discipline. It integrates or rejects approaches based on scientific evidence. The results of rigorous research in CAM will enhance the successful integration of safe and effective modalities into mainstream medical practice. A number of practices, once considered unorthodox, have been proven safe and effective and have been assimilated seamlessly into current medical practice. Practices such as support groups are now widely accepted as important allies in our fight against disease and disability. NCCAM has initiated a series of specific activities to facilitate the successful integration of safe and effective modalities into mainstream medical practice. The activities include conducting research that provides compelling evidence of efficacy and safety and publishing these findings in peer-reviewed journals; studying factors that promote or impede integration; supporting the development of model curricula for medical and allied health schools and continuing medical education programs; and informing the public in a clear and definitive manner. In FY 2001, we launched our intramural research program in which CAM strategies will be explored in patients at the NIH Clinical Center, the world's largest facility dedicated to patient-oriented research. In addition, we mounted a new integration research initiative to study factors that promote or impede integration; determine whether CAM research results can be translated to real-world settings; and support the evaluation of programs that integrate CAM and conventional care. The NCCAM's Intramural Research Program and Specialized Research Centers consider integrative medicine an essential component of their activities.

Research Training. NCCAM's ability to achieve our research goals is dependent on the availability of a critical mass of skilled investigators in both CAM and conventional communities. It is our goal to increase the knowledge, experience, and capacity of CAM practitioners to conduct or participate in rigorous research as well as enhance conventional practitioners' and researchers' knowledge and experience in specific CAM areas. NCCAM has

taken a comprehensive approach to *research training*, making awards at the institutional level, as well as to individuals. Likewise, NCCAM supports mentored and independent trainees, from the predoctoral level through mid-career and senior faculty members. The research spectrum of these trainees is broad, covering the continuum of basic through clinical studies. NCCAM supports all of the major training mechanisms offered by NIH. Research training is also an important component of NCCAM's Intramural Research Program and our specialized Research Centers. Some of NCCAM's Centers spend as much as ten percent of their budget on training.

CAM Research Database. In FY 2001, NCCAM partnered with the National Library of Medicine (NLM) to develop *CAM on PubMed*. This new resource, a subset of the NLM's PubMed, offers consumers, researchers, health care providers and CAM practitioners free, web-based access to journal citations directly related to complementary and alternative medicine.

PubMed provides an easy way to access over 11 million citations and abstracts in the MEDLINE database and additional life science journals. MEDLINE currently covers nearly 4,500 journals published in the United States and more than 70 other countries.

Future Directions

NCCAM will work to facilitate a more integrated practice of medicine by continuing to hold CAM therapies to the highest standards of evidence. We have established two primary goals related to integration:

1. Facilitate development of model health professional curricula that incorporate information about safe and effective CAM practices; and
2. Facilitate coupling of effective CAM and conventional practices within a coordinated, interdisciplinary healthcare system.

Conclusion

NCCAM, in collaboration with the NIH Institutes and Centers and other outstanding government, academic and private sector partners, is building on a foundation of superb science and consumer service. NCCAM is set to emerge as a world leader—not only by researching the safety and effectiveness of complementary and alternative medicine—but by producing research results that will help treat or prevent many of the diseases that affect every American family.

Native American healing practices Methods for restoration of health based on the belief that physical and emotional well-being is interconnected with morality, spirituality, and harmonious relationships with the community and nature. There are approximately 500 Native American Nations (commonly called tribes), each with its own practices and beliefs and some basic rituals and healing practices in common.

Although Native American healers claim to have cured victims of heart disease, diabetes, thyroid problems, skin rashes, asthma, and cancer, as well as emotional and spiritual problems, there is no scientific evidence to support these claims. Practitioners of Native American healing believe illness takes root in the body because of spiritual problems, that a psychologically disturbed person may not be receptive to healing or cannot be healed, and that diseases target individuals who are unbalanced, embrace negative thinking, and lead unhealthy lifestyles. Many Native American healers also believe that birth defects and other hereditary conditions result from the parents' immoral behavior. Native American healing practices attempt to restore balance and wholeness in an individual in order to retrieve physical and spiritual health.

The most common aspects of Native American healing include the use of herbal remedies, purifying rituals, shamanism, and spiritual healing to treat illnesses of both the body and the spirit. Herbal remedies treat many physical problems, and purifying rituals cleanse the body; practitioners claim that such rituals make the person more receptive to other Native American healing techniques. When it is believed that angry spirits caused an illness, a Native American healer called a shaman is often relied on for invoking spiritual healing powers to treat the person and appease the spirits. Symbolic healing rituals that may involve family and friends of the sick person help invoke the spirits to participate in healing the sick person.

One of the most common forms of Native American healing involves the use of herbal remedies, including teas, tinctures, and salves. For example, willow tree bark is a remedy for arthritis. Purifying and purging the body are also important techniques used in Native American healing. Not unlike steam baths or saunas, sweat lodges and special teas that induce vomiting may be part of a healing regimen. Smudging—cleansing a place or person with the smoke of sacred plants—is also done to induce an altered state of consciousness and sensitivity, making a person more receptive to the healing. Prayer is also a major component of Native American healing practices.

Another practice of Native American healing, symbolic healing rituals, can involve a shaman and even entire communities. These ritual ceremonies include chanting, singing, body painting, dancing, exorcisms, sand paintings, and even the use of mind-altering substances, such as peyote, to persuade the spirits to heal the sick person.

Native American healing has been practiced in North America for thousands of years and has roots in Ayurvedic, Chinese, and other traditions, but the greatest influence continues to emanate from Native American knowledge of nature, plants, and animals. The migration of tribes and contact with other tribes along trade routes allowed for exchanges of information and techniques. The tribes gathered many herbs from the surrounding environment and sometimes traded over long distances. Contemporary Native American Indian community-based medical systems offer traditional healing modalities and rituals.

According to information on the Native American website, "One recent clinical trial examined 116 people with a variety of ailments (such as infertility, chest and back pain, asthma, depression, diabetes, and cancer) who were treated with traditional Native American healing. More than 80 percent showed some benefit after a seven- to 28-day intensive healing experience. Five years later, 50 of the original participants said they were cured of their diseases while another 41 said they felt better. Another nine showed no change, five were worse, and two had died. However, the comparison group who received different treatments also showed benefits. More clinical studies are needed to confirm the benefits of the specific healing methods."

Native American healing is said to be able to improve the quality of a person's life and reduce stress through prayer, introspection, meditation, and communal support. Because Native American healing is based on spirituality and mysticism, there are very few scientific studies to support the validity of the practices. Discrepancies among Nations, shamans, and types of ailments and individual considerations make it almost impossible to study Native American healing under accepted scientific standards. Moreover, certain Native Americans conceal their practices and techniques because they do not want their sharing to exploit their culture and weaken their healing powers.

Individuals with catastrophic illnesses such as cancer often seek complementary therapies such as Native American practices, which may be used in relieving certain symptoms of cancer and side effects of cancer treatment. People with cancer and other chronic conditions are advised to consult their physician before pursuing purification rituals or herbal remedies as primary or sole treatment.

A combination of religion, spirituality, herbal medicine, and rituals to treat medical and emotional problems, Native American healing has no scientific evidence it can cure cancer or any other disease, but the communal support provided by this approach to health care does offer the possibility of significant benefits.

See also AYURVEDA; FAITH HEALING; SWEAT LODGE.

naturopath A licensed naturopathic physician (N.D.) who attends a four-year graduate level naturopathic medical school and is educated in all of the same basic sciences as a medical doctor but also studies holistic and nontoxic approaches to therapy with a strong emphasis on disease prevention and optimization of wellness. In addition to a standard medical curriculum, the N.D. is required to complete four years of training in clinical nutrition, acupuncture, homeopathic medicine, botanical medicine, psychology, and counseling (to encourage people to make lifestyle changes to support their personal health). A naturopathic physician takes rigorous professional board exams so that he or she may be licensed by a state or jurisdiction as a primary care general practice physician.

See also NATUROPATHY.

naturopathy Health practices also known as naturopathic medicine. The word *naturopathy* was coined in America a century ago from the Greek words meaning "nature" and "disease." The healing power of nature—*vis medicatrix naturae*—had been espoused by the ancients, including the Greek "father of medicine," Hippocrates, perhaps one of the world's earliest naturopathic and homeopathic physicians. The concept of invoking nature's healing power by using herbs, water, fasting, diet, and other noninvasive, gentle treatments is now seeing a renaissance, particularly in the United States. Modern naturopathic physicians still employ treatments that do not override the body's innate ability to heal itself, and they advocate preventive measures to promote optimal health and functioning. In addition, N.D.s conduct and make practical use of the latest biochemical research involving nutrition, botanicals, homeopathy, and other natural treatments.

For many diseases and conditions (ulcerative colitis, asthma, menopause, flu, obesity, and chronic fatigue, among others), treatments used by naturopathic physicians can be primary and even curative. Naturopathic physicians also function within an integrated framework, for example, by referring patients to appropriate conventional medical specialists. Naturopathic therapies complement the treatments used by conventionally trained medical doctors. The result is a team-care approach that recognizes the need of the patient to receive the best overall treatment most appropriate to his or her specific medical condition.

Naturopathic medicine was popular and widely available throughout the United States well into the early part of the 20th century. During the 1920s there were a number of naturopathic medical schools, thousands of naturopathic physicians, and thousands of patients using naturopathic therapies. But the rise of "scientific medicine," the discovery and increasing use of new pharmaceuticals including antibiotics, and the establishment of a wide-ranging medical system primarily based (both clinically and economically) on high-tech and pharmaceutical treatments put naturopathic and other natural healing methods into a temporary decline.

By the 1970s, however, the American public felt the impact of the costs, problems, and limitations of conventional medicine and began to explore other methods now referred to as integrative, alternative, and complementary medicine.

According to the Internet article "What Is the History of Naturopathic Medicine?" by Peter Barry Chowka: "Today, licensed naturopathic physicians are experiencing noteworthy clinical successes, providing leadership in innovative natural medical research, enjoying increasing political influence, and looking forward to an unlimited future potential. Both the American public and policy makers are recognizing and contributing to the resurgence of the comprehensive system of health care practiced by NDs. In 1992, the National Institutes of Health's (NIH) Office of Alternative Medicine, created by an act of Congress, invited leading naturopathic physicians (educators, researchers, and clinical practitioners) to serve on key federal advisory panels and to help define priorities and design protocols for state-of-the-art alternative medical research. In 1994, the NIH selected Bastyr University as the national center for research on alternative treatments for HIV/AIDS. At a one-million-dollar level of funding, this action represented the formal recognition by the federal government of the legitimacy and significance of naturopathic medicine. Meanwhile, the number of new N.D.s is steadily increasing, and licensure of naturopathic physicians is expanding into new states. By April of 1996, eleven of fifty states had naturopathic licensing laws (Alaska, Arizona, Connecticut, Hawaii, Maine, Montana, New Hampshire, Oregon, Utah, Vermont, and Washington). A number of other states are likely to enact naturopathic licensing in the near future."

In October 1996, the Natural Medicine Clinic, which is the first medical facility in the nation to offer natural medical treatments to the community, opened in Kent, Washington, funded by the King County (Seattle) Department of Public Health. Bastyr University, one of the three American naturopathic colleges, was selected to operate the clinic.

Naturopathy, wrote Chowka, "is as old as healing itself and as new as the latest discoveries in biochemical sciences. In the United States, the naturopathic medical profession's infrastructure is based on accredited educational institutions, pro-fessional licensing by a growing number of states, national standards of practice and care, peer review, and an ongoing commitment to state-of-the-art scientific research. Modern American naturopathic physicians (N.D.s) receive extensive training in and use therapies that are primarily natural (hence the name naturopathic) and non-toxic, including clinical nutrition, homeopathy, botanical medicine, hydrotherapy, physical medicine, and counseling. Many N.D.s have additional training and certification in acupuncture and home birthing. These contemporary N.D.s, who have attended naturopathic medical colleges recognized by the U.S. Department of Education, practice medicine as primary health care providers and are increasingly acknowledged as leaders in bringing about progressive changes in the nation's medical system."

Naturopathy is also useful in the treatment of animals. More information on animal homeopathy is available through Diana Hayes, DIHom Dip Animal Homeopathy- Registered Holistic Animal Practitioner and vice president and national publicity officer of the Holistic Animal Therapy Association of Australia, Inc. (HATAA), telephone 011 1300 132 966 (Australian only),and international fax 011 6 1 8 9201 0282. Hayes is located in Victoria, Australia.

See also HIPPOCRATES; HOMEOPATHY.

near-death experience The state described by individuals as between life and death, usually an out-of-body feeling that one is floating above and looking down on his or her own body and all the goings-on around it before returning into the body and being revived. During this experience, which has infinite variations according to the individual's perception, a healing or other restorative or enlightening vision, knowledge, or sensory experience may occur and foster a major change in one's thinking and approach to life.

negative energy A component of natural forces that may cause adverse effects on the body and mind. Negative thinking, pessimism, anger, fear, and the like, are believed to induce many disorders, including cardiac arrhythmias and emotional disturbances. Alternative practitioners often advocate releasing negative energy and fostering relaxation through meditation, exercise, yoga, chanting, dance, breathwork, bodywork, and other techniques. The goal is to develop a healing consciousness through positive energy.

neural therapy The injection of anesthetics into a site of the autonomic nervous system (which regulates breathing, heartbeat, digestion, and all body processes), acupuncture points (acupoints), scars, glands, and other bodily tissues in order to unblock energy flow, restore dysfunctional neural balance, increase the flow of lymphatic fluids, detoxify tissues, and reverse the cumulative effects of trauma. Particularly popular in Europe, including its native Germany, neural therapy is reported to be beneficial to individuals who have asthma, allergies, arthritis, kidney disease, gallbladder disease, headaches, depression, chronic pain, emphysema, hormonal imbalance, glaucoma, liver disease, prostate disease, thyroid disorders, muscle and sports injuries, multiple sclerosis, chronic fatigue syndrome, and other ailments.

Neural therapy was developed in 1952 by two German physicians, Ferdinand Huneke and Walter Huneke, who based their successful treatment of their patients on the idea they called *Sterfelder*, meaning "fields of interference." The procedure corresponds with the concept of the "ground system," a theory that states that disturbances in the connective tissues between cells are the cause of disease. In the United States, Dietrich Klinghardt, M.D., Ph.D., has established the American Academy of Neural Therapy, which offers training to aspiring neural therapy practitioners. Neural therapy is also applicable to dentistry. More information is available at www.neuraltherapy.com.

neurolinguistics A system of studying certain functions of the brain in order to promote physical and emotional healing effects. Neuro-Linguistic Programming (NLP) was developed in 1975 and provides a powerful technology for creating healthier interpersonal and intrapersonal relationships. NLP helps one aim to nonjudgmentally identify the ways in which he or she has been "programmed" to think, act, and feel. It is designed as a tool for learning how to release unwanted limiting habits and beliefs.

The study of this science began with the modeling of experts in the field of interpersonal and intrapersonal communication and change including Virginia Satir, a renowned family therapist, Fritz Perls, the developer of Gestalt therapy, and Milton Erickson, developer of Ericksonian hypnosis. Ericksonian hypnosis helps individuals develop deep trance states used for relaxation and stress-reduction, problem-solving, and accessing the inner resources necessary for coping with life's ongoing challenges. Milton Erickson's hypnotic language patterns can be used in everyday communication as well as in formal trance inductions. NLP includes many of these hypnotic language patterns and underlying presuppositions of

Erickson's work, although it is in itself a distinct field of study. The two fields are complementary, working with both the conscious and the unconscious mind. More information is available at http://www.nlptraining.com.

Neurolinguistic programming may also help treat learning disabilities. According to an article by Lise Menn, of the University of Colorado: "Where in your brain is a word that you've learned? If you know two languages, are they stored in two different parts of your brain? Is the left side of your brain really the language side? If you lose the ability to talk because of a stroke, can you learn to talk again? Do people who read languages written from left to right (like English) think differently from people who read languages written from right to left (like Hebrew and Arabic)? What about if you read a language that is written using some other kind of symbols, like Chinese or Japanese? If you're dyslexic, is your brain different from the brain of someone who has no trouble reading?

"All of these questions and more are what neurolinguistics is about. Techniques like Functional Magnetic Resonance Imaging (FMRI) and event-related potential (ERP) are used to study language in the brain, and they are constantly being improved. We can see finer and finer details of the brain's constantly changing blood flow—where the blood flows fastest, the brain is most active. We can see more and more accurate traces of our electrical brain waves and understand more about how they reflect our responses to statements that are true or false, ungrammatical or nonsense, and how the brain's electrical activity varies depending on whether we are listening to nouns or verbs, words about colors, or words about numbers. New information about neurolinguistics is regularly covered in national news sources.

"Brain activity is like the activity of a huge city. A city is organized so that people who live in it can get what they need to live on, but you can't say that a complex activity, like manufacturing a product, is 'in' one place. Raw materials have to arrive, subcontractors are needed, the product must be shipped out in various directions. It's the same with our brains. We can't say that all of language is 'in' a particular part of the brain; it's not even true that a particular word is 'in' just one spot in a person's brain. But we can say that listening, understanding, talking, and reading each involve activities in certain parts of the brain much more than other parts.

"Most of these parts are in the left side of your brain, the left hemisphere, regardless of what language you read and how it is written. We know this because aphasia (language loss due to brain damage) is almost always due to left hemisphere injury in people who speak and read Hebrew, English, Chinese, or Japanese, and also in people who are illiterate. But areas in the right side are essential for communicating effectively and for understanding the point of what people are saying. If you are bilingual, your right hemisphere may be somewhat more involved in your second language than it is in your first language.

"The organization of your brain is similar to other peoples' because we almost all move, hear, see, and so on, in essentially the same way. But our individual experiences and training also affect the organization of our brains—for example, deaf people understand sign language using just about the same parts of their brains that hearing people do for spoken language.

"What is aphasia like? Is losing language the reverse of learning it? People who have lost some or most of their language because of brain damage are not like children. Using language involves many kinds of knowledge and skill; some can be badly damaged while others remain in fair condition. People with aphasia have different combina-tions of things they can still do in an adult-like way plus things that they now do clumsily or not at all. Therapy can help them to regain lost skills and make the best use of remaining abilities. Adults who have had brain damage and become aphasic recover more slowly than children who have had the same kind of damage, but they continue to improve over decades if they have good language stimulation.

"What about dyslexia, and children who have trouble learning to talk even though they can hear normally? There probably are brain differences that account for their difficulties, and research in this area is moving rapidly. Since brains can change with training much more than we used to think, there is renewed hope for effective therapy for people with disorders of reading and language." (Menn, Lise, Obler, L.K., and Holland, Audrey L., *Non-fluent aphasia in a multilingual world*. Amsterdam: John Benjamins, 1995), pp. xvii–212.

Nightingale, Florence   A British nurse and phil-anthropist (1820–1910), who established the profession of secular nursing and revolutionized hospital care and documentation of care as we know it today. A proponent of public health, she advocated in her writings and practice that the whole person—body, mind, and spirit—be considered treatable, and that illness may be caused by and affected by one's state of mind. In her book *Notes on Nursing* (London: Harrison and Sons, 1859), Nightingale wrote: "[H]ow much more extraordinary is it that, whereas what we might call the coxcombries of education—e.g., the elements of astronomy—are now taught to every school-girl, neither mothers of families of any class, nor school-mistresses of any class, nor nurses of children, nor nurses of hospitals, are taught anything about those laws which God has assigned to the relations of our bodies with the world in which He has put them. In other words, the laws which make these bodies, into which He has put our minds, healthy or unhealthy organs of those minds, are all but unlearnt. Not but that these laws—the laws of life—are in a certain measure understood, but not even mothers think it worth their while to study them—to study how to give their children healthy existences. They call it medical or physiological knowledge, fit only for doctors. . . . Pathology teaches the harm that disease has done. But it teaches nothing more. We know nothing of the principle of health, the positive of which pathology is the negative, except from observation and experience. And nothing but observation and experience will teach us the ways to maintain or to bring back the state of health. It is often thought that medicine is the curative process. It is no such thing; medicine is the surgery of functions, as surgery proper is that of limbs and organs. Neither can do anything but remove obstructions; neither can cure; nature alone cures."

nonlocal mind   The term coined by Larry Dossey, M.D., author of several books on mind-body medicine and related topics, including *Reinventing Medicine: Beyond Mind-Body to a New Era of Healing* (HarperSanFrancisco, 1999), to describe unbounded consciousness. Nonlocal happenings, Dossey writes on page 9, are unmediated by a sensory experience or other intermediate signal or stimulus, and nonlocal events are unmitigated: that is, their magnitude or power does not diminish as a result of distance. Nonlocal phenomena are immediate, he says, and take place outside time and space. His use of the word *nonlocal* maintains the concept of infinitude and unlimited. Nonlocal medicine, Dossey says, involves a totally free mind in which to explore all possibilities for healing.

"Imagine that . . . a part of your mind is not present in your body or brain or even in this moment. Imagine that this aspect of your consciousness spreads everywhere, extending billions of miles into space, from the beginning of time into the limitless future, linking us with the minds of one another and with everyone who has ever lived or will live. This is the infinite piece of your consciousness.

"This picture of your mind outside your head may at first seem foreign. But as we shall see, 'nonlocal' or 'infinite' describes a natural part of who we are. Its expressions include sharing of thoughts and feelings at a distance, gaining information and wisdom through dreams and visions, knowing the future, radical breakthroughs in creativity and discovery, and many more. And this part of your mind

can be used today in healing illness and disease in what I call Era III healing."

See also DOSSEY, LARRY; PRAYER, POWER OF.

nosode   A homeopathic remedy extracted from diseased material, such as tuberculinum from tissue infected with *Mycobacterium tuberculosis*.

nursing, holistic   Professional nursing with a deliberate focus on treating the entire individual—physical, emotional, and spiritual.

See also Appendix I; NIGHTINGALE, FLORENCE.

nutritional therapy   Any food substance or diet geared toward the repair or rejuvenation of the body or prevention of potential illness. It is the consensus of experts that the general American diet, which includes saturated fats, refined starches, white flour, feedlot-fattened beef and pork, pesticides, preservatives, chemical additives, excessive sugar, irradiation, genetic engineering, fish from polluted waters, toxins in the food chain, and repetition, as opposed to variety, in the daily foods, has a significant ill effect on our health. A poor diet can contribute to the risk of heart disease, stroke, diabetes, certain forms of cancer, and other problems such as obesity and allergies.

Among common food nutrients used in nutritional therapy are acidophilus culture complexes; activated charcoal; aloe vera; amaranth; amazake; arrowroot; astragalus; barley flour; barley grass; barley malt syrup; basmati rice; bee pollen; bee propolis; bentonite; black beans; bran; brewer's yeast; buckwheat; canola oil; carob powder; cheese; chlorella; chromium picolinate; coenzyme Q10; chondroitin sulfate A; cream of tartar; daikon radish; dashi; date sugar; dulse; egg replacer; ethylenediaminetetraacetic acid (EDTA); electrolyte drinks; essene bread; essential fatty acids; flax seed oil; fructose; garlic; ginger; ginkgo biloba; ginseng; glycerine (vegetable); gomashio; green magma; guar gum; gum guggul; gymnema sylvestre; kashi; kefir; kuzu; lecithin; millet; miso; mochi; molasses; mushrooms; Nutrasweet; oats and oat bran; octacosanol; oils (natural vegetable); omega 3-oils; pasta; psyllium husks; pycnogenol; quercetin; quinoa; rice; rice syrup; royal jelly; sea vegetables; soy milk and cheese; spirulina; spelt and kamut;

sprouts; sucanat; tahini; teas (black and green); tempeh; tofu; tortillas; triticale; turbinado sugar; umeboshi plums; vinegars; wheat germ and wheat germ oil, and wheat grass.

Various alternative and complementary medicines—Ayurveda, homeopathy, osteopathy, among them—advocate certain types of foods and food regimens believed to promote and restore health, such as low-salt diet.

See also AYURVEDA; DETOXIFICATION THERAPY; FOOD THERAPY; HOXSEY THERAPY; JUICING; MACROBIOTIC DIET.

obeah   The science of traditional medicine and herbs according to African bush medicine.

See also FOLK MEDICINE.

oils, essential   Herbal extracts used in flavoring, medication, perfume, massage, therapeutic baths, compresses, and aromatherapy. Essential oils are absorbed by the skin and are not meant to be taken orally unless under the supervision of a trusted aromatherapist or other practitioner. Essential oils have various effects, including bactericidal properties and psychological benefits for individuals being treated for anxiety, depression, stress, and other problems. Plants produce essential oils in the form of globules in or on the surface of the plant tissues as a way to ensure their environmental safety. The oils may attract beneficial insects and ward off harmful ones; the evaporated oil gives off a vapor barrier that may protect the organism from excessive heat or cold, and the oil's fragrance may also be a subtle means of communication between plants. Some healers believe the oil is the essence of the plant and therefore its vital force, or energy, which can be used therapeutically.

The essential oils of a plant are extracted through various methods, including distillation, and the cold-press method, enfleurage method, chemical solvent method, resinoid method, and carbon dioxide method. There is evidence of distillation devices used more than 5,000 years; ancient Egyptians, for example, used essential oils for many purposes, such as mummification and cosmetics. Ancient Babylonians, Chinese, Asian Indians, Greeks, and Romans documented their use of essential oils, which may be blended for intensified effects. Synthetic oils are not considered for use by healers because they lack the energy of a living organism. Among the many oils are the following:

- Ajowan: herbaceous, spicy; Trachyspermum ammi (family, Apiaceae [Umbelliferae]), from fruits or seeds or whole aerial plant, India; production method: steam distillation; avoid during pregnancy, possible dermal; sensitization irritant

- Allspice berry: spicy, *Pimenta officinalis* (family, Myrtaceae); used in potpourris and flavoring of beverages, sweets, and other foods; warming, cheering, sense-enhancing; avoid use in sun; also known as pimento, *P. dioica*; from fruits, Cuba, Mexico, and the United States; production method: steam distillation; aphrodisiac; blends well with ginger, geranium, lavender, labdanum, ylang ylang, patchouli, orris; may irritate skin

- Almond: sweet; *Prunus amygdalus*, *P. dulcis* (family, Rosaceae); from the nut of the tree and native to Asia and the Mediterranean, a carrier oil for aromatherapy blends; also a skin moisturizer

- Ambrete seed: spicy; *Abelmoscyhus moschatus*; also known as *Hibiscus abelmoschus* (family, Malvaceae); sweet, floral, musky aroma that intensifies and improves after a few months of storage; blends well with other oils; for muscular aches and pains related to fatigue and poor circulation, also an antidepressant; from seed, France; production method: steam distillation; balancing, calming; emollient aphrodisiac; blends well with neroli, olibanum, rose, sandalwood, other floral oils

- Amyris: woodsy; *Amyris balsamifera, Schimmelia oleifera* (family, Rutaceae); for stress relief, muscle relaxation, and a meditation aid; also known as sandalwood amyris; from wood, West Indies; production method: steam distillation; blends well with lavandin, citronella, cedarwood

- Angelica root: earthy, musky; *Angelica archangelica, A. officinalis, A. glauca* (family, Apiaceae [Umbelleferae]); for depression, anxiety; production method: steam distillation; from the root, France, India, Germany, Hungary; blends well with patchouli, clary sage, citrus oils, frankincense; avoid during pregnancy and in sunlight

- Aniseed: sweet; *Illicium verum* (family, Illiciaceae); for indigestion, cramping, spasmodic cough; production method: steam distillation; from India, China, Spain; blends well with lavender, orange, pine, bay; should be avoided by pregnant women

- Anise: sweet; *Pimpinella anisum, Anisum officinalis* (family, Apiaceae [Umbelliferae]); for relaxation, deodorant; from China; production method: steam distillation; blends well with amyris, bay, cardamon, caraway, cedarwood, coriander, fennel, galbanum, mandarin; may cause slight dermal toxicity; use recommended dilution or less

- Apricot kernel: nut oil; *Armeniaca vulgaris, Prunus armeniaca* (family, Rosaceae); for improving skin

- Arjowan: *Trachyspermum ammi, T. copticum* (family, Apiaceae [Umbelliferae]); for circulatory and muscular problems; may irritate sensitive skin

- Armoise: aromatic; *Artemisia vulgaris*; from France; production method: steam distillation; used as an emollient, soothing agent, muscle relaxant; blends well with patchouli, rosemary, lavandin, sage, clary sage, cedarwood, cedar leaf; should be avoided by pregnant women

- Avocado: oil; *Persea americana, P. gratissima* (family, Lauraceae); added to carrier oils, up to 20 percent as an aid to skin moisturizing; may be toxic in large amounts

- Babassu: nut oil; *Orbignya barbosiana* (family, Arecaceae); from the Amazon; used for stretch marks

- Balsam Peru: earthy aroma; *Myroxylon balsamum* or *pererae* (family, Fabaceae [Legumunosae]); to soothe chafed skin; added to perfumes

- Basil: licorice-like aroma; *Osimum basilicum* (family, Labiatae); used to refresh concentration, counteract fatigue and stress; blends well with lavender, bergamot, clary sage, and geranium; not for use during pregnancy; can irritate skin; also East Indian basil (*O. gratissimum*) and hairy basil (*O. canum*); from Madagascar, France; production method: steam distillation; used as deodorant, insect repellent, muscle relaxant; blends well with bergamot, black pepper, clary sage, geranium, hyssop, lavender, marjoram, neroli; use recommended dilution or less; contains citronella

- Bay leaf: spicy; *Pimenta racemosa* (family, Myrtaceae); hair and scalp tonic, aphrodisiac, stimulant to memory, and for depression and respiratory problems; also known as West Indian bay and laurel sweet bay; *Laurus nobilis* is also a bay; from the West Indies; production method: steam distillation; blends well with coriander, eucalyptus, ginger, juniper berry, lavender, lemon, marjoram, orange, rose, rosemary, thyme, ylang ylang; may irritate skin; use half of recommended dilution or less; can cause skin irritation

- Beechnut: nut oil; *Fagus grandifolia, F. sylvatica* (family, Fagaceae [Legumunosac])

- Ben: seed oil; *Moringa oleifera, M. pterygosperma* (family, Moringaceae); for skin care

- Benzoin tincture: oil; *Styrax benzoin, S. tonkinensis* (family, Styracaceae); for soothing, stimulating, and warming chapped skin; also known as friars balsam

- Bergamot: citrus, calming; *Citrus bergamia* (family, Rutaceae); for flavoring in Earl Grey tea; for oily and blemished skin and in vaporizer as room deodorizer; increases susceptibility to sunburn; do not apply to the skin before sun exposure; bergapten-free bergamot reduces photosensitivity; from fruit peel, Italy, Ivory Coast; production method: expression; for use as antiseptic, deodorant, perfume, soothing agent, skin conditioner; blends well with chamomile, coriander, cypress, geranium, juniper, lavender, lemon, neroli, ylang ylang; may be phototoxic

- Birch, Sweet: sweet, bracing; *Betula lenta, B. capinefolia* (family, Betulaceae); stimulates circulation and used for arthritic and muscular pain; may be toxic

- Birch, white: woodsy; *Betula alba* (family, Betulaceae); for soothing and clearing the skin of psoriasis and eczema, relaxing muscles, and stimulating circulation; from wood and bark, France; production method: steam distillation; blends well with patchouli, vetiver, copaila; pregnant women should avoid birch

- Black currant seed and bud: oil; *Rives nigrum* (family, Grossulariaceae); from Asia and Europe; a carrier oil addition and bud oil; for use in perfume and foods; for premenstrual syndrome and rich source of vitamin C

- Black pepper: spicy; *Piper nigrum* (family, Piperaceae); stimulates, warms, and tones; for abdominal and muscle massage, especially before sports or dance activity; for perfume and as aphrodisiac; blends well with rose, rosemary, marjoram, and lavender; may irritate skin; use in small amounts; from India and Indonesia; production method: steam distillation; blends well with olibanum, sandalwood, lavender, rosemary, marjoram

- Borage: seed oil; *Borago officinalis* (family, Boraginaceae); high content of gamma-linoleic acid (GMA), may slow skin aging process; also used as a carrier oil

- Brazil nut: nut carrier oil; *Bertholletia excelsa* (family, Lecythidaceae); from the Amazon; becomes rancid quickly; store in dark, cool place

- Cabreuva: oil; *Myrocarpus fastigiatus* (family, Fabaceae [Legumunosae]); from a South American tree; warming, calming, and aphrodisiac properties; for increasing alertness

- Cade: smoky; *Juniperus oxycedrus* (family, Cupressaceae); from wood, France; production method: steam distillation; for veterinary parasitic skin problems (lice, etc.), for men's perfume, and as smoky flavoring in food

- Cajaput: camphoraceous; *Melaleuca cajaputi* (family, Myrtaceae); for improving mood and building resistance to infections, as steam inhalation, and as treatment for oily skin and spots; stimulant and irritant; use carefully; from leaves and stems, Indonesia; production method: steam distillation; also for use as antiseptic, deodorant, insect repellent; blends well

with bergamot, birch, cardamom, clove, geranium, lavender, myrtle, nutmeg, rose, thyme

- Calendula: *Calendula officinalis* (family, Asteraceae); for skin infections, wounds, rashes, bites, and inflammations including hemorrhoids and rheumatism (See also MARIGOLD)

- Calamint (catnip): mood elevator; *Calamintha clinopodium, C. grandiflora, C. officialis, Nepeta cataria, Saurreja calamintha* (family, Lamiaceae); also for pain reduction

- Calamus (sweet flag): *Acorus calamus, Calamus aromaticus* (family, Araceae); ancient herb that has been used for more than 4000 years; from India; high component of asarone, which may be toxic and carcinogenic; plants that do not contain asarone grown in North America and Russia.

- Calophyllum: thick nut oil; *Calophyllum inophullum* (family, Guttiferae); from Asia; for use as carrier oil

- Camphor white: camphoraceous; *Cinnamomum camphora* (family, Lauraceae); for oily or spotty skin, as aphrodisiac, and as insect repellent, in detergents, soaps, disinfectants, deodorants, and room sprays; from wood, Japan, China; production method: steam distillation; toning, cooling properties; blends well with olibanum, ylang ylang, orange, mandarin; use sparingly; not for individuals who are pregnant or have epilepsy

- Canola (rapeseed): seed oil; *Brassica napus* (family, Brassicaceae); used in cooking and as a carrier; original species contained up to 40 percent erucic acid, harmful to the thyroid, kidneys, and other internal organs; the genetically altered species contains only about 1 percent of the toxic acid

- Cananga: floral, calming, euphoric; *Cananga odorata* (family, Annonaceae); muscle relaxant; antidepressant properties; from flowers, Java; production method: steam distillation; also used as deodorant, skin conditioner; blends well with bergamot, lavender, lemon, neroli, palmarosa, sandalwood, vetiver, ylang ylang

- Caraway: minty; *Carum carvi, Apium carvi* (family, Apiaceae [Umbelliferae]); aids circulation and intestinal problems, muscle tension, skin care; reduces effects of contusions; from seeds, Holland; production method: steam distillation; blends well with galbanum, eucalyptus, rosemary; may cause slight dermal toxicity

- Cardamom seed: spicy, warming; *Elettaria cardomum* (family, Zingiberaceae); used by ancient Egyptians used as perfume and incense; also aids digestion, for muscle relaxant, skin conditioner, tonic bath oil, perfumes, and in foods; from seeds, Central America; production method: steam distillation and CO_2; blends well with coriander, olibanum, galbanum, geranium, juniper berry, lemon, myrtle

- Carnation (clove pink): aromatic oil; *Dianthus caryophyllus* (family, Caryophyllaceae); most fragrant in evening; aphrodisiac properties; may irritate sensitive skins

- Carrot seed and root: spicy; *Daucus carota* (family, Apiaceae [Umbeliferae]); for dry, mature skin types; restores elasticity to skin; root oil used in yellow food coloring and in tanning lotions; from seeds, India; production method: steam distillation; blends well with bergamot, juniper berry, lavender, lemon, lime, neroli, orange, petitgrain, rosemary

- Cashew nut: carrier oil; *Anacardium occidentale* (family, Anacardiaceae); from Latin America and Asia

- Cascarilla bark: *Croton eleuteria* (family, Euphorbiaceae); for stress reduction and meditation, fragrance, and in soaps, detergents, foods, drinks, and cigarettes; not for use as a strong purgative

- Cassia: spicy; *Cinnamomum cassia, C. aromaticum, Laurus cassia* (family, Lauraceae); like cinnamon bark, for flavoring foods, toothpaste, mouthwash, and chewing gum; very irritating and potentially allergenic to the skin

- Cassie: *Acacia farnesiana, Cassia ancienne* (family, Mimosaceae); for perfume, rheumatic symptoms, and chest ailments

- Castor: *Ricinus communis* (family, Euphorbiaceae); from India; ingestion of nuts potentially lethal; oil extracted at low temperature to eliminate content of ricin from oil; for analgesia, clearing of blackheads, and dandruff treatment

- Catnip (many varieties): *Nepeta cataria;* from aerial parts, France, United States, Yugoslavia

- Cedar leaf: calming, aromatic; *Thuj, occidentalis;* from leaves and stems, United States; production method: steam distillation; for use as deodorant, astringent, soothing agent; blends well with lavender, lavandin, rosemary, armoise

- Cedarwood: woodsy, balsamic; *Juniperus mexicana scheide* (family, Pinaceae); for perfumes; Cedarwood Virginia used therapeutically

- Cedarwood (Atlas): aromatic; *Cedrus atlantica* (family, Pinaceae); for clearing breathing passages and hair and skin care

- Cedarwood Virginia: woodsy; *Juniperus virginiana, J. communis* (family, Cupressaceae); therapeutic oil from ancient times; astringent useful for protection and care of oily and blemished skin, as an inhalant relieves coughs and colds, as moth repellent, for cellulite, and as Tibetan temple incense; use in moderation during pregnancy; from wood, United States; production method: steam distillation; also used as antiseptic, skin conditioner, deodorant, insect repellent, soothing agent; blends well with patchouli, vetiver, sandalwood

- Celery seed: sweet, spicy; *Alpium graveolens* (family, Apiaceae [Umbelliferae]); may stimulate milk flow, balance hormones, relieve liver and elimination system problems; from seeds, India; production method: steam distillation; blends well with basil, cajeput, chamomile, grapefruit, guaicwood, lemon, orange, palmarosa, rosemary

- Chamomile, German: fruity, an absolute; *Matricaria chamomilla* or *M. recutia* (family, Asteraceae [Compositae]); also known as blue chamomile or chamomile matricaria (blue color is from azulene formed during distillation of the oil); for massage oils and herbal mixtures; from flowers, Germany; production method: steam distillation; also used as muscle relaxant, soothing agent, skin conditioner, aphrodisiac; blends well with bergamot, jasmine, labdanum, neroli, clary sage, rose

- Chamomile, Roman: fruity; *Chamaemelum nobile* or *Anthemis nobilis* (family, Asteraceae [Compositae]); for soothing effect, protection of dry skin, treatment of nervous headache, insomnia, menstrual disorders; except for individuals sensitive to ragweed, oil comfort during high-pollen seasons; one of the few essential oils for use on inflamed skin conditions; blends well with lavender, bergamot, jasmine, neroli, clary sage; from flowers, Europe; production method: steam distillation

- Chamomile Moroc (Sauvage): calming, aromatic; *Anthemis mixta, Ormenis mixta, O. multicaulis* (family, Asteraceae [Compositae]); not a true chamomile; for soothing intestinal symptoms; from blossoms, Morocco; production method: steam distillation; blends well with cypress, labdanum, lavandin, lavender, vetiver, cedarwood, olibanum

- Champaca flower and leaf: calming, euphoric; *Michelia alba, M. champaca* (family, Magnoliaceae); also known as frangipani; for mental clarity and alertness

- Cinnamon (bark and leaf): spicy; *Cinnamomum zeylanicum, C. verum, Laurus cinnamomum* (family, Lauraceae); strong, warming antiseptic, comforting oil during cold season, room fragrance; from leaves and stems, Sri Lanka; production method: steam distillation; also used as anti-inflammatory agent, aphrodisiac, skin conditioner, deodorant; blends well with caraway, citrus oils, clove, myrtle, nutmeg, olibanum; may irritate skin

- Citronella: citrus; *Cymbopogon nardus, Andropogon nardus* (family, Poaceae [Gramineae]); from Java; natural deodorizer, insect and cat repellent; production method: steam distillation; blends well with bergamot, lemon, orange, lemongrass

- Clary sage: herbaceous; *Salvia sclerea* (family, Lamiaceae [Labiatae]); contains hormone-like compound similar to estrogen; for massage on muscles and on abdomen before and during menstruation; induces feeling of well-being, may induce vivid dreams; for oily hair and skin, dandruff, treatment of wrinkles; has sensual properties; from flowering tops, Morocco; production method: steam distillation; also used as skin conditioner, astringent, soothing agent, aphrodisiac, muscle relaxant; blends well with cedarwood, labdanum, citrus oils, lavender lavandin; not for use during pregnancy; do not drink alcohol or drive

- Clove (bud, leaf, and stem): spicy; *Syzygium aromaticum, Eugenia caryophyllata, E. aromaticia, E. caryophyllus* (family, Myrtaceae); antiseptic and stimulating oil used in mouthwash and gargle, applied topically to gums to relieve toothache; also used as mosquito repellent; potent skin irritant; use carefully; not for use during pregnancy; from flowers, Madagascar; production method: steam distillation; blends well with basil, black pepper, cinnamon, citronella, grapefruit, lemon, nutmeg, orange, peppermint, rosemary, rose

- Coffee: stimulant; *Coffea arabica* (family, Rubiaceae); adrenal gland and nervous system stimulant; use with caution

- Copaiba: *Copaifera officinalis* (family, Fabaceae [Legumunosae]): a resinoid and essential oil; from the tree; for boosting circulation, stress reduction, clearing of air passages, and perfume fixative

- Coriander: sweet, spicy; *Coriandum sativum* (family, Apiaceae [Umbelliferae]); for massage to relieve stiffness and muscle ache; also used as bath oil; may be slightly toxic; use sparingly; from seeds, France; production method: steam distillation; blends well with bergamot, black pepper, cinnamon, citronella, cypress, galbanum, ginger, jasmine, lemon, neroli, orange

- Cornmint: minty; *Mentha arvensis* (family, Lamiaceae [Labiatae]); for clearing of air passages, boosting of metabolism, and refreshing and sharpening of senses; may irritate skin and overstimulate the nervous system

- Costus: calming; *Saussurea costus, S. lappa* (family, Asteraceae [Composite]); for flavorings and perfume

- Cubeb: spicy; *Cubeba officinalis, Piper cubeba* (family, Piperaceae); for increasing circulation, improving digestion, clearing out sinuses and breathing passages, relieving aches and pains

- Cumin: sharp, spicy; *Cuminum cyminun, C. odorum* (family, Apiaceae [Umbelliferae]); for stimulating metabolism of obese or edemic individuals, or those mentally or physically exhausted; may be slightly photosensitizing or irritating to skin

- Cyperus (Cypriol): *Cyperus scariosus* (family, Cyperaceae); sedge grass used to make papyrus, cloth, and fragrances; also used as insect repellent and a tonic for the digestive system

- Cypress: coniferous; *Cupressus sempervirens* (family, Cupressaceae); astringent oil for refreshing oily and blemished skin, deodorant, antiperspirant, massage on cellulite and on abdomen during menstruation; blends well with lavender and sandalwood; from leaves and stems, France; production method: steam distillation; flammable

- Dill: *Anethum graveolens* (family, Apiaceae [Umbelliferae]); reduces appetite, with fennel and baking soda, a constituent of "Gripe Water" (British term for anticolic water)

- Elecampane: *Aster officinalis, Hellenium grandiflorum, Inula helenium* (family, Asteraceae [Compositae]), also known as inula; used for mood elevation; also breathing aid for some asthma patients

- Elemi: *Canarium commune, C. luzonicum* (family, Burseraceae); for immune system stimulation, especially for debilitated persons; also an expectorant and aid in clearing airways; also for insomnia, meditation, and during counseling sessions

- Eucalyptus: camphoraceous; *Eucalyptus globulus* (family, Myrtaceae); powerful antiseptic, used in baths and massage during cold season, as chest-rub oil and in vaporizer as air purifier; blends well with lavender and pine; other eucalyptus oils include Australian eucalyptus (*E. australina*); lemon eucalyptus (*E. citriodora*); dives or broad-leaved peppermint (*E. dives*); peppermint eucalyptus (*E. piperita*); blue mallee (*E. polybractea*); grey peppermint (*E. radiata*); cully gum (*E. smithii*); from leaves and stems, Spain; production method: steam distillation; also for use as deodorant, antiseptic, soothing agent, skin conditioner, insect repellent; blends well with coriander, juniper berry, lavender, lemon, lemongrass, thyme

- Evening primrose: *Centhera biennis*; high gamma-linoleic acid (GLA), vitamin, and mineral content; for face and body massage blends, especially to combat dry skin and eczema

- Fennel: anise; *Foeniculum vulgare, F. officinale, Anethum foeniculum* (family, Apiaceae [Umbelliferae]); sweet aniseed-like aroma; for skin care, massage where cellulite is present; also used for digestion in breast-firming massage and promotion of milk production, use sparingly; can be a skin irritant; not for young children, pregnant women, or epilepsy patients; from fruits, Italy; production method: steam distillation; also for use as antiseptic, aphrodisiac, soothing agent, muscle relaxant; blends well with basil, geranium, lavender, lemon, rose, rosemary, sandalwood; slight dermal toxicity

- Fir needle: fresh, spicy; *Abies alba* (family, Pinaceae); dilute well; may irritate skin; other firs include Canadian balsam, (*A. balsamea*); Siberian fir (*A. siberica*); hemlock, (*Tsuga canadensis*); and black spruce (*Picea mariana*)

- Frankincense: balsamic; *Boswellia thurifera* or *B. carteri* (family, Burseraceae); also known as olibanum (*B. papyrifera*); used for centuries; soothes, warms, and aids meditation; used as incense on altars and in temples; slows breathing, controls tension, sharpens mental focus; also for toning and caring for mature/aging skin (used by Egyptians in face masks for its rejuvenating properties); related to elemi (*Canarium luzonicum*); from resin, India and France; production method: steam distillation; also for use as skin conditioner, soothing agent; blends well with basil, black pepper, galbanum, geranium, grapefruit, lavender, orange, patchouli, sandalwood

- Galangal: *Alpina officinarum, Languas officinarum* (family, Zingiberaceae); a general stimulant with stress-reducing properties

- Galbanum: green; *Ferula galbaniflua, F. cummosa, F. rubicaulis* (family, Apiaceae [Umbelliferae]); used in food flavoring, but also for mature skin care and clearing airway congestion; from resin, Middle East and France; production method: steam distillation; also for use as skin conditioner, muscle relaxant; blends well with citronella, elemi, olibanum, jasmine, palmarosa, geranium, ginger, rose, ylang ylang

- Gardenia: absolute oil; *Gardenia grandifloria* (family, Rubiaceae); mood-elevation effects; from flowers

- Garlic: *Allium sativum* (family, Liliaceae); antihypertensive, among other therapeutic and nutritive properties; not for use by individuals with eczema or psorisis; external application may irritate skin; may cause colic in babies if used by breast-feeding mothers

- Geranium: floral; *Pelargonium graveolen* (family, Geraniaceae); balancing oil for mind and body; sweet-smelling; relaxes, restores, and maintains emotional stability; astringent for all skin types (in skin-care products for fragrance and cleansing); also as insect repellent, for massage where there is cellulite, and treatment of eczema and psoriasis; blends well with other floral oils; used as a room deodorizer if mixed with lavender and bergamot; from leaves and stems, China; production method: steam distillation; also for use as skin refresher, astringent; blends well with cedarwood, citronella, clary sage, grapefruit, jasmine, lavender, lime, neroli, orange, petitgrain, rose, rosemary, sandalwood

- Ginger: spicy; *Zingiber officinalis* (family, Zingiberaceae); fortifying, astringent, comforting oil for muscle massage and nausea; blends with orange for warming winter baths, and with other citrus oils; from roots, China; production method: steam distillation; also used as aphrodisiac

- Goldenrod: *Solidago canadensis, S. odora* (family, Asteraceae [Compositae]); calming, warming; for bee stings and for encouragement of communication and meditation

- Grapefruit: citrus; *Citrus paradisi, C. racemosa* (family, Rutaceae); refreshing, uplifting, for nervous exhaustion, relief of cellulite, oily skin, toning effect on skin and tissues; do not apply to skin in direct sunlight; from fruit, United States; production method: expression; also for use as soothing agent, astringent, skin conditioner; blends well with citrus oils, especially bergamot, orange

- Guaiac wood: green, woody; *Bulnesia sarmientoi* (family, Zygophyllaceae); no aromatherapy uses

documented, but appropriate for herbal uses; from wood, Paraguay; production method: steam distillation

- Helichrysum (Italian everlasting or immortelle): *Helichrysum angustifolium, H. italicum* (family Asteraceae [Compositae]); one of approximately 500 species of helichrysum; species used as an antidepressant; freshens air, mind, and body; clears chest and sinus congestion; relieves aches, pains, and menstrual discomfort; from flower, France, Spain, Yugoslavia; production method: steam distillation; also *Helichrysum: Helichrysum stoechas* (family Asteraceae); from flower, France, Spain Yugoslavia; production method: steam distillation

- Henna (Hina): *Lawsonia inermis* (family, Lythaveae); from flower, India; production method: steam distillation and absolute

- Hops: *Humulus lupulus* (family, Moraceae); calming, sleep aid, and use in sleep pillows; mild pain reliever; may be slightly toxic; use sparingly

- Hyssop: herbaceous; *Hyssopus officinalis, H. decumbens* (family, Lamiaeae [Labiatae]); sacred to ancient Greeks and Hebrews, who used hyssop brooms to clean sacred places; warm, vibrant; promotes alertness and clear thinking; also used as air purifier and fragrance, and in treatment of colds, flu, and bruises; from roots, India, Egypt, and Europe; production method: steam distillation; also used as soothing agent, skin conditioner; blends well with celery, fennel, lavender, orange, rosemary, tangerine; not for use by pregnant women or individuals with epilepsy or hypertension

- Jasmine absolute: floral; *Jasminum officinale* or *J. grandiflorum* (family, Oleaceae); emotionally warming; relaxes, soothes, uplifts, and aids self-confidence; for stress and general anxiety; as perfume and skin-care oil; for hot, dry skin; sensual properties, aphrodisiac; use very small amount; large number of blossoms (gathered at night when scent is optimal) required to produce only a few drops of oil; from flowers, Egypt; production method: solvent, extraction; also antiseptic; blends well with floral absolutes

- Juniper: fresh, coniferous; *Juniperus communis* (family, Cupressaceae); tones, stimulates; antiseptic and astringent for bath and massage of cellulite; said to restore "psychic purity" and strengthen immune system; cleansing effect used in many men's perfumes, after-shaves, and colognes; calming effect on emotions; from flowers, Yugoslavia; not to be used during pregnancy; production method: steam distillation; blends well with elemi, cypress, clary sage, lavandin; flammable

- Khella: *Ammi visnaga* (family, Umbelliferae [Compositae]); rarely available commercially; from seeds, Egypt and Morocco; production method: steam distillation; no formal testing; not for use if pregnant or if photosensitive

- Labdanum (cistus or rock rose): balsamic; *Cistus ladanifer* (family, Cisgaceae); used as fixative in perfumes, for meditation and counseling sessions; calming, stress-reducing, and mood-elevating properties; from resin, Morocco and Spain; production method: steam distillation; also used as skin conditioner; blends well with clary sage, juniper berry, bergamot, cypress, vetiver, sandalwood, patchouli, olibanum, lavender, labdanum

- Labrador tea: *Ledum groenlandicum* (family, Ericaceae); relaxing, soporific; used for meditation and as expectorant; from aerial parts, Canada; production method: steam distillation; not to be used before driving or using equipment because of soporific properties

- Lantana: *Lantana camara* (family, Verbenaceae); rare on commercial market; from aerial parts, Madagascar; production method: steam distillation; no traditional uses as oil; avoid during pregnancy because of ketone content

- Lavender: herbaceous; *Lavendula augustifolia, L. officinalis, L. vera* (family, Lamiaceae [Labiatae]); versatile uses; relaxes, restores, balances body and mind; refreshes tired muscles, feet, and head; for treatment of burns and scarring (use with caution); blends with many other oils; from flowering tops, France; production method: solvent extract for the absolute or steam distillation for essential oil

- Lavandin: *Lavandula hybrida, L. fragrans, L. hortensis* (family, Lamiaceae [Labiatae]); hybrid plant (combining true lavender and spike lavender); camphoraceous, herbaceous, floral aroma; refreshing, purifying; used in perfumes, soaps, and detergents; blends well with many other oils, including cypress, geranium, citronella, clove, cinnamon leaf, pine, thyme, and patchouli; from leaves, France; production method: steam distillation

- Lavender spike: herbaceous; *Lavandula latifolia*; from leaves and stems, Spain; production method: steam distillation; for use as muscle relaxant, soothing agent, skin conditioner, astringent; blends well with lavender, lavandin, rosemary, eucalyptus, petitgrain, neroli

- Lemongrass: citrus; *Cymbopogon citratus* (family, Poaceae [Gramineae]); sweet, refreshing, cleansing, and stimulating tonic; in shampoo acts as shine agent; antiseptic, astringent oil; deodorizing room fragrance; may irritate skin; from aerial parts, Guatemala; production method: steam distillation; also used as insect repellent; blends well with geranium, jasmine, lavender; may irritate skin

- Lemon: citrus; *Citrus limonum* (family, Rutaceae); used in cosmetics; cleanses, refreshes, cools, and stimulates; astringent and antiseptic used to lighten dull, stained hands or to condition nails and cuticles; blends well with other oils; do not use on the skin in direct sunlight; from fruit peels, United States; production method: expression; some steam-distilled

- Lemon verbena: *Aloysia citriodora, A. triphylla, Lippia citriodora, L. tripohylla, Verbena triphylla* (family, Verbenaceae); used in perfume and liqueurs; mood-elevating, warming properties; photosensitizer; do not apply to skin before going into the Sun

- Lime: citrus; *Citrus aurantifolia* (family, Rutaceae); like lemon and other citrus oils, not for use in direct sunlight unless lime oil has been distilled rather than expressed (distillation eliminates the phototoxic effect); from fruit peels, West Indies; production method: cold expression but some steam distillation; may irritate skin; blends well with clary sage, citronella, lavender, lavandin, neroli, rosemary

- Linden blossom: floral absolute; *Tilia europaea. T. vulgaris* (family, Tiliaceae); for stress reduction and as tonic for nervous system; not for use over long period
- Litsea cubeba: *Litsea citrata, L. cubeba* (family, Lauraceae); cooling oil; for digestion and restful sleep; may irritate skin
- Lovage: *Angelica levisticum, Levisticum officinale, Ligusticum levisticum* (family, Apiaceae [Umbelliferae]); known in Europe as "love parsley"; aphrodisiac, purification properties, and aid in reducing cellulite
- Lovage root: earthy; *Levisticum officinalis* (family, Umbelliferae); rare on commercial market; from root, Europe; production method: steam distillation CO_2; may be irritating or allergenic
- Mandarin: citrus; *Citrus noiblis* (family, Rutaceae); fruits once traditional gifts to Chinese mandarins; calming, for oily skin; known in France as "the children's remedy" because of gentleness; for digestive system and, like lavender, as massage oil to help prevent stretch marks; not for use in direct sunlight; from fruit peel, India; production method: expression; blends well with basil, bergamot, camomil, clary sage, olibanum, geranium, grapefruit, lavender, lemon, lime, neroli, orange, rose
- Manuka (leptospermum or New Zealand tea tree): *Leptospermum scoparium, L. ericoides* (Kanuka) *L. petersonii, L. coparium* (Manuka) (family, Myrtaceae); used by the Maoris; properties similar to tea tree oil's; reduces stress and muscular tension; relieves aches and pains, healing to skin; from leaf and branch, New Zealand; production method: steam distilled
- Marigold (tagetes): *Tagetes glandulifera* (or *T. minuta* or *T. putuh*) [family, Asteraceae (Compositae)]; antifungal, especially for foot odor
- Marjoram (Spanish and sweet): herbaceous; *Origanum majorana, Majorana hortensis* (sweet), *Thymus mastichina* (Spanish) [family, Lamiaceae (Labiatae)]; used by ancient Greeks; soothes tired muscles; for massaging on abdomen during menstruation, to regulate nervous system, treat insomnia, as after-sports rub and as hot bath; not for use during pregnancy; sedating proper-

ties; from flowering tops, Spain; production method: steam distillation; blends well with cedarwood, chamomile, cypress, lavender, mandarin, orange, nutmeg, rosemary, ylang ylang, eucalyptus, thyme
- Marjoram, wild: *Thymus masticina* (family, Lamiacea; [Labiatae]); massage oil for sensitive skin; (*Marjoram hortensis*, or sweet marjoram, used for cooking; not for use during pregnancy)
- Massoia bark: *Cryptocarya massoia* (family, Lauraceae); for circulation; aphrodisiac properties; may irritate skin
- Melissa: *Melissa officinalis* (family, Labiatae); garden herb known also as "Lemon balm"; calming, warming, mood-elevating effect; not for use in direct sunlight; lemony aroma and sharp, floral-lemon flavor
- Mimosa: floral; *Acacia dealbata, A. decurrens* (family, Mimosaceae); antidepressant and anti-inflammatory; skin moisturizer; from flowering tops, India; production method: solvent extraction; blends well with lavandin, lavender, ylang ylang, violet, citronella
- Monarda: *Monarda fistulosa* (family, Lamiaceae [Labiatae]); for stress reduction and promotion of breathing comfort; leaves used as a substitute for black tea during Boston Tea Party era; may irritate skin
- Menthe pouliot: minty; *Mentha pulegium* (family, Labiatae, also called Pennyroyal); from aerial parts, Africa; production method: steam distillation; for toning and stimulating; not for use during pregnancy
- Mugwort (Armoise): *Artemisa vulgaris* (family, Asteraceae [Compositae]); thought to cause vivid dreams and psychic ability; for regulating female cycles
- Myrrh: smoky, balsamic; *Commiphora abyssinica, C. molmol, Balsamodendrom myrrha* (family, Burseraceae); not a true essential oil but sap or resin from a tree; centering, meditative properties; one of oldest perfumes; for chafing and chapping caused by cold; also for use as gargle, mouthwash, insect repellent, antiseptic, fixative in perfume; from resin, Somalia; production method: steam distillation; use in moderation,

not during pregnancy; blends well with clove, olibanum, galbanum, lavender, patchouli, sandalwood

- Myrtle: camphoraceous; *Myrtus communis* (family, Myrtaceae); for meditation and mood elevation; clears sinus and breathing passages; from flowering tops, Mediterranean; production method: steam distillation; blends well with bergamot, cardamon, coriander, lavender, lemon, lemongrass, rosemary, spearmint, thyme, tea tree

- Narcissus: floral; *Narcissus poeticus* (family, Amaryllidaceae); from flowers, France; production method: solvent extraction; blends well with clove bud, jasmine, neroli, ylang ylang, rose, mimosa, sandalwood

- Neroli absolute: citrus; *Citrus aurantium* (family, Rutaceae); relaxes, elevates mood; skin-care oil; sensual, antiseptic properties; aids sluggish circulation, relieves tension, stress, anxiety, apprehension; from flowers, France and Italy; production method: solvent extraction; blends well with citrus oils, rose, jasmine, ylang ylang

- Niaouli: sweet; *Melaleuca viridiflora, M. quinquenervia* (family, Myrtaceae); strong antiseptic for acne, boils, and skin irritations; as chest rub, and in a vaporizer

- Nutmeg: spicy; *Myristica aromata, M. fragrans, M. officinalis, Nux moschata* (family, Myristicaceae); antiseptic and for digestion, calming, aphrodisiac, and restful sleep with dreams; in large quantities oil is toxic; from fruits, West Indies; production method: steam distillation; blends well with lavandin, bay, orange, geranium, clary sage, rosemary, lime, petitgrain, mandarin, coriander

- Orange: citrus; *Citrus sinensis* (family, Rutaceae); considered winter oil; warming, soothing, astringent; as massage oil or in baths; not for use on skin in direct sunlight; from fruit peels, West Indies, Israel, and United States; production method: expression; blends well with citrus oils, petitgrain, neroli, orange flower

- Oregano: *Origanum vulgare* (family, Lamiaceae [Labiatae]); warming; helps improve circulation, digestion, mental clarity, and alertness; relieves muscle aches; helps increase physical endurance, energy, perspiration; may reduce cellulite; can irritate skin

- Orris root: floral; *Iris florentina, I. pallida* (family, Iridaceae); used as fixative in perfumes, potpourri, and cosmetics, and as flavoring in toothpastes and candies; may be irritating, toxic, or allergenic; from roots, Morocco; production method: solvent, extraction

- Osmanthus: *Osmanthus fragrans* (family, Oleaceae); perfume with antidepressant, sedative, stress-reducing properties

- Palmarosa: floral; *Cymbopogon martinii,* (family, Graminaceae [Poaceae]); aids clear thinking; also used for moisturizing skin care when mixed with sweet almond and as insect repellent; believed to stimulate cellular regeneration; from aerial parts, India; production method: steam distillation; blends well with geranium, cananga, amyris, guaiac wood

- Parsley seed: *Petroselinum sativum, P. hortense, Apium petroselinum, Carum petroselinium,* (family, Apiaceae [Umbelliferae]); warm, spicy; used as diuretic and for urinary tract problems; do not mistake parsley oil for parsley seed oils, which can have different effects

- Patchouli: woodsy; *Pogostemon patchouli, P. cablin* (family, Lamiaceae [Labiatae]); musky, mood-elevating; sensual, anti-inflammatory, antiseptic, nerve-stimulating properties; used for skin care and dandruff; used in the East to scent linen and clothes and to repel fleas and lice; from leaves, Indonesia; production method: steam distillation; blends well with labdanum, vetiver, sandalwood, cedarwood, geranium, clove, lavender, rose, neroli, bergamot, myrrh, clary sage

- Peppermint: minty; *Mentha piperta* (family, Lamiaceae [Labiatae]); cools, stimulates, refreshes, restores; used as insect repellent, antiseptic, and as massage blend for the digestive system and tired head and feet; may be sniffed from bottle or one drop on a handkerchief to revive during travel; from aerial parts, United States; production method: steam distillation; not for use during pregnancy; may irritate sensitive skin; blends well with bergamot, geranium, lavender, marjoram, rosemary, sandalwood

- Petitgrain: citrus; *Citrus aurantium, C. bigaradia* (family, Rutaceae); from same trees as neroli/orange blossom, but distilled from the leaves and stems, instead of petals; Europe; relaxes, restores, cleanses, elevates mood; similar properties to neroli's, has deodorant properties and helps relieve anxiety and stress; also used as hair rinse; production method: steam distillation; blends well with rosemary, geranium, lavender and bergamot, orange, neroli

- Pine: *Pinus sylvestris* (family, Pinaceae); from needles, young twigs, and cones of pine tree; stimulates, refreshes, cleanses; strong antiseptic and deodorant properties; may irritate skin

- *Ravensara anisata* (and *R. aromatica*): *Cinnamonum camphora, Ravensara anisata, R. aromatica* (family, Lauraceae); *R. anisata* from tree bark, *R. aromatica* from leaves; both used for clearing sinuses and airways, relaxing tight muscles, and relieving menstrual discomfort, aches, and pains

- Rose absolute: floral; *Rosa damascena* (family, Rosaceae); known as "queen of oils," soothing, cleansing, sensual, aphrodisiac, feminine properties; used as skin-care oil; becomes sticky at room temperature and solid at relatively high temperatures; expensive and seldom used in commercial products; not for use during first four months of pregnancy; from flowers, Bulgaria and Morocco; production method: solvent extraction

- Rose Otto: floral; *Rosa damascena* (family, Rosaceae); warm, intense, astringent; one of oldest and best known essential oils; used in all types of perfumes, for skin creams, powders, and lotions; not for use during first four months of pregnancy; from flowers, Morocco and Turkey; production method: steam distillation; blends well with floral oils, especially jasmine

- Rosemary: camphoraceous; *Rosmarinus officinalis, R. coronarium* (family, Lamiaceae [Labiatae]); warms, stimulates, revitalizes, and restores tired muscles, feet; said to promote concentration; used also as antiseptic, hair tonic, before- and after-sports rub; helps fight water retention,

fatigue, stuffy room, and cellulite; not for use by pregnant women and individuals with hypertension or epilepsy; may irritate skin; from leaves, Tunisia; production method: steam distillation; blends well with olibanum, lavender, lavandin, citronella, thyme, basil, peppermint, labdanum, elemi, cedarwood, petitgrain, cinnamon

- Rosewood: *Aniba rosaeodora* (family, Lauraceae); also known as Bois de Rose; relaxing, deodorizing; used in massage oil for tired muscles, for nerve balance, as antidepressant; may fight migraine and ward off general malaise; use oil from Waste Plantation–grown wood to save hardwood rain forests

- Sage: camphoraceous; *Salvia officinalis* (family, Lamiaceae [Labiatae]); regulates central nervous system; used for menstrual and digestive disorders; not for use by pregnant women or individuals with epilepsy; from leaves, Spain; production method: steam distillation; blends well with lavandin, rosemary, citrus oils

- Sandalwood Mysore: woodsy; *Santalum album* (family, Santalaceae); calming, grounding, musky, rich; traditionally burned during meditation and in religious ceremonies; sensual, aphrodisiac, astringent, antiseptic properties; for skin and hair care and as insect repellent and fragrance; from wood, East India; production method: steam distillation; blends well with rose, violet, clove, lavender, black pepper, bergamot, geranium, labdanum, vetiver, patchouli, mimosa, myrrh, jasmine

- Spearmint: minty; *Mentha spicata, M. viridis* (family, Lamiaceae [Labiatae]); energizing, cooling; for use in bath water, facial steam, and as insect repellent, astringent, emollient; from flowering tops, United States; production method: steam distillation; blends well with bergamot, jasmine, lavender, sandalwood

- Spikenard: *Nardostachys jatamansi* (family, Valerianaceae); promotes restful sleep, stress reduction, and relaxation; may help reduce inflammation

- St. John's wort: *Hypericum perforatum* (family, Guttiferae); antidepressant, calming, stress-reducing, mood-elevating; reduced aches, pains, and menstrual discomfort; do not use before going out in the Sun

- Styrax (liquidambar Levant storax, or Storax): *Balsam styracis, Liquidambar orientalis,* (family, Steracaceae); believed to help remove cellulite and break down lymphatic deposits, reduce inflammation, and enhance mood

- Tangerine: citrus; *Citrus reticulata* (family, Rutaceae); sweet, tangy; used as astringent for oily skin, and in drinks and desserts; not for use in the Sun

- Tarragon: citrus; *Artemisia dracunculus* (family, Asteraceae [Compositae]); energizing; said to relieve aches, pains, and menstrual discomfort and improve mental alertness; also used as astringent; from fruit peels, United States; production method: expression; blends well with basil, bergamot, chamomile, clary sage, olibanum, geranium, grapefruit, lavender, lemon, lime, neroli, orange, rose

- Tea tree: camphoraceous; *Melaleuca alternifolia, M. linariifolia, M. uncintata* (family, Myrtaceae); energizing; strong antiseptic, antifungal, and antiviral; for acne, cold sores, foot odor, athlete's foot, warts, and burns; also used as cleaning agent and for soothing skin of dogs with flea allergy dermatitis; may irritate skin; from leaves and stems, Australia; production method: steam distillation; blends well with lavandin, lavender, clary sage, rosemary, cananga, geranium, marjoram, clove, nutmeg

- Thyme (sweet): spicy; *Thymus vulgaris* (family, Lamiaceae [Labiatae]); ancient medicinal and culinary herb; for use as vaporized household disinfectant, deodorant, antiseptic; believed also to ward off rodents and get rid of fleas; not for use by pregnant women or individuals with hypertension; may irritate skin; from flowering tops, Spain; production method: steam distillation; blends well with bergamot, lemon, rosemary, lavender, lavandin, marjoram

- Vanilla absolute: balsamic; *Vanilla plantifolia;* (family, Vanilla); from seeds, Madagascar; production method: solvent extraction; emollient, aphrodisiac; aroma type: balsamic; blends well with sandalwood, vetiver

- Vetivert: woodsy; *Vetivera zizanoides, Andropogon muricatus* (family, Poaceae [Gramineae]); also known as vetiver; relaxing, grounding, sensual, earthy, smoky; helps reduce blood pressure; from roots, Haiti; production method: steam distillation; blends with lavender, sandalwood, and jasmine

- Violet leaves: herbaceous; *Viola odorata*; calming (family, Violaceae); used as soothing agent, skin conditioner; from leaves, France and Egypt; production method: solvent extraction; blends well with clary sage, basil

- Wintergreen: minty; *Gaultheria procumbens* (family, Ericaceae); cleansing; harmful or fatal if taken internally; may irritate skin; not for use during pregnancy

- Yarrow: *Achillea millefolium* (family, Asteraceae [Compositae]); sedative properties; used for chest infections, digestive problems, nervous exhaustion, menstrual problems, rheumatism, acne, scarring, burns, cuts

- Ylang Ylang: floral; *Cananga odorata* (family, Annonaceae); often called the "flower of flowers" and often "the poor person's jasmine"; sweet; long used for sensual, soothing properties, as perfume, skin care, and hair rinse; from flowers, Indonesia; production method: solvent extraction; blends well with bergamot, lavender, lemon, narcissus, neroli, palmarosa, sandalwood, vetiver

- Zanthoxylum: *Zanthoxylum alatum, Z. americum, Z. rhesta* (family, Rutaceae); also known as prickly ash; from berries of the native North American tree; used in stress and nervous tension reduction and for restful sleep

oils, herbal   See OILS, ESSENTIAL.

oja   The Ayurvedic term referring to the ultimate vital force or energy that runs throughout the body. See also AYURVEDA.

Options Institute   A teaching and training organization founded in 1983 by Barry Neil Kaufman on the premise that autism and other developmental disorders may be treated alternatively and integratively. Kaufman is the author of *Happiness Is A Choice* (New York: Fawcett Columbine, 1991), and other books. He and his wife, Samahria (Suzi Lyte) Kaufman, operate the Institute in Sheffield, Massachusetts.

organ remedies   In Chinese traditional medicine, homeopathy, and Ayurvedic medicine, herbal remedies corresponding to the body's organs and their disease or dysfunction and to the whole individual's status. For example, ginseng or astragalus may be prescribed for disorders of the spleen and lungs; hawthorn berries or night-blooming cereus (cactus), for heart problems; rehmannia (Chinese foxglove), sarsaparilla, marshmallow root, or nettle, for kidney and bladder disorders; blue cohosh or shepherd's purse, for uterine disorders; saw palmetto, for prostate problems; and bupleurum, dandelion root, or chelidonium, for liver diseases. The idea that "the herbs are organs" is derived from the writings of the Swiss alchemist and physician Paracelsus (Theophrastus Bombast von Hohenheim), 1493–1541.

Orloff, Judith   American board-certified psychiatrist, assistant professor of psychiatry at UCLA Medical School, and author of books including *Dr. Judith Orloff's Guide to Intuitive Healing: Five Steps to Physical, Emotional, and Sexual Wellness* (Pittsburgh, Pa.: Three Rivers Press, 2001).

Ornish, Dean   American physician; assistant clinical professor of medicine and attending physician at the School of Medicine, University of California, San Francisco; and attending physician at the California Pacific Medical Center in San Francisco. Ornish is also president and director of the Preventive Medicine Research Institute in Sausalito, California. A graduate of Baylor College of Medicine, he was a clinical fellow in medicine at Harvard Medical School and an intern and medical resident at Massachusetts General Hospital. Ornish is the author of books including *Dr. Dean Ornish's Program for Reversing Heart Disease* (New York: Ballantine Books, 1990). The Preventive Medicine Research Institute (PMRI) address is 1001 Bridgeway, Box 305, Sausalito, CA 94965.

orthomolecular medicine   The practice of preventing and treating disease by providing the body with optimal amounts of substances that are natural to it. The term *orthomolecular* was first used by Dr. Linus Pauling in 1968 in his famous paper in the journal *Science*. In nine reports, Pauling provided a rational basis for the use of optimal, even if large, doses of nutrients. His theory explained how evolution was shaped by the loss of the chemical machinery required to make essential nutrients. His first paper appeared in 1970, his last one in 1992. Abram Hoffer, M.D., Ph.D., was Pauling's coauthor for the two vitamin C/cancer reports. Hoffer wrote, "Until his death in 1994, Dr. Pauling contributed perhaps his most important clinical contribution, the work showing the important relationship between vitamin C levels and cardiovascular disease. If everyone were to take optimum amounts of this vitamin, many of the world's major diseases would vanish. The National Academy of Sciences refused to accept Dr. Pauling's valuable reports."

Orthomolecular medicine maintains that genetic factors are pivotal to both the structure of the body and its biochemicals. Genetically biochemical pathways vary significantly in terms of transcriptional potential and individual enzyme concentrations, receptor-ligand affinities, and protein transporter efficiency. In the presence or event of a biochemical anomaly, diseases including atherosclerosis, cancer, schizophrenia, and depression may be caused or aggravated. Correcting the amount of vitamins, amino acids, trace elements, or fatty acids in order to correct the biochemical abnormality is a major goal of orthomolecular therapy.

Hoffer also wrote in *The Journal of Orthomolecular Medicine and its Development* 1967–1996, "In 1967, shortly after the formation of the Canadian Schizophrenia Foundation, and in the USA, the American Schizophrenia Association, we published the first issue of a journal called the *Journal of Schizophrenia*. We had to create our own journals because it was impossible to obtain entry into the official journals of psychiatry and medicine. Before 1967 I had not found it difficult to publish reports in these journals, and by then I had about 150 articles and several books in the establishment press. The subsequent difficulty, therefore, did not arise from the quality and style of my writing since it has probably improved since then.

"It was pretty obvious to those of us practicing nutritional psychiatry, later orthomolecular psychiatry, that it was the content of our material which was found to be not acceptable. This was proven by the attempt of the American Psychiatric Association to censor our work even several years after papers had been published. Dr. Osmond and I appeared before the Committee of Ethics of the APA to answer why we were publicizing a treatment not acceptable to standard psychiatry called xenobiotic psychiatry by Dr. Bernard Rimland. One of the assistant editors of the *American Psychiatric Association Journal* announced that he would never allow any article from our group to appear in his journal. He had been the chairman of the task force which had out of hand condemned any of this work. This new journal was to become the forum available to practitioners of the new psychiatry which official psychiatry found so unacceptable. The peer reviewed journals did their job very effectively, i.e., they prevented any of these new ideas from appearing in their journals. Even today the Medical Index will not abstract our journals using the excuse that they do not have enough money. Peer reviewed journals do not protect the public from research reports of inferior quality, nor do they protect the public from dangerous ideas they protect the establishment from ideas that run counter to their own.

"After two years we shortened the title to 'Schizophrenia' for three years. In 1972 the title was changed to the *Journal of Orthomolecular Psychiatry* to reflect the widening use of nutrition in the treatment of many physical and psychiatric disorders. Dr. Linus Pauling in 1968 had proposed the term orthomolecular psychiatry which we recognised as the correct word to define the total interest in nutrition, clinical ecology, and the use of supplements. There were 14 volumes.

"In 1986 the name was changed to the *Journal of Orthomolecular Medicine*, to reflect the growing interest by physicians in this approach, and the fact that psychiatrists remained singularly disinterested in anything having to do with nutrition and psychiatric disease."

osteopathy A medical discipline founded on the premise that the normal body's structural and functional states are equally important, and with proper nourishment and environment the body can combat disease and dysfunction and heal itself. An osteopathic physician (O.D. or D.O.) seeks to rid the system of either internal or external abnormalities through procedures that include manipulation, medicine, and surgery. Established by Dr. Andrew Taylor Still (1828–1917), osteopathy is considered both conventional and alternative medicine.

According to Dr. I. M. Korr, osteopathy is "a complete system of health care, based on broad principles that offer a way of thinking and acting in relation to questions of health and disease." Osteopathic diagnosis and treatment are geared to promote healthy functioning by correcting mechanical imbalances within and between the structures—muscles, bones, ligaments, organs, and fascia (thin layers of tissue under the skin)—of the body. The goals of the osteopath are to restore, maintain, and improve the functions of the nervous and musculoskeletal systems.

The name *osteopathy*, derived from the Greek *osteon* (bone) and *pathos* (to suffer), that is, "disease or suffering of the bone," although the condition is not confined to bone disease, as its name may imply, but rather refers to the entire musculoskeletal system. As did Dr. Still, who viewed the musculoskeletal system as the vital mechanism of the body, osteopaths observe patients to determine the causes of disease in a holistic way. The physical integrity of the whole body is seen as one of the most important factors in health and disease. Osteopathy and conventional medicine both embrace the scientific knowledge of anatomy and physiology and clinical methods of investigation. However, conventional medicine focuses on illness, and treatment usually involves prescribing drugs or surgery to correct illness. The osteopathic approach attempts to trace anomalies or changes in function that may have occurred over a period that could have altered the relationship between structure and function. Excerpted from the book *Discovering Osteopathy* (Berkeley, Calif.: Ulysses Press, 1997) one Internet article ("Discovering Osteopathy," by osteopaths Peter Sheddon and Paolo Cosechi, http://www.articleindex.com/Health/discovering_osteopathy) recounts that an example might be "a six-year-old boy who, while playing, falls very hard on his bottom. He cries bitterly and complains of pain over his sacrum for a week or so. A kiss and 'rub it better' console him. During a sudden growth spurt as a teenager, the same boy complains of low backache. By the age of eighteen, he has his first attack of sciatica, which is helped by anti-inflammatory and muscle relaxant medicine. He gives up his favorite sport, rowing, because it seems to aggravate the problem. In his late twenties, married with a young child and a stressful job, he begins to have an irritable colon and attacks of cystitis. He takes antibiotics and changes his diet. At the age of forty, he has a major attack of low back pain and sciatica and is in bed for two weeks. At this point, hoping to avoid surgery, he visits an osteopath."

Since the time of Hippocrates, the belief in the self-healing capacity of the body has been acknowledged. Dr. Still resurrected the innate healing concept before the discovery of the law of homeostasis. *Homeostasis,* a scientific term for balance, is the process by which every living thing adapts in order to keep itself stable and function to the best of its ability. Homeostasis is a self-regulating activity, with preset limits such as, in the blood there must be a precise quantity of dissolved oxygen within maximal and minimal levels that keeps body tissues working. The human body is constantly readjusting to maintain this and other chemical and physical forms of balance. When homeostasis is thwarted by disease, injury, or other disruptive influences, osteopathic treatment helps restore balance.

The osteopatic systems theory explores the structure-function relationship in every cell of the body. This is not limited to the cell—it involves the functioning of the whole of the physical body—and it gives us an insight into our mechanisms for survival and goal of well being. A "total body memory" contained by bodily cells, according to osteopathic theory, leads to the idea of the body's requirement for the least possible therapeutic or medical intervention.

Seddon and Cosechi also write, "Osteopaths believe that health, and not disease, is the natural heritage of humans. The human body has inside itself—within certain limits—the capacity for self-repair and correction. It can create its own remedies, provided that good circulation is maintained, a balanced diet is eaten, a positive attitude is held, and—as far as possible—the individual lives in a pollution-free environment. The self-healing mechanism is the backbone and sustainer of the principles and application of osteopathy. Osteopaths believe that disease primarily originates in the individual, and so they concentrate on the person who is suffering rather than on the microorganisms that are thought to cause disease. There are, however, some stages of disease when the changes it has brought about have passed the point of return. In these cases, osteopathy can help people to function to the best of their ability, given the circumstances. Where necessary, an osteopath will refer a patient for further specialist examination and treatment."

See also HIPPOCRATES.

out-of-body experience   See NEAR-DEATH EXPERIENCE.

overheating therapy   See HYPERTHERMIA; ISSELS'S FEVER THERAPY.

Palmer, Daniel David   The American founder of chiropractic (1845–1913), who was born near Toronto, Canada, but practiced and taught chiropractic in Davenport, Iowa. His work was carried on and extended by his son, Bartlett J. Palmer. "I was a magnetic healer for nine years previous to discovering the principles which comprise the method known as Chiropractic," Palmer wrote in his autobiography. "During this period much of that which was necessary to complete the science was worked out. I had discovered that many diseases were associated with derangements of the stomach, kidneys and other organs. In the dim ages of the past when man lived in rude huts and rocky eaves, even up to the present time, he resorted to charms, necromancy and witchcraft for the relief of mental and physical suffering. His whole object was to find an antidote, a specific for each and every ailment which could and would drive out the intruder, as though the disorder was a creature of intelligence. In his desire to free himself from affliction and prolong his existence, he has searched the heavens above, he has gone into the deep blue sea, the bowels of the earth and every portion thereof. He has tried animal and mineral poisons, penetrated the dark forest with superstitious rite and with incantations, has gathered herbs, barks and roots for medicinal use. In his frenzy for relief, trusting that he might find a panacea, or at least a specific, he has slaughtered man, beast and bird, making use of their various parts alive and dead. He has made powders, ointments, pills, elixirs, decoctions, tinctures and lotions of all known vegetables and crawling creatures which could be found, giving therefor his reasons according to his knowledge.

"One question was always uppermost in my mind in my search for the cause of disease. I desired to know why one person was ailing and his associate, eating at the same table, working in the same shop, at the same bench, was not. Why? What difference was there in the two persons that caused one to have pneumonia, catarrh, typhoid or rheumatism, while his partner, similarly situated, escaped? Why? This question had worried thousands for centuries and was answered in September, 1895.

"Harvey Lillard, a janitor, in the Ryan Block, where I had my office, had been so deaf for 17 years that he could not hear the racket of a wagon on the street or the ticking of a watch. I made inquiry as to the cause of his deafness and was informed that when he was exerting himself in a cramped, stooping position, he felt something give way in his back and immediately became deaf. An examination showed a vertebra racked from its normal position. I reasoned that if that vertebra was replaced, the man's hearing should be restored. With this object in view, a half-hour's talk persuaded Mr. Lillard to allow me to replace it. I racked it into position by using the spinous process as a lever and soon the man could hear as before. There was nothing 'accidental' about this, as it was accomplished with an object in view, and the result expected was obtained. There was nothing 'crude' about this adjustment; it was specific, so much so that no Chiropractor has equaled it.

"If no other discovery had been made, this, of itself, should have been hailed with delight. It was the key which has ultimately unlocked the secrets of functional metabolism; it is the entering wedge destined to split the therapeutical log of superstition wide open, revealing its irrational and ignorant construction.

"Shortly after this relief from deafness, I had a case of heart trouble which was not improving. I examined the spine and found a displaced vertebra pressing against the nerves which innervate the heart. I adjusted the vertebra and gave immediate relief—nothing 'accidental' or 'crude' about this. Then I began to reason if two diseases, so dissimilar as deafness and heart trouble, came from impingement, a pressure on nerves, were not other disease due to a similar cause? Thus the science (knowledge) and art (adjusting) of Chiropractic were formed at that time. I then began a systematic investigation for the cause of all diseases and have been amply rewarded."

Palmer founded chiropractic on principles of osteology, neurology, and functions of bones, nerves, and the manifestations of impulse, and originated the art of adjusting vertebrae and the knowledge of every principle included in the construction of chiropractic science.

"The amount of nerve tension determines health or disease," Palmer wrote. "In health there is normal tension, known as tone, the normal activity, strength, and excitability of the various organs and functions as observed in a state of health. The kind of disease depends upon what nerves are too tense or too slack."

See also CHIROPRACTIC.

Palmer Method   See PALMER, DANIEL DAVID.

palmistry   The art of reading an individual's character and divining the future by interpreting lines on the palm of the hand. Palmistry may have originated in ancient India, and it was probably from their original Indian home that the traditional fortune-telling of the Gypsies was derived. It was also practiced in China, Tibet, Persia, Mesopotamia, Egypt, and ancient Greece. In medieval Europe it was used to discover witches, who were thought to have pigmentation spots as signs of a pact with the devil.

Though palmistry is still practiced, there is no known scientific basis for it. http://education.yahoo.com.

panchakarma   The Ayurvedic term for the five types of therapeutic internal cleansing: vomiting, purging, two kinds of enemas, and nasal inhalation. These therapies are meant to restore balance and prevent disease.

See also AYURVEDA.

Paracelsus   The pseudonym of the German-Swiss physician and alchemist Philippus Aureolus Theophrastus Bombast von Hohenheim (1493–1541), who claimed to have received his doctoral degree at the University of Ferrara. He adopted the name *para-Celsus*—meaning "beyond Celsus" (the Roman authority on medicine)—and wandered throughout Europe and the Middle East, studying with alchemists. He valued the common sense of common people more than the dry teachings of Aristotle, Galen, and Avicenna and stressed nature's healing power. He gave open lectures in German at the University of Basel and was eventually forced to flee the city as his broadmindedness scandalized authorities. His written works include *Der grossen Wundartzney* (Great surgery book, 1536). He anticipated by centuries the treatment of syphilis by mercury compounds, the realization that inhaled dust causes miners' silicosis, and homeopathy and was the first to connect goiter with minerals in drinking water. http://education.yahoo.com.

particulars   Symptoms described in homeopathic medicine as personal to the patient and expressed as "My ———," as opposed to generals, which relate to the whole person.

See also HOMEOPATHY.

past-life regression therapy   A combination of hypnosis and psychiatric analysis that can reveal experiences in past lives thought to influence illness and wellness in the present lifetime of an individual. Most recently, this technique of psychotherapy/psychiatry has been popularized by Brian Weiss, M.D., psychiatrist, head of the Weiss Institute in Florida and author of several books, including *Many Minds, Many Masters* (New York: Fireside, 1988). *Through Time Into Healing* (New York: Simon & Schuster, 1992), and *Messages from the Masters,* (New York: Warner Books, 2000).

According to Denise Linn in *Past Lives, Present Dreams* (New York: Ballantine Books, 1997), "Past-life therapy can sometimes give answers that neither traditional medicine nor traditional therapy provides. Of course, there can be many contributing reasons for our problems in life, and it can be all too easy to blame these on past-life behavior. Nevertheless, past-life exploration has proved incredibly powerful in many cases where other types of therapy have failed. Past-life exploration can assist the process of gradually realizing our full potential as conscious, loving beings." Linn claims also that past-life therapy may result in positive treatment for problems of health, relationships, emotions, finances, talents and abilities, forgiveness, guilt, and fear of death, among others.

See also INTERIOR REALIGNMENT.

Peale, Norman Vincent The American author, senior minister of the Collegiate Reformed Protestant Dutch Church of the City of New York (Marble Collegiate Church), 1898–1993, who was one of the earliest proponents of the mind-body connection through his theories of positive thinking and positive imaging. Born in a rural Ohio town, Peale grew up helping to support his family by delivering newspapers, working in a grocery store, and selling pots and pans door to door. For half a century, Dr. Peale was one of the most influential Protestant clergymen in the United States. He applied Christianity to everyday problems and had a keen understanding of human psychology. He was a reporter on the Findlay, Ohio, *Morning Republic* before entering the ministry and went on to write 40 books. With his wife, Ruth, Peale founded the Foundation for Christian Living in 1945.

As a young boy, Peale battled strong inferiority feelings. Over the years he developed and refined the message that anyone could put the principles of positive thinking and strong faith into practice and improve his or her own life dramatically. At age 34 Peale accepted a call to Marble Collegiate Church in Manhattan, where he remained for 52 years as one of New York City's most famous preachers. Membership grew from 600 when he arrived to well over 5000 today. In 1945 Dr. Peale, his wife, Ruth Stafford Peale, and Raymond Thornburg, a Pawling, New York, businessman founded *Guideposts* magazine. With little money and a strong vision they managed to raise $1,200 from Frank Gannett, founder of the Gannett newspaper chain, J. Howard Pew, the Philadelphia industrialist, and Branch Rickey, owner of the Brooklyn Dodgers. *Guideposts* was designed to be a nondenominational forum for people to relate their inspirational stories to provide a spiritual lift to all readers. Today, the 48-page magazine, under the direction of Ruth Peale, is the 13th largest paid-circulation magazine in the United States with a circulation of more than 4 million.

Peale's fourth book, *The Power of Positive Thinking*, was published in 1952—when he was 54—and has sold nearly 20 million copies and has been printed in 41 different languages. He was the author of 46 inspirational books, including *The Art of Living, A Guide to Confident Living, The Tough-Minded Optimist*, and *Inspiring Messages for Daily Living*.

For 54 years, Peale's weekly radio program, *The Art of Living*, was on the air. His sermons were said to be mailed to more than 750,000 people per month, and in 1964 a movie was made of his life, *One Man's Way*.

With the educator Kenneth Beebe in 1947 Peale cofounded the Horatio Alger Association, dedicated to honoring contemporary Americans who have achieved success and excellence in the face of adversity. The *Guideposts* family of nonprofit organizations includes the Peale Center, the Positive Thinking Foundation, and Guideposts Publications. Their mission is to be the world leader in communicating positive, faith-filled principles that empower people to reach their maximal personal and spiritual potential. Peale died on December 24, 1993, at age 95.

See also FAITH HEALING; PRAYER, POWER OF.

peculiars The homeopathic description of odd and rare symptoms that correspond to the individual rather than to the typical symptoms of a disease.

See also HOMEOPATHY.

pets, alternative healing methods for See NATUROPATHY; PET THERAPY.

pet therapy A combination of all the forms of holistic medicine used in animal healing, which are almost identical with the forms used for human health. Professionals in both fields often study together and learn from one another. Veterinary practices differ only in that the humans responsible for the animal must make all the choices for healing and provide the options for health to the pet. Currently animals can have almost every type of healing that is available to humans. The concept of alternative medicine for pets begins with the prevention of illness by designing and maintaining a healthy lifestyle with diet, exercise, stress reduction, and a nontoxic home and finding the most effective, least invasive, least expensive, and most nontoxic method of curing. Systems of healing from all over the world are available to animals. www.virtualvet.com/petowners/holistic/Holisthrp01.htm; http://education.yahoo.com

Philippine healing methods   See PSYCHIC SURGERY.

Phoenix Rising yoga   See YOGA.

physical therapy   Developed by Sister Elizabeth Kenny after the polio epidemic in the 1940s, a discipline of rehabilitation geared toward the restoration of function to parts of the body injured by trauma, disease, or loss of the body part. Exercise, massage, and applications of cold, heat, electricity, and ultraviolet radiation are included in physical therapy to help revitalize range of motion and muscular strength and ability in order that patients may perform activities of daily living. A physical therapist, who must complete an accredited physical therapy educational program and pass a licensing examination, is legally responsible for evaluating and treating patients or supervising physical therapy plans of care and programs for patients. A physical therapy diagnosis refers to the decisions made by a physical therapist concerning the appropriate treatment and rehabilitation for each patient after he or she has been treated by a medical doctor or had a pathologic diagnosis made by a physician.

phytotherapy   Another term for the practice of herbal medicine, or the herbal treatment of disease.

Pilates   A method of exercise developed by Joseph H. Pilates that has been very popular with dancers since the 1940s. Pilates was born in Germany in 1880 and died in New York in 1967. He developed a fitness regimen bearing his name and used it successfully to overcome his disabilities as a frail and sickly child. Pilates devised a series of controlled movements that engage the mind and body in developing strong, flexible muscles, without building bulk. Emphasis was placed on developing

deep torso strength and flexibility, or "centering," to ensure proper posture and to reduce risk of injury. The lithe musculature and ease of movement possessed by a cat were the image he used to illustrate the technique's objectives. The Pilates method places emphasis on correct posture and technique and does not rely upon high numbers of repetitive exercises.

See also www.stottpilates.com/pilinfo.html.

pitta   One of the three *doshas,* or basic body types, and the representation of the "Sun force," as opposed to the "Moon force," in Ayurvedic medicine.

See also AYURVEDA; *DOSHAS*; YIN-YANG.

placebo   From the Latin word meaning "I shall please," a "sugar pill" or otherwise inactive substance given as medicine to a patient who believes it is actually medicine. Used in study groups, particularly in the double-blind study technique, placebos are known to work and have the same effects (called the placebo effect) in some cases that a medication would have. The placebo is a prime example of how the mind influences the body's reactions and status. Spontaneous remission that sometimes occurs in individuals with catastrophic disease may be attributed to the placebo effect. Also, detractors of homeopathy may claim that homeopathic remedies are placebos.

See also HOMEOPATHY; SPONTANEOUS HEALING.

plant-spirit healing   The use of bioenergetic healing techniques, such as Therapeutic Touch, on plants. In experiments performed by Dr. Thelma Moss, medical psychologist at UCLA's Neuropsychiatric Institute, Kirlian photographs were taken of a plant whose leaf was severely damaged. Then Moss requested that renowned bioenergetic healer Olga Worrall hold her hand over the leaf in an effort to transfer healing energy. Another Kirlian photograph, taken afterward, showed the leaf had undergone significant energetic changes toward improvement.

See also BIOENERGETICS; KIRLIAN PHOTOGRAPHY.

polarity therapy   A hands-on technique of bodywork consisting of manipulation of pressure points and joints, stretches, breathing exercises, massage, reflexology, hydrotherapy, and nutritional and emotional counseling developed by Randolph Stone, D.C., D.O., N.D., who based his technique on the concept that illness is created by blockages of energy flow throughout the body. Stone also believed that the use of the hands—one electromagnetically positive, the other electromagnetically negative—helps release the blocked energy, and that release in turn promotes better physical, mental, and emotional status. The American Polarity Therapy Association was established in 1984.

See also BIOENERGETICS.

poultice, herbal A moist "pad" of fresh herbs used as a therapeutic topical application to relieve pain and promote circulation.

prakruti The human constitution consisting of one or more of the primary body/personality types—*vata*, *pitta*, and *kapha*, according to Ayurvedic medicine.

See also AYURVEDA; *DOSHAS*.

pranayama Yogic breathing exercises.

See also YOGA.

pranic healing Restoration of health and balance by using prana, the Ayurvedic word meaning breath, life force, or vital energy that goes through the body.

See also AYURVEDA; YOGA.

prayer, power of The belief that prayer has a direct and positive effect on people afflicted with illness. Studies have been conducted in which one group of ill individuals has been prayed for and another group has not been prayed for; the group of people who were prayed for had a better and faster recovery rate, indicating that prayer, particularly when it is done by large groups of people, has beneficial effects.

See also DOSSEY, LARRY; FAITH HEALING.

primal scream therapy A psychotherapeutic technique geared toward releasing old and intense emotional burdens carried subconsciously that may be causing illness. According to a winter-spring

1994 International Primal Association (IPA) Newsletter article by Larry King (H. Lawrence King) adapted by him from material he wrote for *Behavior Today* and read as an introduction to his 1993 convention workshop, "Primal 101": "Psychotherapy is the art and science of easing emotional problems. Many forms of psychotherapy are designed to help the client know and understand what is in their unconscious. Very few are designed to actually change *what is in the unconscious*. However, if the material in the unconscious is not changed, it retains its enormous power to occasionally override even the most powerful of egos. When it does that, we call it 'neurosis.' In one way or another, it always results in emotional pain. The unconscious is primarily a record of the past *and* a storehouse of past physical and emotional tensions. These tensions can be triggered by present events so that they are felt in the present. In fact, because their origin is from the unconscious, and we are thus unaware of their actual source, these powerful tensions seem to originate in the present, and the person or situation triggering them appears to be their primary cause—when they may, in fact, be only a very minor part of the cause.

"My understanding of the object of psychoanalysis," King continued, "is that it helps the client discover these unconscious origins of present-day tensions (and their accompanying but misplaced ideations) and to analyze and use the knowledge consciously to change present and future behaviors."

Another IPA article, by John Rowan in the fall 1999 IPA Newsletter, explained primal integration as opposed to primal scream therapy or primal therapy: "Primal integration is a form of therapy brought over to Britain by Bill Swartley, one of its main originators, although it was also pioneered here by Frank Lake. It is not to be confused with Primal Therapy, coming from Arthur Janov; it is a parallel development occurring at about the same time. It lays the major emphasis upon early trauma as the basic cause of neurosis, and enables people to regress back to the point in time where the trouble began, and to relive it there. This often involves a cathartic experience called a 'primal.' But some people using this approach do not like this language, and instead call what they do regression-integration therapy. It is strongly influenced by the research of Stanislav Grof, who pointed particularly to the traumas often associated with the experience of birth.

"In primal integration therapy the practitioner uses a variety of techniques taken from body therapies, feeling therapies, analytic therapies and transpersonal therapies, because a lot of stress is laid on the unity of body, feelings, thought and spirituality. Grof has recently written very well about this, and his holotropic therapy is close to what we call primal integration. Because of the emphasis of primal integration on early trauma, people sometimes think it is going to put all neurosis down to one trauma, happening just once in one's life. But of course traumas are seldom as dramatic as this. The commonest causes of neurosis are simply the common experiences of childhood—all the ways in which our child needs are unmet or frustrated. This is not necessarily a single trauma, in the sense of a one-off event—that is much too simplistic a view. Rather would we say with Balint that the trauma may come from a situation of some duration, where the same painful lack of 'fit' between needs and supplies is continued."

Rowan added that the goal of primal integration is straightforward: to contact and release the real self. "Once that has been done," he wrote, "enormously useful work can be done in enabling the person to work through the implications of that, and to support the person through any life changes that may result. But until the real self has been contacted, the process of working to release it will continue. Obviously the main technique is regression—that is taking the person back to the trauma on which their neurosis is based. Laing has argued that we should also talk about recession—the move from the outer to the inner world. Primal integration agrees with this, and finds that recession and regression go very well together. One of the clearest statements of the case for doing this comes from Grof: he talks about the COEX system, a set of emotional experiences which hang together for a person, and appear or disappear as a whole. It is a gestalt which keeps on reappearing in the person's life."

The International Primal Association, 18 Cedar Hill Road, Ashland, MA 01721, or 1-877-PRIMALS

(1-877-774-6257) or info@primals.org, "fosters deep personal healing, which in turn fosters the healing of our larger communities. Now, more than ever, we are committed to spreading the word about healthy emotional living," according to its website. "Many of our projects and activities, such as the newsletter, Internet support group, membership directory, peer group development, and certification program are focused on enriching our community life. Other initiatives such as our website, world-wide contact list, therapist referral list, annual conventions, and regional retreats are intended to bring more primal people closer together, and make primal life more available to those in need."

See also PAST-LIFE REGRESSION THERAPY.

psychic surgery   An alternative, highly controversial therapy that originated in the Philippine Islands. Psychic surgeons (shamans) who practice there may be located through local hotels. Psychic surgery is performed through the mind and spirit of the healer, who through a vision has proclaimed to have been given the gift of healing and psychic surgery by the Holy Spirit. While in a semitrance or meditative state, the healer' hands, guided by the spirit, "detect" parts of the body that are diseased and "inject" spiritual energy into them. Practitioners and individuals who have undergone this experience say blood, tissue, pus, cartilage, bone, worms, stones, or other substances may materialize on the patient's body. At times, it is also claimed, the spirit causes the healer's hands to enter the body and extract diseased tissue without leaving a wound or scar. The tissue closes as the hands are "taken out" of the body.

Energy projected from the healer's hands "opens" body tissue and is considered similar to a scalpel by enthusiasts of this procedure: energy appears to harmonize with the patient's body as the body is entered, and the healer's semitrance has been said to alter cosmetic appearance as well as reduce tumors and effect change in deep tissue. After psychic surgery, in many circumstances, the organs remain, but free of disease, or "cleansed," say psychic surgeons and their patients. Spiritual energy, instead of an anesthetic, as might be used in conventional surgery, is said to heal and enhance injury caused by emotional, mental, physical, dietary, or chemical trauma. The relaxation response of the patient carries the quick, painless process; no recovery period is necessary, and enthusiasts say there are no complications or risks involved. However, the psychic surgeon's hands, acting as a scalpel, are reported to create to observers a straight line perforating the skin over the diseased or injured area that causes little or no bleeding. It is said a patient is conscious throughout the procedure and able to get off the healing table without discomfort.

Psychic surgical procedures of approximately 15 to 30 minutes may include spinal adjustment, removal of tumors or cancerous growths, alignment of bones, and adjustment of internal organs such as uterus, ovaries, kidneys, liver, pancreas, and heart. The patient may have a nearly invisible mark at the area of psychic incision, which may feel slightly tender for 24 hours, according to reports of patients of Reverend Gregorio, a psychic surgeon of the Philippines.

According to Dr. Donald McDowall, author of *Psychic Surgery—A guide to the Philippines Experience*, (self-published, 1992), "It is estimated that there are more than 400 psychic surgeons in the Philippines. There is one in every big hotel in Manila. Reverend Tony Agpaoa was the most famous. *Warning:* If you choose to undergo this type of healing, determine the credentials of the surgeon you are using, believe in his healing ability and your soul's willingness to be healed. Psychic surgery is a modern expression of traditional Filipino shamanism, calling upon the Holy Spirit and other cosmic energy to achieve the healing. Practiced also in North America by visiting Filipino shamans, psychic surgery often involves the extraction of 'tumors' from the body through a bloody but painless and invisible 'incision' in the patient's abdomen. This is not a physically invasive process, and the patient is able to leave the operating table without discomfort. A highly controversial method, psychic surgery is an option for those who have faith in God."

See http://www/crystalinks.com/psychic_surgery.html.

In "Impression on observing psychic surgery and healing in Brazil which appear to incorporate (+) qi gong energy & the use of acupuncture points" (*Acupuncture & ElectroTherapeutics Research* 1997; 22:17–33), Y. Omura writes: "Most patients received injections of a dark-brown solution, which, some of the visiting doctors speculated, may be an iodine solution mixed with either alcohol or a local anesthetic. In many patients, he injected this solution near the pathological area or at an acupuncture point near the pathological area. When the needle of the syringe was in the acupuncture point, he twirled it with his fingers several times and then withdrew it. Minor surgery was performed in about $1/5$ of the patients with whom the author observed. Most of the surgical incisions were made on the midline of the tissue over the spine near the pathological area. The clamping of blood vessels and the closings of the surgical wounds were performed by licensed surgeons or licensed nurses. The main treatment appears to be the application of external Qi Gong energy through the fingers of the right-hand, in combination with Shiatsu Massage and a manual procedure resembling chiropractic manipulation."

The late Reverend Agpaoa, who operated an international travel agency, was indicted for fraud associated with psychic surgery in 1967. He forfeited a $25,000 bond when he jumped bail and returned to the Philippines. The controversy of psychic surgery does not deter the surgeons, who claim that the patient's mind and willingness are the components of the healing and that the drama provided by the procedure gives patients greater confidence.

In two articles published in *Vancouver Magazine* ("No anesthetic, no knife; bail-jumping Reverend Antonia Agpaoa will heal you with his bare hands," 1978 July: 45–47, and "Trick or treatment?" 1978 July: 47), G. Marchant writes: "A recent Yukon Medical Association report on psychic surgery notes that some individuals with chronic, non-specific disorders who had undergone psychic surgery showed marked subjective improvement." The Philippine Medical Association (PMA) claims: "[The surgeons] take advantage of the gullibility of people. We know that they are fooling the people, but it is hard to do anything about it. Patients won't complain. Either they are ashamed that they have been made fools of, or they have died—so we usually have no proof against faith healers." Marchant added: "The Canadian Embassy in Manila had signed three death certificates for people who would never return alive from their miracle tours (although not from Agpaoa's tours). Of more than 20 known cancer cases who went to Baguio from Vancouver three and fours years ago, not one is still alive according to the BC Cancer Agency. . . . In 1974, Donald F. Wright and Carol Wright testified before a U.S. Federal Trade Commission hearing in Seattle investigating travel agents promoting tours to visit the Philippine healers. The Wrights, from Iowa, students and believers of ESP and magnetic healing, traveled to the Philippines in 1973 to study psychic surgery. Eventually they were convinced that what they saw was not surgery but trickery, and they learned the methods from their surgeon teacher. They were taught how to shop for animal parts used to make up a 'bullet.' A bullet is actual animal tissue or a clot of animal blood and cotton, which is made to appear like tissue coming from inside the body. They were taught how to make the bullet, wrap it, prepare the tissue, how to hide the bullet and then how to transfer it onto the patient." (Source: http://www.bccancer.bc.ca/PPI/UnconventionalTherapie)

In his essay "Unraveling the Enigma of Psychic Surgery" (http://www.ca-sps.org/HarveyJMartinIII.html, 1999), Harvey J. Martin III wrote: "While the persecution of the Filipino healers was getting into gear, the Institute of Noetic Sciences published a report on aspects of the placebo effect that were known only to a select group of medical researchers. One of the topics covered in the report was the little known subject of placebo surgery. In the 1950s, several American doctors conducted an experiment designed to determine the merits of the surgical procedure for angina pectoris. In the experiment, three of five patients received the operation. The other two were merely placed under anesthesia, and given a surface incision, which was then sutured. Once awakened, the five patients were monitored during their recovery from the operations. To the amazement of the physicians, a significant percentage of the patients who had received placebo operations were cured. In 1961, Dr. Henry Beecher reviewed two double-blind studies of the placebo operations. These studies convincingly demonstrated that the actual operation produced no greater benefit than the placebo operation. In a separate study conducted by Dr. Leonard Cobb and his associates, placebo surgery proved to be more effective than the real thing. Cobb reported that fully 43% of the patients who received placebo surgery reported both subjective and objective improvement. In the patients who had received the real operation, only 32% reported satisfactory results. What this research established is that the mere form (metaphor) of surgical procedures can produce the same results as the actual surgical procedures." (Source: http://www.metamind.net/enigmaipsysur.html)

The National Council against Health Fraud (NCAHF) Consumer Information Statements on Faith Healing and Psychic Surgery (1987) offer guidelines on psychic surgery and other alternative healing methods: "(1) 'Faith healing' refers to the apparently beneficial outcomes of rituals or religious activities on behalf of the afflicted. Unless such outcomes are clearly miraculous (e.g., the restoration of an amputated body part) they may simply be regarded as fortuitous and probably involving psychological mechanisms. This does not deny the value of faith healing for psychological conditions but places limitations upon its usefulness for the purpose of minimizing unnecessary harm and maximizing its possible therapeutic value. (2) Faith healing should never be done publicly or in such a manner that the afflicted must demonstrate his/her faith by discontinuing needed medications, removing supportive braces, or performing potentially trauma-inducing acts. (3) Faith healers should provide their 'gift of healing' without fee or acceptance of donations (i.e., in the example of Christ, in whose name they often claim to heal). (4) Potential healees should be psychologically prepared to accept null effects to prevent them from taking such results as a sign of divine rejection or punishment. (5) The alleged removal of diseased tissue from the body without leaving an incision as has been practiced in the Philippines for some years is denounced as a complete fraud; not only does it waste money and cause psychological harm through promoting false hope, it can prevent people from seeking valuable health care before it becomes too late for effective therapy."

NCAHF is a private nonprofit, voluntary health agency that focuses on health misinformation, fraud, and quackery as public health problems. Its positions are based upon the principles of science that underlie consumer protection law. NCAHF advocates: (1) adequate disclosure in labeling and other warranties to enable consumers to make truly informed choices; (2) premarketing proof of safety and effectiveness for products and services claimed to prevent, alleviate, or cure any health problem; and (3) accountability for those who violate the law.)

See also Appendix I; FAITH HEALING; SHAMAN.

Azuma N, Stevenson I. "Psychic surgery" in the Philippines as a form of group hypnosis. *American Journal of Clinical Hypnosis* 31, no. 1 (July 1988):61–67.

Cassileth BR. *Alternative medicine handbook: the complete reference guide to alternative and complementary therapies.* New York: W. W. Norton & Co., 1998, p. 316.

Dein S. "The management of illness by a Filipino psychic surgeon: a western physician's impression." *Social Science & Medicine* 34, no. 4 (February 1992):461–464.

Hafner AW, editor. *Reader's guide to alternative health methods.* Milwaukee, Wisc.: American Medical Association, 1993, pp. 69, 335.

psychosomatic disease   Physical symptoms and illness originating from emotional disturbances or fears, the result of mind-body connection. Psychosomatic illnesses are not considered mental illnesses but rather are treated both conventionally and alternatively, because the symptoms and suffering are real and present.

pulse analysis   Also called *Nadi*, a diagnostic procedure in Ayurvedic medicine based on characteristics of the radial pulse, including fast, narrow, feeble, cool, irregular, jumping, excited, prominent, hot, moderate, regular, slow, strong, steady, soft, broad, and warm.

See also TONGUE ANALYSIS.

purifying fruit drinks   See DETOXIFICATION; JUICING.

purvakarma   An oil and steam bath cleansing therapy used in Ayurvedic medicine.

See also AYURVEDA.

qi (ch'i)   The Chinese word (pronounced chee) for "vital energy," or "life force." According to Harriet Beinfeld, L.Ac., and Efrem Korngold, L.Ac., O.M.D., authors of *Between Heaven and Earth: A Guide to Chinese Medicine* (New York: Ballantine Books, 1991), *qi's* "can be understood as the creative or formative principle associated with life and all processes that characterize living entities. All animate forms in nature are manifestations of Qi. Qi is an invisible substance, as well as an immaterial force that has palpable and observable manifestations.

"Qi has its own movement and also activates the movement of things other than itself. Qi begets motion and heat. Within the context of the human person, Qi is that which enlivens the body and is differentiated according to specific functional systems. All physical and mental activities are manifestations of Qi: sensing, cogitating, feeling, digesting, stirring, propagating. . . . Qi governs the shape and activity of the body and its process of forming and organizing itself. Qi also means the totality of Blood, Moisture, and Qi, earth, sea, and air, the total summation of the life of the organism, body, or world."

Zheng qi refers to the normal flow of energy through the meridians and body organs. *Zong qi* refers to the energy that accumulates in the thorax, or gathering qi. *Wei qi*, known as defensive *qi*, flows under the skin and protects against environmental or external bacteria and other potential pathogens.

qigong   Also rendered *chi gong* or *ch'i kung*, *qigong* is a physical and spiritual Chinese discipline geared toward helping energy (*qi* or *ch'i*) move throughout the body for optimal functioning. Often referred to as a branch of energy medicine, the *qigong* philosophy is that clogged, impure, or polluted *qi* causes disease or dysfunction and that it can be removed or cleansed so the body may be restored to health. *Qigong* is reported to relieve stress and anxiety, improve general fitness, counter insomnia, and relieve migraines. In addition, *qigong* has been reported as beneficial to individuals with cancer, asthma, heart disease, acquired immunodeficiency syndrome (AIDS), arthritis, hypertension, prostate problems, impotence, diabetes, hemorrhoids, constipation, myopia, and presbyopia.

The practice of *qigong* may involve breathing exercises, meditation, and hands-on manipulation of energy (or laying on of hands) along the body's meridians, energy pathways that in traditional Chinese medicine are represented as a sort of road map. "Medical" *qigong* may be used as a self-healing technique and as an aid to help others heal. *Qigong* masters, as they are known, make a conscious effort through focused mental intent, meditation, or prayer to send healing *ch'i* to ailing individuals, or in a technique called "external *qi* healing" or external *qigong* they draw excessive energy, which may also be damaging, away from an individual who is experiencing dysfunction or pain. Internal *qigong*, a practice with 3000 or more variations (including t'ai ch'i) centered on self-healing, involves exercises that are easily adapted to an individual's condition, strength, and circumstances.

In *Reinventing Medicine: Beyond Mind-Body to a New Era of Healing* (HarperSanFrancisco, 1999), Larry Dossey, M.D., wrote of two *qigong* masters, Ronger Shen and Yi Wu, who "were among the first in China to learn a technique called Soaring Crane *qigong*, which was introduced to the public in China in the 1980s and which soon attracted more than 20 million adherents. When the masters came to the United States they collaborated with a research team at Mt. Sinai School of Medicine to test the effects of qigong in a sophisticated, well-controlled experiment published in 1994. In addition to the *qigong* practitioners, the Mt. Sinai team was composed of David J. Muehsam, M. S. Markov, Patricia A. Muehsam, and Arthur A. Pilla. As their 'subject,' they chose a biochemical reaction involved in the contracting of muscles that line the blood vessels and intestinal tract. The biochemical reaction is highly complex and occurs in stages. It requires the binding of calcium to a protein called calmodulin, which then activates an enzyme called myosin light chain kinase. This activated enzyme then causes phosphorus to attach to molecules called myosin light chains. The end result is the production of energy required for the contraction of muscle tissue.

"The researchers asked the *qigong* practitioners to treat the tissue samples, which were taken from animals, as they would treat a patient in real life. They stood two to five feet away from the test tubes during treatment, which lasted for six minutes for each sample. In all of nine trials, the *qigong* masters were able to modify the biochemical reaction by an average of 15 percent, which is an effect size seen in many clinically significant biological reactions in the body. The odds against a chance explanation of the outcome were less than one in twenty."

Regular *qigong* practice is said to initiate the relaxation response, that is, a decrease in heart rate and blood pressure and the optimal flow of oxygen to body tissues; alter chemicals in the brain called neurotransmitters that can moderate pain, depression, and addictive cravings; boost the immune system by increasing the rate and flow of lymphatic fluid and help the body resist disease and infection.

More information is available by contacting the National Qigong Association (NQA), P.O. Box 540, Ely, MN 55731, or (218) 365-6330, or www.nqa.org.; and the Qigong Institute, 561 Berkeley Avenue, Menlo Park, CA 94025, or www. qigonginstitute.org.

See also ACUPUNCTURE; Appendix I.

qi ni   *Qi*, or energy, that flows in the wrong direction, sometimes called "rebellious *qi*."

See also QI.

qi xian   Deficient, or decreasing, *qi*, which results in less than optimal body functioning.

See also QI.

qi zhi   Stagnant or sluggish *qi*.

See also QI.

radical healing An integrated approach to healing and healing traditions set forth by Rudolph M. Ballentine, M.D., author of several books, including *Radical Healing: Integrating the World's Great Therapeutic Traditions to Create a New Transformative Medicine* (New York: Harmony Books, 1996). The approach combines theories, techniques, and remedies from Ayurveda, homeopathy, traditional Chinese medicine, European and Native American herbology, nutrition, and psychotherapeutic bodywork.

"Besides its relation to the Latin *radix* (which means root), the term radical has a less well-known and more technical botanical significance," Ballentine wrote. "It denotes the tiniest, hairlike terminals of a plant's root, which extend its action into the depths of the soil, and, by finding and entering cracks and crevices in the bedrock, slowly fracture it and split it open. Some of the beliefs and assumptions about our reality that sustain and promote our suffering are the deepest and most resistant to change. It is those assumptions that can make diseases seem untreatable or 'incurable.' The *modus operandi* of radical healing is to penetrate the strongholds of human limitation and rend them asunder, opening the possibility of a transformation and evolution that conventional medicine has not ventured to approach. Without that probing thoroughness, that radical intensity, we will not be able to heal the profound disorders that are now plaguing us, individually and collectively."

radionics An alternative health care system and type of vibrational medicine that involves the use of special devices and a substance from a patient (a lock of hair, nail clipping, or a drop of blood, for example) to analyze and diagnose an illness. The American neurologist Albert Abrams in the 1920s experimented with cancer patients. As he tapped each one's abdomen just above the navel, he found that there was a dull sound instead of the typical hollow sound of a healthy patient's abdomen. He found the same phenomenon in patients with other diseases as well. After further investigations, Abrams came to believe that disease was actually a form of radiating energy and manifestation of an imbalance of electrons throughout the body, and on this premise he devised a variable resistance meter, or biodynamometer, to measure a patient's energy. He placed a patient's blood sample or lock of hair (referred to as "witnesses") in a container he called a dynamizer, which was then attached to the biodynamometer. He would then palpate the abdomen of a healthy individual and make a diagnosis. According to Richard Gerber, M.D., in *A Practical Guide to Vibrational Medicine* (New York: HarperCollins Publishers, 2000): "Radionics is one of the few areas in vibrational medicine capable of providing tools that allow a trained radionics operator to measure and quantify the energy characteristics of the physical body, its organs, the chakras, the etheric body, and the higher spiritual bodies. So bizarre and irrational to the left-brain, analytical, scientific mind are some of the phenomena observed in radionics that its detractors have claimed that radionics is not truly science but something more akin to magic. To the uninformed, it actually appears as if something magical is taking place during radionics therapy. But to those who are better informed about the nature of radionics and what it is capable of, this developing science provides a whole new understanding of the far-reaching potentials of human consciousness and the hidden healing capabilities of the multidimensional human being. . . . Only in the age of quantum physics and laser holography have scientific models begun to evolve that may help explain radionics."

The American chiropractor Dr. Ruth Drown took up Abrams's work after his death, but she was prosecuted for fraud and medical quackery. The British engineer George De La Warr also did research based on Abrams's theory; in 1924 a study of what Abrams dubbed radionics was funded and subsequently endorsed by the Royal Society of Medicine. Radionics remains controversial. The general concept is that a person can be diagnosed through his or her body's energy-field vibrations, evident in all parts of the body, with the aid of technological devices. The basic principles of radionics include that (1) every disease may be characterized by unique energy or frequencies; (2) humans react to the frequency, specifically detectable by a certain abdominal reflex, when they are facing geomagnetic west; (3) disease frequencies may be conducted along metallic wires; (4) radionic instruments known as variable-resistance devices serve as "tunable" electronic filters to detect one disease frequency at a time, and (5) a psychic link, even at a distance, develops between the radionics operator and the patient through the blood spot or "witness."

The radionics practitioner requests a medical and lifestyle history and a "witness," and after analyzing its vibrations with the help of a new automatic computerized treatment system (ACTS), the practitioner offers findings and recommendations for treatment.

See also VIBRATIONAL MEDICINE.

rajasic　In Ayurvedic medicine, anything that produces energy. *Rajas*, the Sanskrit word for movement, is one of the three *gunas*, the three attributes of primordial physical energy in the cosmos. In Ayurvedic medicine, *rajas* is an active, kinetic force in the body.

See also AYURVEDA.

rakta moksha　The Ayurvedic term for bloodletting as a treatment for toxic conditions of the body, such as urticaria, acne, scabies, hives, certain blood and bone disorders, enlarged liver or spleen, and gout.

rasa　A concept in Ayurvedic medicine referring to the initial stage of taste. *Rasa* is experienced as sweet, sour, salty, pungent, bitter, or astringent.

See also AYURVEDA.

rasayana　The Ayurvedic term for rejuvenation.

rebirthing　Various techniques performed on adult clients to simulate birth in order to help an individual overcome anxiety and other emotional problems.

reconstructive therapy　A treatment modality geared toward healing torn, injured, or weak joints, ligaments, tendons, and cartilage by injections of natural irritants into the joints. Used to treat degenerative arthritis, epicondylitis (tennis or golfer's elbow), carpal tunnel syndrome, bursitis, and low back pain, reconstructive therapy injections combine lidocaine or other local anesthetic with an irritant that boosts the healing process at the site of the injury or damage. Irritants are natural substances, which include sodium morrhuate (made from cod liver oil), dextrose, phenol, and various minerals. The irritant solution helps blood vessels dilate and summons fibroblasts, or healing cells, to the injured area. The fibroblasts then produce the protein known as collagen, which forms new connective tissues, facilitating the reconstruction of the impaired structure. Studies and clinical trials have shown reconstructive therapy to be effective in some cases and an alternative to surgery for some orthopedic problems.

More information is available by contacting the American Association of Orthopedic Medicine, 90 South Cascade Avenue, Suite 1230, Colorado Springs, CO 80903, or (719) 475-0032; or the American Osteopathic Academy of Sclerotherapy, 107 Maple Avenue, Wilmington, DE 19809, or (302) 792-9280.

See also Appendix I.

reflexology　Originally called "zone therapy" in the early 1900s by the American physician William Fitzgerald, an energy healing method with similar attributes to Reiki, acupressure, and acupuncture, and massage that uses the soles of the feet as a map of the entire body's zones. The nerve endings in these zones are reported to correspond to body systems, structures, and organs and therefore to impairments in any of them. The reflexologist stimulates the nerve endings in specific areas of the feet to reduce blockages of energy that may be the cause of problems elsewhere in the body. For example, the reflexology foot chart shows that the toes correspond to the head and neck, the ball of the foot to the thorax, the arch of the foot to internal organs, the heel to the sciatic nerve and pelvis, and so on. The right foot represents the right side of the body; the left foot represents the left side. Acupressure applied on the foot's reflex points may help alleviate such conditions as tension and migraine headaches, gastrointestinal problems, asthma, acne, eczema, arthritis, sciatica, premenstrual syndrome, and neurological disorders. Although reflexology generally has no adverse effects, caution is indicated for pregnant women, who may experience uterine contractions when certain areas of the feet are stimulated. Also, individuals who have pacemakers, gallstones, kidney stones, phlebitis, thrombosis, lower-limb vascular problems, ulcers, foot injury, or blood clots should consult a physician before choosing reflexology.

Reflexology as it is practiced today was adapted from Dr. Fitzgerald's zone therapy by the nurse and physiotherapist Eunice Ingham in the 1930s. The author of a book on the reflexology theory, Ingham created the foot chart and identified the reflex points. Her nephew, Dwight Byers, continued Ingham's work and became known as the leading authority on reflexology. More information is available by contacting the American Reflexology Certification Board and Information Service, P.O. Box 620607, Littleton, CO 80162, or (303) 933-6921.

See also Appendix I; ZONE THERAPY.

refrigerant In Ayurvedic medicine, foods or herbs that are categorized as cooling, or capable of reducing body temperature. Examples of cooling substances are dandelion root, rhubarb, pomegranate, unsalted butter, unsalted cheese, ghee (milk or butter fat clarified by boiling), goat's milk, mother's milk, coconut oil, maple syrup, lentils, garbanzos, soybeans, broccoli, cabbage, carrots, celery, cauliflower, cucumber, lettuce, okra, white potato, spinach, sprouts, zucchini, apple, banana, figs, grapes, melon, pears, saffron, coriander seeds, barley, basmati rice, wheat, and white rice. Cooling foods are usually prescribed for individuals with a *pitta* constitution, that is, a general body type described as a moderate frame and body

weight; soft, oily, warm, fair skin; aggressive, intelligent personality; sharp memory; fiery or violent dreams; moderate financial status; fanatic faith; irritable, jealous nature; excessive thirst; and good appetite. Refrigerants help balance the "fiery" type of body and personality. Refrigerants are also used in homeopathic medicine.

See also AYURVEDA; HOMEOPATHY.

Reich, Wilhelm Twentieth-century medical doctor and former student of Sigmund Freud who developed Reichian therapy, a system of bodywork and breathing exercises that helps unblock repressed emotions that may be causing muscle tension, pain, and misalignment, which Reich referred to as "armoring." In addition to breathing techniques, Reichian therapy includes movement such as kicking to release emotional tension.

Reiki A branch of energy medicine involving intense mental focus and the laying on of hands, named from the Japanese words *rei* and *ki*, meaning "universal life energy." Reiki's main premise is to direct or infuse healing energy to the body in order to rebalance blocked energies, release toxins, and activate innate healing capabilities. Unlike students of other energy healing methods and disciplines, Reiki students are given "attunements," processes similar to rites of passage in religious practices, by Reiki masters, rendering them open and able to draw upon healing energy from the universe and channel it in a therapeutic way. Some Reiki practitioners believe they are helped by healing spirit guides or by a higher spiritual force.

The modern practice of Reiki is attributed to Dr. Mikao Usui, who in the early 1900s was principal of Doshisha University in Kyoto, Japan, and a Christian minister as well. Incorporating Japanese symbols that are said to summon a higher power and adapting ancient healing techniques used by Jesus and Buddha, Usui developed a safe, non-invasive therapy that works on physical, mental, and spiritual levels for both the practitioner and the Reiki recipient. Now a mainstream course offered to nurses and other health care professionals, Reiki is credited for its ability to relieve pain, reduce stress and anxiety, mitigate the nausea and vomiting associated with chemotherapy and radiation, and produce other positive effects. There are various schools of Reiki, including White Light Reiki, and each practitioner may develop his or her own personal style.

The actual Reiki sessions, which may last from 45 minutes to more than an hour, involve a laying on of hands working with all seven chakras, or energy zones, of the body, and meditation, prayer, or intense focus of the practitioner. The practitioner (who serves merely as a conduit) directs healing energy through his or her hands to each of the body's seven chakras. Reiki has been shown to be beneficial as a complementary treatment for chronic and acute ailments, including back pain, migraines, sinusitis, stress-related and menstrual problems, arthritis, asthma, eczema, depression, insomnia, cystitis, sciatica, malfunctions of the endocrine system, and chronic fatigue syndrome. Reiki is also used to assist in the healing process for patients recovering from surgery. Although Reiki is generally considered safe, individuals with diabetes must be informed that Reiki can affect the body's insulin level and must be monitored carefully if they choose to receive Reiki treatments. Furthermore, individuals with pacemakers may be unpredictably affected by Reiki energy, and it is recommended that treatments be either refused or performed with extreme caution. Reiki may be used safely on plants, foods, animals, environments, and life in general. Essentially giving Reiki heightens the energy level of a living organism or an inanimate object, such as a computer or car engine, and may be given directly or as distance healing.

See also CHAKRAS.

rejuvenation therapy   Any treatment modality or technique that helps restore health, vitality, and optimal level of functioning. Rejuvenation according to Ayurvedic medicine requires physical, mental, and spiritual approaches to restoring balance, health, and longevity.

See also AYURVEDA.

relaxant   Any substance or agent that induces muscular or psychological tranquility.

Relaxation Response   A phrase coined by the author and physician Herbert Benson to describe the opposite of the body's "fight-or-flight" reaction

to a stressor. The relaxation response, which involves lowered blood pressure, respirations, metabolic rate, and heart rate, has long-term beneficial effects on health and well-being and may be accomplished through the use of meditation, various mental focusing techniques, and breathing exercises.

According to Benson, regular elicitation of the relaxation response has the ability to counteract the cumulative, negative effects of stress and rebalance the body back into a healthy state. Achieving the relaxation response (which is a general term for any technique or method that induces relaxation) may involve repeating a word, sound, prayer, phrase, or muscular activity, thus clearing one's mind of the daily "clutter." Focus words can include *love, peace, relax, calm, ocean, one, om, insha'allah,* or whatever word or phrase, one chooses. The key steps are repetition of the word or words and passive disregard for intrusive thoughts. When doing the repetitions, one should sit quietly, eyes closed, in a comfortable position; relax the muscles; breathe slowly and naturally, saying the focus word silently upon exhalation; and assume a passive attitude. Stay seated for at least a minute before stopping the exercise and rising. Benson recommends practicing this technique once or twice a day for 10 to 20 minutes each time.

Many relaxation techniques have been set forth as complementary treatments for illness, including yoga, Reiki, Therapeutic Touch, meditation, and bodywork. Relaxation aids patients before and after surgery and has been shown to help counteract the effects of hypertension, chronic pain, sleep-onset insomnia, unexplained infertility, premenstrual syndrome, cancer, acquired immunodeficiency syndrome (AIDS), cardiac arrhythmias, anxiety, depression, hostility, migraine and cluster headache, asthma, and other ailments. Relaxation is considered a major factor in the practice of mindbody medicine.

See also BENSON, HERBERT.

remedy picture   The set of symptoms that characterize or dictate a certain remedy, or treatment, also known as the total symptom picture, in homeopathic medicine. As opposed to treating one symptom at a time, the remedy picture is similar to the use of a broad-spectrum antibiotic when a specific pathogen may not be identified. A homeopathic combination remedy may be considered if the individual's symptoms correspond to homeopathic substances and their potency.

remission A period in which a disease process subsides or seems to disappear. Disciplines of mind-body medicine are now studying cases of spontaneous remission of catastrophic illnesses to determine what physical and emotional changes have occurred to cause remission or in some cases complete recovery from a life-threatening illness.

ren In traditional Chinese medicine, the meridian, or energy channel or pathway, that extends down the front of the body from the lower lip to the genitals.
See also ACUPUNCTURE.

restorative A substance or agent that strengthens and helps heal the body.

Rishis Hindu seers, said to be incarnations of the god Vishnu, who through meditation gathered and set forth the knowledge base for what is known as Ayurveda, or Indian medicine. The most famous rishis were Gotama, Viswamitra, Jamad-agni, Vasistha, Kasyapa, Atri, Bhrigu, and Daksha. See http://www.clubi.ie/ov.lestat/ofgodsr.html.
See also AYURVEDA.

Rolfing A form of deep-tissue massage geared toward relieving stress and increasing energy and mobility, particularly for individuals with whiplash, chronic back pain, and muscle and spinal problems. Developed by the biochemist and physiologist Ida P. Rolf, Rolfing is based on the concept that the body should be aligned with gravity lest there be excess strain upon movement. Rolfing treatments involve vigorous, possibly painful, manipulation and pressure to break up "knots" and realign muscles. Rolfing is not recommended for individuals who have cancer, rheumatoid arthritis, and other inflammatory ailments. However, studies have shown that people who received Rolfing treatments experienced a variety of benefits, such as improved posture, greater physical strength, greater range of motion, improvements in spine curvature, and improved nervous-system response. Also, some children with cerebral palsy benefited from Rolfing.

In 1970 Rolf founded the Rolf Institute for Structural Integration, 205 Canyon Boulevard, Boulder, CO 80302, or (303) 499-5903, or http://www.rolf.org, and wrote the book *Rolfing: The Integration of Human Structures* (New York: Harper & Row, 1977).

root chakra Another term for the first chakra, located at the base of the spine and symbolizing survival and prosperity.
See also CHAKRAS.

Rosen, Marion German physical therapist who developed the Rosen Method for the treatment of chronic tension caused by unconscious memories and belief systems. The method includes breathing exercises, relaxation techniques, massage, and psychotherapy.

Rosenthal Center for Complementary and Alternative Medicine See Appendix I.

rubefacient A substance that is slightly irritating and causes redness of the skin. Examples are knotweed and smartweed, used for therapeutic purposes in homeopathic medicine.

Rubenfeld Synergy Method A body-mind energy system, incorporating components including bodywork, intuition, psychotherapy, talk, movement, awareness, imagination, humor, and compassionate touch, developed in the 1960s by Juilliard graduate and former music conductor Ilana Rubenfeld, Ph.D. The author of several books, including *The Listening Hand, Psychotherapy Handbook, Ushering in a Century of Integration, Gestalt Therapy: Perspectives and Applications*, and *Beginner's Hands: Twenty-five Years of Simple Somatics*, Rubenfeld is considered a somatic psychology pioneer. She founded the Rubenfeld Synergy Center (877-776-2468), where professional training programs are offered to those who wish to become synergists. The basic philosophy of the method focuses on awareness as the key step toward positive change, and on the body as a physical, emotional, and spiritual whole. In addition, the method integrates the idea that stored emotions and memories may cause imbalance or distress, and exercises involving verbal expression, movement, gentle touch, Gestalt therapy, Ericksonian hypnotherapy, Alexander Technique, the Feldenkrais Method, and breathing patterns, among others, are geared toward helping the individual relax, heal, and reach higher levels of self-awareness and self-esteem.

See also ALEXANDER TECHNIQUE; ENERGY MEDICINE; FELDENKRAIS METHOD; FREUD, SIGMUND.

saints, healing powers attributed to See CASEY, THE REVEREND SOLANUS.

salve In folk and other herbal remedies, a mixture of beeswax and vegetable oil for preserving herbs and spices.

samagni The Ayurvedic term for the balance of appetite, digestion, and metabolism.

See also AYURVEDA.

sangoma A male or female shaman, or healer, of southern Africa. In the Zulu culture, for example, the *inyanga* treats physical disease; the *sangoma* is concerned with the psychic world but may use similar media. After a calling to their roles by ancestors and a training period of either several months, five to seven years, or up to 25 years, *sangomas* (also called diviners) try to diagnose illness and its cause and to ward off evil spirits and antisocial individuals. The *sangoma*, who may otherwise lead a normal life and perhaps have a second job, uses various diagnostic methods, such as "throwing the bones." Part of the diviner's attire is a "swatch" made from the hair of an animal's tail. In the past, when a distant friend or relative became ill, the *sangoma* known and trusted by the family was consulted in respect of absent healing. Also, a wooden or leather doll would be created, named, and dressed for the ill person. Any of the ill person's belongings would be added to the doll as a symbol of the link between it and the person, and the *sangoma* would perform healing methods on the doll. The healer would then take the doll, place it in a beautiful model hut, feed it, sprinkle or fill it with medicinal plants, and through it try to communicate with the absent ill person. Not unlike distant Reiki or other energy medicine that may be conducted despite distance between the healer and healee, this form of healing is still viable in many parts of southern Africa and is believed to be particularly effective when the patient is an inmate in a prison or mental institution. The dolls may also be used to call back a runaway spouse.

See also VOODOO.

Selye, Hans The Vienna-born physiologist, physician, and pioneering stress researcher (1907–1982) who developed a theory of stress known as the "general adaptation syndrome" (GAS), which involves the stimulation of the hypothalamic-pituitary-adrenal axis when exposed to stress, or the "flight-or-fight response." Working in Montreal, Canada, for 50 years, Selye maintained that chronic stress experienced by an individual could eventually wear down both physical and emotional defenses, exacerbate aging, and cause illness. In 1979 Selye and Alvin Toffler, D.Sc., founded the Canadian Institute of Stress (CIS), now an international leader in preparing workplaces, communities, and individuals in the risk management strategies required for successful, not stressful transitions to their planned futures. While in his second year of medical school (1926), Selye recognized the influence of stress on people's ability to cope with and adapt to the physical and emotional pressures of injury and disease. He discovered that patients with a variety of ailments manifested many similar symptoms, which he ultimately attributed to their bodies' efforts to respond to the stresses of being ill. He called this collection of symptoms—this separate stress disease—stress syndrome, or the general adaptation syndrome (GAS). Selye continued researching GAS and wrote 30 books and more than 1500 articles on stress and related problems, including *Stress without Distress* (New York: New American Library, 1975) and *The Stress of Life* (New York: McGraw-Hill, 1976). Some have referred to him as "the Einstein of medicine." A physician and endocrinologist with several honorary degrees for his pioneering contributions to science, Selye also served as a professor and director of the Institute of Experimental Medicine and Surgery at the University of Montreal. According to the National Stress Institute, research indicates that stress is related to cardiac, gastrointestinal, skin, neurological, immune system, and emotional disorders.

See also LONGEVITY MEDICINE; NEUROLINGUISTIC PROGRAMMING.

sexual chakra   Another term for the root chakra in Ayurvedic medicine.
See also CHAKRAS.

shad rasa   In Ayurvedic medicine the six basic tastes: salty, sweet, acidic, pungent, bitter, and astringent.
See also AYURVEDA.

shaman   From the Evenki language (the Tungusic language of Siberia), the term for a priest or priestess who acts as a healer through the use of magic based on the belief in gods, demons, and ancestral spirits. Shamanism is a religious practice of people in far northern Europe and Siberia. Women shamans also have a long history in China, India, and other Asian countries and are known to use traditional medicine as well as laying on of hands, rituals, incantation, herbalism, and spiritual healing energy in attempts to cure disease. In Korea a woman shaman is called a *mansin*. A Haitian Voodoo priestess is called a *mambo*. In Hispanic culture she is known as *curandera*.
See also CURANDERISMO; KAHUNA; SANGOMA; VOODOO.

Shealy, C. Norman   A medical doctor and Ph.D., the founder of the American Holistic Medical Association, and a respected neurosurgeon. Shealy is the director of the Shealy Institute, Springfield, Missouri, a center for comprehensive health care and pain and stress management. His books include *Miracles Do Happen* and *The Self-Healing Workbook*, and he served as consulting editor for

The Complete Family Guide to Natural Home Remedies and *The Complete Family Guide to Alternative Medicine* (both published by Element Books, Boston, Mass.)

shen   In traditional Chinese medicine an individual's spirit, or a highly significant aspect of a person's mind or spirit.

shiatsu   A type of massage.
See also MASSAGE.

shivananda   A form of yoga.
See also YOGA.

Siegel, Bernie S.   An American surgeon, teacher, and prominent advocate of holistic healing. Former president of the American Holistic Medical Association, he is the author of the best-selling books *Love, Medicine & Miracles; Peace, Love and Healing: Bodymind Communication and the Path to Self-Healing: An Exploration; How to Live between Office Visits;* and *Prescriptions for Living.* For the last 20 years Siegel, until recently a surgeon at Yale New Haven Hospital, has emphasized the importance of each person's taking responsibility for his or her health and health care. He formed an organization, called EcAP, which has been highly successful in helping people with cancer. On the Internet article "Conscious Healing," Siegel said: "I'd say that the key element . . . probably has to do with group meetings. These are opportunities to get a sharing; a new family; and love. When there is the ability to express all of these feelings, an incredible healing occurs in groups. Then the other components are things like reading, meditating, living in the moment, dealing with feelings and learning to love one's self. But I think underlying all of this while talking to doctors who are dealing with heart disease, with infertility, with cancer and AIDS, is that the group seems to be the unique powerful thing. And again I call it the 'care-frontation/loving discipline.' This is a group where we are here to change. And that's a powerful part of it I think." More information is available at www.ethoschannel.com/personalgrowth/voices/bs_voices.html

In a 1991 interview with Tova Navarra intended for publication in the *Asbury Park Press,* a New Jersey daily newspaper, Siegel revealed many of his own feelings and how his practice of holism evolved. The article reads as follows:

> In the early 1970s, Dr. Bernie S. Siegel found his job as a surgeon becoming painful. The workdays never ended, it seemed to him, and patients—so many of them—died, making him feel like a failure. On the verge of despair, he decided to listen to a "guide," a voice within him, that urged him to seek a way to go beyond the role of "mechanical" life-saver. After years of personal growth, Siegel wrote in *Love, Medicine & Miracles*: "I tried to step out from behind my desk and open the door to my heart as well as my office. . . . I began encouraging patients to call me by my first name. . . . I committed the physician's cardinal sin: I 'got involved' with my patients."

> Because of this, his patients and practice took on a new meaning, and other books to describe it followed: *Peace, Love and Healing* and *How to Survive Between Office Visits*. In all his books, Siegel spouts mind/body philosophy that contributes to and augments the increasingly popular view of the mind/body connection.

> Along with the influential health professionals including Drs. Deepak Chopra, Dean Ornish, Elisabeth Kübler-Ross, O. Carl Simonton, Wayne Dyer, and many others, Siegel, who also teaches at Yale University, literally operates on the premise that a person's temperament has great impact on his physical state. In addition to being integral to ancient Eastern philosophy, religion, and medicine, the mind/body idea was summarized by Hippocrates, the "father of medicine," who said, "I would rather know what kind of person has a disease than what kind of disease a person has."

Q: What has stopped health care professionals in the past from hooking into the idea of studying spontaneous remission—the mysterious retreat of a catastrophic illness—and other forms of wellness?

Siegel: The training: diagnosis-oriented, mechanistic, not about people. If things such as spontaneous remission happen they don't understand, they say it was either a miracle or a lab error.

Q: What is the impact of your philosophy these days?

Siegel: All impact takes time, but in the past 10 to 15 years, there have been incredible changes and opening. I've been invited to speak at hospitals, medical schools, and on television, and I've received recognition and awards. But what a struggle I had at first telling professionals to see that

their patients have a room with a view and to play music the patients like in the OR! If you gave lectures or sermons and got into the scientific realm, you'd have an argument on your hands, because so much of what we all read and were exposed to was in the specialized academic journals. The medical establishment is now saying let's do research on the value of this mind/body connection. That's truly exciting, because to have gotten to that point, they had to accept the idea.

Q: According to your writing and the general literature, some of it considered "New Age," acceptance plays a big part toward well-being in modern health care and in everyday life. What accounts for the acceptance?

Siegel: That no one is against success. That's the good part, the one that can bring about institutional changes.

Q: Given your own story of how you had felt so hopeless about your profession that you nearly gave up surgery altogether, how did you come to accept the more metaphysical ideas and apply them to your practice?

Siegel: For me, it started with my mother telling me: "It was meant to be. God is redirecting you, and something good will come of it." This way of thinking sets you up to live an intuitive life rather than one based on what's officially "right" or "wrong." I also recognized that children taught me how to take care of adults. Children aren't into failure until adults fill them with it. Children shift into the spiritual realm more easily than adults. For example, children with cancer have said interesting things, such as "Maybe God gave me cancer because I'd write a book and help other people." One child said, "I never want to be a doctor because I don't want to tell people there's nothing I can do," while another child said he wanted to be a doctor "so when their hair falls out, I can say mine did, too, and it will grow back."

Q: Would you say your handle on life, with or without cancer or other disease, is one of keeping the faith?

Siegel: My basic sense is—the basic message is—the way you beat the difficulties in life is not in the cure, but how you live, love, laugh, and have faith. You can find your own way of giving love to the world. I say happiness is a choice, not something given to you. Cancer sometimes wakes people up. Life for everyone is a labor pain and a prison sentence: You can "give birth" to yourself and learn from people imprisoned who are happy people. I learn from them.

Q: What about your detractors?

Siegel: Most of that is their projection of their problem with money, guilt, shame, or blame. At times people will quote me on things I never wrote; they created or saw their own perception, like an artist doing a painting a certain unique way. It's within you to find inspiration. You learn not to be angry with attackers.

Q: What happens when you feel critical of yourself?

Siegel: I might criticize myself for having been ignorant of the upbringing of many people, people who said, "We didn't have [Siegel's] parents," etc. I had to learn to rewrite to the people in pain to clarify. Also, I have to remember that change doesn't mean I've done something wrong.

Q: Which means simply that life is unfair?

Siegel: Most people say that because they don't separate natural disaster from a neighbor burning your house down. They lump adverse effects together. If they use all their resources, however, themselves and spiritual resources, they can build in happiness in the day. Those who are ill can build in a better chance of recovery.

Q: You use the phrase "living in God's country." What do you mean?

Siegel: I mean you can learn to be in God's country where there are no schedules and no clocks. It's part of how to die laughing; people do die with a smile. It's not a fairy tale. They embrace a joy in having lived and contributed. I like to think of the most frequently asked question on earth—"Where's the bathroom?"—and the most frequently asked question in heaven—"Why was I so serious back there?"

See also MUSIC THERAPY.

Simonton, O. Carl   An American radiation oncologist and author of *Getting Well Again* (with Stephanie Matthews-Simonton and James Creighton, Jeremy P. Tarcher, Los Angeles, Calif., 1978). He founded and directed the Simonton Cancer Center, P.O. Box 890, Pacific Palisades, CA 90272, or (800) 459-3424, (310) 459-4434, and www.simontoncenter.com, and pioneered the use of imagery by people with cancer. Simonton believed that stress is the greatest single factor causing lowered immune function and the recurrence of cancer.

six stage patterns   In traditional Chinese medicine a system for diagnosing illness.

solar plexus   The region behind the stomach and between the suprarenal glands (approximately the midtorso from the diaphragm to the upper abdomen), also called the celiac plexus. Two large nerve bundles, the celiac and superior mesenteric ganglia, are housed in the solar plexus and pass sympathetic fibers to the abdominal organs. In energy medicine disciplines such as Reiki, the solar plexus is known as the third chakra (manipura), associated with the color yellow, the element of fire, the pancreas and adrenal glands, and the function of personal power and emotions. A Reiki practitioner often places both palms on a client's solar plexus as a way to make an initial energy connection before the actual Reiki treatment begins.

See also CHAKRAS; REIKI.

solar therapy   Also known as heliotherapy, the treatment of a disorder, such as seasonal affective disorder (SAD), with sunlight. Lack of exposure to sunlight has been shown to cause depression and other illnesses, and in many cases, indoor lighting fixtures with bulbs or light sources that simulate actual sunlight offer relief from symptoms.

sound therapy   The use of music, the voice, and other types of sound as a way to treat anxiety, stress, physical symptoms, and pain; to induce relaxation; and to increase the level of mental, physical, and social functioning. For example, music may help reduce stress and pain and decrease anxiety before and after surgery, in the intensive care unit, and during flexible sigmoidoscopy, cardiac catheterization, and other procedures, and it has been shown to relax infants and children, women in labor, and people with stroke or Parkinson's disease. Other sounds, including rain forest, seashore, and babbling brook, available on CDs and cassette tapes, have recently become popular for creating a certain ambience in a room, for relaxation, and for induction of sleep.

Using sound as a clinical application, the French otolaryngologist Alfred A. Tomatis developed a sound therapy to help repattern a child's auditory range and attention span. The French physician

Guy Berard also developed a sound therapy, the Berard Method, using music to improve impaired hearing. The German physicist Ingo Steinbach created the system called Spectral Activated Music of Optimal Natural Structure (SAMONAS), which was supposed to train the auditory system to process sound normally and thus foster normal speech, language, concentration, and general learning ability. Another sound therapy is toning, which requires an individual to stand with eyes closed and a relaxed jaw and repeat certain vowel sounds in order to release stress, balance mind and body, and improve his or her vocal and listening skills.

According to www.biowaves.com/Info/WhatIsSound.cfm, "Healing has often been affected by such modalities as sound, light, music therapy, and various other energy medicine techniques that alter the frequency patterns of an individual. All matter, including herbs, pharmaceuticals, and even food with its accompanying vitamins, minerals and other nutrients could be examined from a frequency perspective that may explain their biological effects. . . . This is obvious if you consider that electrons are always moving and vibrating. All healing interventions influence the body by somehow altering its frequency resonance. Computer technology such as Bio-Resonance Therapy can measure the specific frequency imbalances in much the same way as one would measure brain wave activity. The voice is a holographic blueprint of the whole body. This allows sound therapy to be more subjective since it does not depend on the skill or orientation of the practitioner. After the assessment, appropriate suggestions can be made and actions taken with respect to the identified energetically stressed issues. This laser like approach is then able to support the body. Once the body is supported, it can then utilize its own innate healing abilities to restore health. We also theorize, that since frequencies are so important to biological well-being, then there may be a correlation between health issues and one's vocal energy pattern. . . . The voice is an accurate map or holograph of the body energetics. Every individual has a unique voice energy print that may be charted with special computer software. When charted, the voice often reveals patterns of sound frequency energy imbalance. Voice frequencies appear to relate to physical, emotional, genetic, and nutritional conditions. Once the frequency energy patterns are measured, missing frequencies may be supplemented externally with a device called a tonebox. Rebalancing the frequency energy patterns supports the individual being tested in a way that helps them heal themselves. This work is analogous to brain wave entrainment. By providing a constant external input into the biological system at a frequency where it is deficient, it eventually rebalances as it learns to resonate at that frequency. For example, the Bulgarian psychiatrist Gorgi Lazanoff was able to show an increased capacity for learning, or superlearning, by playing Baroque music (1700s Bach, Vivaldi, Telemann, Handel) and having his students breathe in rhythm with the beat.

"The audio waveform is analyzed for frequencies in stress which are then compared to our experimental frequency assignments of vitamins, minerals, amino acids, bones, muscles and all manner of substances, including drugs and toxins. Once these frequencies in stress are identified, Bio-Resonance Therapy utilizes low-frequency waveforms generated with a small, "Walkman"-style tonebox and delivered through headphones, sub-woofer or a vibration transducer. Each tonebox can be programmed for up to 12 tracks, with up to 4 very accurate frequencies on each track. These low-frequency waveforms are non-invasively delivered to the body, often resulting in immediate remarkable changes. Research indicates that low-frequency waveforms seem to activate vitamins, minerals, amino acids and other biologic substances, and show promise at being able to detoxify frequencies that correlate with dangerous substances that may be prominent in the voice analysis."

See also MUSIC THERAPY; VIBRATIONAL MEDICINE.

southern African healing methods   See SANGOMA.

spiritual healing   See FAITH HEALING.

spontaneous healing   The abatement of symptoms or disappearance of disease without apparent cause. Some attribute spontaneous healing, also called spontaneous remission, to an act of God or a remarkable change of attitude or events in a person's life. In his article "Spontaneous Remission and the Placebo Effect," Stephen Barrett, M.D., retired psychiatrist and head of the consumer organization called "Quackwatch," wrote: "When someone feels better after using a product or procedure, it is natural to credit whatever was done. However, this is unwise. Most ailments are self-limiting, and even incurable conditions can have sufficient day-to-day variation to enable quack methods to gain large followings. Taking action often produces temporary relief of symptoms (a placebo effect). In addition, many products and services exert physical or psychologic effects that users misinterpret as evidence that their problem is being cured. These 'Dr. Feelgood' modalities include pharmacologically active herbal products, quack formulas adulterated with prescription drugs, colonic irrigations (which some people enjoy), bodywork, and meditation. Scientific experimentation is almost always necessary to establish whether health methods are really effective. Thus it is extremely important for consumers to understand the concepts of spontaneous remission and the placebo effect."

See http://www.quackwatch.org/04ConsumerEducation/placebo.html.

See also FAITH HEALING; PRAYER, POWER OF.

Steiner, Rudolf   The Austrian philosopher (1861–1925) who developed the idea of science of the spirit, which he called anthroposophy. His experience of the reality of the Christ was pivotal in his teachings and vision and soon took a central place in his whole teaching, in his books and lectures. From 1911 he also showed that drama, painting, architecture, eurythmy, and other arts hold creative powers that can be drawn from spiritual vision. In response to World War I (1914–18), Steiner claimed that with insight into humankind's nature, a new social sphere could be established. His ideas added to the body of knowledge in education, agriculture, therapy, and medicine. The book *Anthroposophical Medicine* (Rochester, Vt.: Healing Arts Press, 1984) by Victor Bott, M.D., outlines the medical system Steiner created, which combines concepts of both Christianity and Indian Vedanta.

Still, Andrew Taylor   The American physician (1828–1917) who founded the first school of osteo-pathic medicine in Kirksville, Missouri, in 1892. Still's two major theories were that the human body naturally contains all intelligence and remedies it needs to ward off disease, and that proper alignment of bones, muscles, and nerves is essential to optimal function. He did not believe in dispensing drugs, but as a result of his doctrine, Still's future osteopaths incorporated the use of drugs, vaccines, surgery, and other treatment modalities thought to be appropriate for each case. Today, doctors of osteopathy (D.O. or O.D.) practice alongside and interchangeably with medical (M.D.) doctors.

See also OSTEOPATHY.

stimulant   An agent or substance that intensifies energy, has a warming effect, or increases the functioning level of organs or body systems.

stomach wash   Also known as emesis therapy, *vaman*, or *vamankarm* (therapeutic vomiting), an Ayurvedic method of emptying the stomach of mucus or other excess and undesirable substances called *kapha* in individuals with asthma, bronchitis, swollen glands, diabetes, obesity, sinusitis, skin diseases, chronic cold, edema, epilepsy (between seizures), chronic tonsillitis, and migraines. Three or four glasses of licorice and honey or calamus root tea or two glasses of salt water are to be taken, and afterward one rubs the tongue to induce vomiting—and the release of emotions—until bile appears in the vomitus. Vomiting eight, six, or four times, with a one-quart maximum and a one-pint minimum amount of vomitus, is considered therapeutic. The stomach wash, a gentler treatment than *vamankarm*, involves drinking salt water and tickling the back of the throat with a finger to induce vomiting until the stomach is empty. The method is not recommended for children; elderly, frail, pregnant, grieving, menstruating, or emaciated individuals; or those with anorexia, heart disease, cavities in the lungs, or bleeding problems in the upper airways or organs.

See also AYURVEDA.

stress   From the Old French word *estresse*, meaning "narrowness," the disruption of balance causing strain, pain, or other disturbance in functioning.

Stressors—causes of stress—include fear, anxiety, crisis, joy, injury, disease, gravity, and mechanical force. Some stress is considered necessary in order for biological mechanisms to function optimally. Unmanageable amounts of stress, however, usually result in anomalies or undesirable changes in functioning. *Eustress* refers to good stress, and distress refers to bad or painful stress. Either may have a deleterious effect on the body.

See also SELYE, HANS; SIMONTON, O. CARL.

structural integration See TRAGER INTEGRATION.

subclinical symptoms Precursors of symptoms or predisposition to disease.

See also KINESIOLOGY.

succussion From the Latin *succussio*, meaning a "shaking," the act of shaking an individual in order to hear any internal splashing sounds that indicate the abnormal presence of fluid, particularly in the thoracic area. *Succussion* also refers to the homeopathic method of shaking remedy preparations.

Sufis See ISLAMIC SUFI HEALING PRACTICES.

suggestion, power of See HYPNOTHERAPY; MIND-BODY CONNECTION; NONLOCAL MIND; PLACEBO.

supplements, dietary See NUTRITIONAL THERAPY.

surgery, psychic See PSYCHIC SURGERY.

sweat lodge A Native American healing practice, similar to a steam bath or sauna to induce profuse sweating in order to rid the body of wastes, but with spiritual aspects geared to healing emotional disturbances as well as physical problems. Enthusiasts claim that pollution, artificial environments, synthetic clothing, and lack of regular exercise clog pores and block the body's natural flow of perspiration and can lead to physical and emotional problems. Depending on how hot the sweat bath is and the climate in which it occurs, a 15-minute sauna or sweat induces the heavy metal excretion that normally takes healthy kidneys 24 hours to accomplish. Body sweat flushes toxic metals such as copper, lead, zinc, and mercury from the body. A sauna is often

recommended as a supplement to treatment with dialysis machines.

Sweat can also eliminate excessive salts that often cause hypertension and urea, a metabolic by-product, which can cause headaches, nausea, and in extreme cases, vomiting, coma, and death. Sweat may also draw out lactic acid that causes painful or stiff muscles and general fatigue.

When sweat-lodge heat dilates capillaries, blood flow to the skin and heart rate increases. Impurities in vital organs are flushed out by the flow of fluids. Finnish and German doctors cite studies indicating sweat baths help persons with high blood pressure and heart problems. Congested airways open in the heat, thus relieving colds or minor respiratory problems, but sweat baths are not recommended for persons with pneumonia and major respiratory problems. The heat of a sweat bath and the often rapid cooling afterward are said to condition the body against colds, disease, and infection. Recent tests in Finland validate the practice of splashing water on superheated rocks as a way to produce negative ions, particularly if the rocks are heated by a wood fire instead of electricity. A lack of negative ions and excess of positive ions have been linked to heart attacks, aggravated asthma, migraines, insomnia, rheumatism, arthritis, hay fever, and allergies. Some causes of unhealthy ionic conditions are weather disturbances, central air conditioning, air pollution, and driving in a closed automobile for extended periods.

Spiritual Aspects

The Native American sweat lodge is said to offer spiritual as well as physical benefits. Dr. Rudolph Ballentine, in his book *Radical Healing* (New York: Harmony Books, 1999, p. 333) wrote: "The sweat lodge is a tangible expression of the intricate mingling of being tested, of being reduced to the mere bones of your life before being guided into a rebirth—a re-creation of yourself—through the ordeal of the cleansing crisis. It demonstrates in a humble, yet eloquent way the connection between physical healing and the realm of the spirit. What is released in the experience of the sweat lodge is the confining consciousness of a limited, fearful ego, and the physical encrustations that hold your body in a form that can only express such a constricted consciousness. Then you are free. The shaman used the sweat lodge to move beyond the limited consciousness of the ego to a place where he could seek guidance for those who were suffering, to transport himself to other dimensions of reality where he could retrieve the spirits of those who were lost, or even to call forth a vision of the future. To sum up, the subject of cleansing is of crucial importance, but is widely ignored."

The lodge itself symbolizes communication with the Higher Power, not unlike a church or temple. According to http://curtis collection.com/cheyennesweatlodge.html, "The lodge is often built or restored during the morning of the chosen Sweat Day. People fast while working on the lodge to help their intent remain pure, and prayer and tobacco are offered as willow (the wood of choice) or other saplings are cut, as holes are dug for the placement of saplings and as the pit for the hot rocks is excavated. Sioux sweat leader Bobby Woods said: 'Willow branches used to construct the lodge also taught bathers a lesson. In Fall, leaves of the willow died and returned to earth . . . in Spring, they come to life again. So too, men died but lived again in the real world of Creator where there is nothing but the eternal spirits of deceased things. A foretaste of this true life could be known here on Earth if they purified their bodies and minds, thus coming closer to the Great Spirit who is All-Purity. . . .' Woods also said willows used in the lodge symbolically mark off the four quadrants of the universe—everything of the world and sky was represented within the framework.

"Muskogees use willow extensively for sweat lodges, brush arbors, and medicines. Willow bark contains salicin, an analgesic and ingredient in several aspirin-like compounds. There are many ailments for which willow and aspirin are effective. Cutting or pruning willow encourages additional branches to sprout. In addition, a willow tree's life cycle reflects the human life cycle. The constructed lodge is usually a round or oval-shaped dome, representative of the womb and sometimes called 'Mother Earth's womb'. The door is low to prevent heat from escaping but lessons of humility are easily taught when one must bend low to enter the lodge. Sweats begin in silent darkness inside the lodge. The arrival of glowing rocks is a constant reminder of One-Above's penetrating goodness and radiance. Sakim, Creek spiritual leader, constantly reminds us that Silence is the voice of Creator, One Above. Sometimes, a flute is played; this represents bird song, Creator's first specific gift to the newly created. In the Pine Arbor Creation Story, birds received songs for their part in drying out land when it was covered with water—bird songs are both a form of spiritual silence and an aural blessing."

Other symbols in the sweat lodge include a small altar mound made of dirt in front of the lodge entrance, where participants can place special items, and fire, which represents various concepts according to the nation. For Creeks, for example, fire is a piece of the Sun and perfect symbol of Creator. Saunas and sweat lodges exist throughout the world, largely in North and Central America, Ireland, Finland, and much of Europe, Russia, Africa, Japan, the Mediterranean, and the Middle East. (http://www.memory.lor.gov/ammem/award98/lenhtml/curthome.html)

Edward S. Curtis, photographer and author of *Cheyenne Sweat Lodge*, volume 6 of a 20-volume set entitled *The North American Indian*, wrote: "With the Cheyenne the sweat bath is one of the most essential religious observances. Through its agency their purified minds and bodies are brought in accord with the supernatural powers. Even when it is employed in healing disease the thought is that the power of the spirits, not the steam, will expel the sickness. Certain medicine men have the right to build sweat lodges and conduct the ceremony, and they can impart the prerogative to others. In this way alone can a man obtain the sweat lodge medicine, that is, the right to have a sweat lodge built and then to preside at the ceremony. After the promise of valuable presents the medicine man instructs the novice, while his wife teaches the wife of the latter her duties. The transfer of the medicine of healing and fighting is also involved in the transaction. . . . The origin of the sweating ceremony is ascribed to the buffalo, and buffalo skull is always placed in front of and looking toward the lodge." Tobacco is smoked as well during the sweat-lodge ceremony.

See also NATIVE AMERICAN HEALING; HYDROTHERAPY.

t'ai ch'i (t'ai ch'i chuan)   A combination of meditation and martial art, which originated in ancient China. The discipline is named in the Chinese words for "Supreme Ultimate Force" and based on first learning to feel and then to direct an energy known as *chi* (or *qi*). It is said that "where mind goes, *ch'i* follows." The t'ai ch'i theories are generally taught after one has mastered the external, dancelike moves. The practical exercises follow Taoism, a reflective, mystical Chinese philosophy first associated with the scholar and mystic Lao Tzu (Laozi), an older contemporary of Confucius. Lao Tzu wrote and taught in the province of Hunan in the sixth century B.C. and authored the seminal work of Taoism, the *Tao Te Ching*.

Although Taoism has many elements, the major concept is that the world is steeped in beauty and should be viewed and treated with great reverence. T'ai ch'i also has, particularly among Eastern practitioners, a long connection with the *I Ching*, a Chinese system of divination. There are associations of the eight basic *I Ching* trigrams and the five elements of Chinese alchemy (metal, wood, fire, water, and earth) with the 13 basic postures of t'ai ch'i created by Chang San-feng. There are also other associations with the full 64 trigrams of the *I Ching* and other movements in the t'ai chi form. The notion of "supreme ultimate" is often associated with the Chinese concept of yin-yang—the dynamic duality (male/female, active/passive, dark/light, forceful/yielding, etc.) in all things. Force (or, more literally, fist) can be thought of here as the means or way of achieving this yin-yang, or "supreme-ultimate" discipline.

Dating to the third century A.D., t'ai ch'i chuan consists of two schools, Wu and Yang. Depending on the school, the number of exercises varies from 24 to more than 100. Movements are performed slowly, softly, and gracefully with smooth, even transitions between them. Many practitioners say practicing t'ai ch'i offers improved posture, alignment, and/or movement patterns, all of which, when impaired, can contribute to tension or injury. (See www.chebucto.ns.ca/Philosophy/Taichi/what.html; and www.taichinetwork.org.)

See also FENG SHUI; QI; YIN-YANG.

tea, herbal   Beverage made from various herbs, such as chamomile tea to induce relaxation and calm an upset stomach.

See also INFUSION.

Thai massage   Dating back to ancient times and originating in northern India, a combination of yoga, meditation, acupressure, exercise movement, and reflexology. Thai massage is worked on a floor with the client dressed in comfortable loose clothing. It is performed in gentle, rhythmic movements designed to energize and balance the body. Similar to acupressure and shiatsu, it has been nicknamed "yoga for the lazy." This method focuses on the major meridians, also called energy lines or Nadis, which run throughout the body. It aims to harmonize the body, to loosen blocks, and to recoup deficiencies along the energy lines. In contrast to traditional Chinese medicine, which uses acupuncture to manipulate the pressure points, Thai massage stimulates these points with healing touch and allows life energy, or prana, to circulate. It can prevent illness by dissolving blocks before they are manifested psychologically or physically. Injured athletes may recover and experience increased flexibility. More information is available at www.ancientmassage.com.

therapeutic baths　See HYDROTHERAPY.

Therapeutic Touch (TT)　Based on ancient healing practices involving the body's electromagnetic energy fields, a scientific nursing intervention formally developed in the early 1970s by Dolores Krieger, Ph.D., R.N., professor emerita of New York University, and the natural healer Dora Van Gelder Kunz, to assist in balancing the flow of human energies by directing or manipulating them with the hands. The Therapeutic Touch practitioner seeks to repattern the recipient's weakened or compromised energy flow and stimulate the immune system to boost its innate ability to foster healing.

Therapeutic Touch (TT) was the first of human bioenergetic field therapies to receive funding for further study from the National Center for Complementary and Alternative Medicine (NCCAM), which was established by the National Institutes of Health. In one study conducted by the University of Alabama at Birmingham (UAB) Center for Nursing Research, Therapeutic Touch was shown to have a positive impact on acquired immunodeficiency syndrome (AIDS) patients' immune system function and to reduce stress. In another UAB study, funded by the U.S. Department of Defense, TT was shown to be beneficial in reducing pain and anxiety in burn patients, and a more recent study suggested that TT also helps patients who are bereaved. It has also been reported that neonates and anesthetized or comatose patients may also benefit from TT, which is intended to create a feeling of integration and equilibrium through mobilizing the body's own healing energies.

The principles of TT are centering, assessment, balancing, and reassessment. Centering refers to the practitioner's summoning and maintaining a peaceful mindset before a TT session with a patient. This may be accomplished through deep-breathing or other relaxation or meditative technique, which is chosen by the individual. Once centered, the practitioner "scans," or assesses, the patient's energy field in order to perceive cues, that is, indicators of imbalance in the energy field. Usually the patient is lying down as the practitioner uses the palms of his or her hands to "connect" with the energy that surrounds the outside of the body. In general TT, the patient's body is not touched by the practitioner; TT differs from a laying-on of hands or other direct-contact therapies. Instead, the practitioner focuses on the few inches beyond the body, where the energy field may be manipulated. Energy field cues may be perceived by the practitioner as sensations such as heat, cold, tingling, or whatever is intuited. After the practitioner gains that intuitive knowledge about the patient's energy field, balancing involves several techniques: *modulating* refers to tempering the outflow of energy, *directing* refers to the transfer of energy between the patient and practitioner, *unruffling* is a clearing or smoothing of the energy field, especially in areas that are distressed. The law of opposites also applies, in that an energy field may be rebalanced by the practitioner's intuitive projection of an opposite cue.

Upon completion of Therapeutic Touch, the practitioner then must reassess the patient's energy field to determine the outcome of the session. Practitioners agree that a consistently beneficial outcome may be the result of many years of practice and development of the therapist's own sensitivity. Training in TT consists of a minimum of 12 hours of education with a qualified TT educator who meets specific guidelines of the Nurse Healers-Professional Associates International Inc. (NH-PAI), the official organization of Therapeutic Touch.

Therapeutic Touch is taught at New York University by Dr. Krieger as well as in more than 200 facilities, including medical centers, universities, and massage therapy schools, and in more than 78 countries. The NH-PAI offers a national credential, along with policies, procedures, and guidelines for scope of practice and teacher/mentor/practitioner. A variation of TT, Healing Touch, was developed by Janet Mentgen, R.N., in 1981; it uses TT in addition to other bioenergetic techniques.

See also BIOENERGETICS; KRIEGER, DOLORES; KUNZ, DORA VAN GELDER.

Thomson, Samuel　Leader of a movement of herbalists who patented his system of herbal medicine in 1813 and sold the rights to others who wished to practice it. They became known as Thomsonian practitioners, and by 1839, there were 100,000 in the United States. Thomsonians formed the Eclectic Medical Institute in 1845, on the premise of combining European herbal medicine and the herbal practices of several Native American tribes. The Eclectics, who established many schools in major American cities, published an official pharmacopoeia in 1854, which by 1909 reached its 19th edition, but because of the emergence of new drugs and a growing pharmaceutical industry, the last of the Eclectic schools, in Cincinnati, Ohio, shut down in 1939. Today's schools of naturopathy provide courses in natural and holistic medicine practices including traditional Chinese medicine, homeopathy, Ayurveda, nutrition, and herbal medicine.

Thomsonian practitioners   See THOMSON, SAMUEL.

tincture   A liquid homeopathic remedy, usually with an alcohol base.
    See also HOMEOPATHY; MOTHER TINCTURE.

tissue remedies   See CELL SALTS.

tongue analysis   Also called *jihva*, a system of diagnosis in Ayurvedic medicine based on observing characteristics of the tongue. The tongue is "mapped" according to other parts of the body (similar mapping of the soles of the feet is seen in reflexology); ailments that include sensitive colon, delicate heart, kidney disorder, bronchitis, pneumonitis, delicate lungs, unabsorbed nutrients, toxins in the colon or gastrointestinal tract, and deep-seated fear or anxiety, may be determined by markings, colorations, moisture, and other states of the tongue. Face, lips, nail, and eye evaluations are also used in Ayurvedic diagnostic measures.
    See also AYURVEDA.

tonic, hot   Folk medicine or herbal remedies for illnesses such as colds and flu and for energization and warming of the body, especially in the event of chills and achiness. Tonics may be served hot or cold, depending upon the ingredients, which may include honey, various juices, cloves, cinnamon, herbs, hot mustard powder, turmeric, cilantro, cumin, and black pepper.
    See also JUICING.

tonification   An Ayurvedic and homeopathic term for any treatment that is geared to fortifying the body and promoting a sense or state of well-being.

Trager Integration   A gentle, rhythmic, shaking massage technique, as opposed to massages that involve pressure, oils, or forceful manipulation, that helps release tension in joints. The method was developed by Dr. Milton Trager, who spent 50 years expanding his theories. Born in Chicago in 1908 with a congenital spinal deformity, Trager overcame his disability and improved his body to athletic status. When he was in his late teens his family had moved to Miami Beach, Florida, where he trained to be a boxer. After each boxing session, his trainer would give him a massage. Young Milton offered to give the trainer a massage when he looked particularly tired one day. His trainer was so impressed by the results that Milton was encouraged to treat his father, who had sciatica, which after two sessions was healed. From that point on, Trager worked on many people and a variety of conditions. At age 42 he applied to 70 medical schools before being accepted by Universidad Autonoma de Guadalajara in Mexico, where a clinic was set up for him to continue his work in psychophysical integration. In 1955 he received his M.D. degree. He continued to practice and teach for the next 20 years and cofounded the Trager Institute in 1980. There are now thousands of certified practitioners around the world. At the age of 88 Dr. Trager died in January 1997. More information is available at www.trager.com; www.magnoliaspa.com

Transcendental Meditation   Practiced by 5 million people worldwide, a simple, natural, effortless technique of centering one's body and mind in a restful state for approximately 20 minutes a day. Transcendental Meditation (TM) was founded by Maharishi Mahesh Yogi in 1957 and was first taught in Great Britain in 1960. Over 4 million people around the world have learned Transcendental Meditation (160,000 in Britain), and the first published research on this technique appeared in 1970. In 1980 Maharishi introduced Maharishi Ayur-Veda, a thorough and comprehensive revival of the world's most ancient system of health care. The TM technique requires no belief or lifestyle change, is nonreligious, is not time-consuming, and can be learned by anyone regardless of age, level of education, or cultural background.

Transcendental Meditation gives a unique quality of rest to mind and body. It allows stress and tiredness to be released in a natural way, resulting in greater energy, clarity, and enjoyment of life. Benefits include the following:

- Unfolds one's personal effectiveness and mind potential
- Reduction of stress
- Improvement of physical and mental health
- Reduction of negative effects of aging
- Improvement of relationships
- Helps in gaining self-knowledge in order to fulfill life's deepest need
- Improvement in the environment and creation of world peace
- Reduction of hospital admissions and doctor visits
- Reduction of medical expenditure
- Lowering of blood pressure
- Reduction of atherosclerosis (hardening of the arteries)
- Promotion of more positive health habits
- Decrease in cigarette, alcohol, and drug abuse

Maharishi's Vedic Approach to Health is the name given to the integrated system of health care that includes both Transcendental Meditation and Maharishi Ayur-Veda, as parts of a spectrum of approaches to improving health and well-being. Transcendental Meditation is practiced for about 20 minutes twice daily, sitting comfortably with eyes closed.

Transcendental Meditation has been taught extensively around the world over the past 40 years. Instruction involves a standard seven-step course given by qualified teachers who have undergone an extensive and systematic training program, ensuring high professional standards worldwide. Many British doctors have learned the technique and recommend it to their patients, in a number of cases the National Health Service has paid for instruction in Transcendental Meditation when it has been recommended by a doctor. Transcendental Meditation has many applications in the field of health and supports the highest ideals of modern health care. Its teachers, however, do not replace the services of a doctor in any way and always advise people to follow the recommendations of their doctor on health matters.

Research on Transcendental Meditation has been conducted at more than 200 universities, hospitals, and research institutions in 27 countries. As a result, more than 500 research and review papers covering a wide variety of physiological, psychological, and sociological effects have been written. These have been collected in six volumes of research papers, of which over 150 are reprinted from scientific journals.

Transcendental Meditation allows mental activity to settle down in a natural way while alertness is maintained and indeed enhanced. After Transcendental Meditation, individuals report feeling refreshed physically and mentally. The mind is calmer and more alert, thinking is clearer, and energy levels are increased. Benefits are cumulative with regular practice. More can be accomplished with less effort. Those with busy schedules note that Transcendental Meditation produces increased efficiency in activity; time is used more effectively. When mental and physical well-being are enhanced, personal relationships also improve; such improvement is a commonly reported and valued benefit of Transcendental Meditation.

Physiological research has shown that Transcendental Meditation gives rise to a unique state of deep rest characterized by marked reductions in metabolic activity, increased orderliness and integration of brain functioning, increased cerebral blood flow, and features directly opposite to the physiological and biochemical effects of stress, including skin resistance changes, and reductions in plasma cortisol and arterial blood lactate. Several other neuroendocrine changes have also been observed during Transcendental Meditation. Taken together, these studies clearly distinguish the physiological characteristics of Transcendental Meditation from those of sleep or simple relaxation. The most important contribution of Transcendental Meditation to health would appear to be in primary prevention. Research in the United States examined health care utilization over five consecutive years among 2000 people practicing Transcendental Meditation, as compared to control groups (from a total sample of 600,000) who were closely comparable with regard to age, gender, occupation, and health benefits. Over the five-year period the Transcendental Meditation participants consistently had fewer than half the number of doctor visits and days in hospital when compared to controls. Of considerable interest was the fact that the Transcendental Meditation group showed relatively little increase in need for health care with increasing age, whereas the opposite trend was clearly seen in controls, as would usually be expected. Hospital admission rates for medical and surgical conditions were 60–70 percent lower in the Transcendental Meditation group, with reductions in all 17 disease categories studied. For example, numbers of hospital admissions were 87 percent lower for diseases of the heart and blood vessels, 55 percent lower for tumors, 73 percent lower for respiratory disorders, 87 percent lower for neurological problems, and 30 percent lower for infections.

Reduced requirements for health care are consistent with research showing that Transcendental Meditation reduces a variety of important risk factors for disease, including those for coronary heart disease and cancer. These findings include reductions in high blood pressure; elevated cholesterol levels; cigarette smoking, alcohol consumption, and drug abuse; overweight; cardiovascular reactivity to stress; physiological and psychological stress levels; and anxiety, depression, and hostility. Transcendental Meditation also enhances potential protective factors such as job satisfaction and overall psychological health and well-being.

A number of studies have shown that Transcendental Meditation leads to clinically beneficial reductions in blood pressure. Randomized controlled trials have found that Transcendental Meditation is significantly more effective in reducing mild high blood pressure than any of the following: a relaxation technique (progressive muscular relaxation), a pseudomeditation procedure (which attempted to imitate the Transcendental Meditation technique), or a "usual care" program consisting of advice on weight loss, salt restriction, exercise, and reduced alcohol intake.

Transcendental Meditation produced reductions in systolic and diastolic blood pressure comparable to those commonly found with antihypertensive medication, but without any adverse side effects.

Further analysis showed that Transcendental Meditation produced significant reductions in systolic and diastolic blood pressure for men and women in both high- and low-risk groups on six measures of hypertension risk: psychosocial stress, obesity, alcohol use, physical inactivity, dietary sodium-potassium ratio, and a composite measure of these risk factors. Nonpharmacological methods are now recognized as crucial to therapy for hypertension, especially in patients below 60 years. For example, the United States Joint National Committee on the Detection, Evaluation, and Treatment of High Blood Pressure has recommended that nonpharmacological, behavioral approaches "should be used both as definitive intervention and as an adjunct to pharmacologic therapy and should be considered for all antihypertensive therapy."

A review of research on behavioral therapy for hypertension concluded that Transcendental Meditation provides an optimal nonpharmacological treatment and preventive program for high blood pressure because the technique

- Produces rapid, clinically significant blood pressure reductions
- Is distinctly more effective than other meditation and relaxation procedures
- Is continued by a high proportion of subjects (in contrast to lower continuation rates for relaxation techniques and the frequent problem of poor compliance with use of prescribed antihypertensive drugs)
- Has documented acceptability and effectiveness in a wide range of populations
- Is effective in reducing high blood pressure both when used as sole treatment and when used concurrently with medication
- Reduces high blood pressure in "real-life" environments outside the clinic
- Is free of harmful side effects or adverse reactions
- Reduces other cardiovascular risk factors and improves health in a general way as well

In addition, a recent analysis found that Transcendental Meditation may be more cost-effective in treating mild hypertension than medication.

A systematic review of 144 studies found that Transcendental Meditation was more effective in reducing anxiety than other techniques (including progressive muscular relaxation, methods claimed to induce a Relaxation Response, and other forms of meditation). The superiority of Transcendental Meditation remained highly significant when only the strongest and most rigorous studies were included in the analysis. Transcendental Meditation has also consistently been found to reduce depression, hostility, and emotional instability, indicating the growth of a more stable, balanced, and resilient personality.

Transcendental Meditation has been found to lead to decreased use of alcohol, cigarettes, and nonprescribed drugs. A statistical meta-analysis summarizing 19 studies on the effects of Transcendental Meditation found the technique produced substantial and highly significant reductions in alcohol, cigarette, and illicit drug use, with larger effects than other treatments, including standard therapies and other techniques of meditation and relaxation. Over an 18- to 24-month period abstinence ranged from 51 percent to 89 percent for Transcendental Meditation compared to 21 percent for good conventional substance abuse programs.

A controlled, randomized study conducted at Harvard University found that elderly individuals who learned Transcendental Meditation showed significantly greater improvements in a variety of age-related aspects of mental and physical health and well-being than subjects taught other techniques or a no-treatment control group. Those who learned a relaxation procedure that attempted to imitate Transcendental Meditation showed no improvement on any measure. Most subjects practicing Transcendental Meditation rated their technique as useful and easy to practice, in contrast to lower rates for the other techniques. Furthermore, after three years, all those who had learned Transcendental Meditation were still alive, in contrast to significantly lower survival rates for the other three groups and for the remaining inhabitants of the institutions where the study was conducted.

Individual health affects the collective health of a society. More than 40 controlled studies have now shown that about 1 percent of the population of a community practicing Transcendental Meditation, or an even smaller fraction practicing the advanced TM-Sidhi program, can lead to reduction of problems such as violence, crime, accidents, disease, and suicides and to general improvement in economic prosperity and well-being for the whole society.

See also YOGA.

trauma remedies In homeopathic medicine, potentized remedies such as *Arnica montana* administered to individuals who have experienced a catastrophic illness, injury, or event.

See also HOMEOPATHY.

tribal healing practices See NATIVE AMERICAN HEALING PRACTICES.

tridoshas In Ayurvedic medicine the three body or constitutional types known as *vata, pitta,* and *kapha* (Sanskrit terms). The *doshas* reveal many characteristics and tendencies of an individual, who may be a combination of two or all the *doshas*. *Vata* relates to the elements ether and air, *pitta* represents fire, and *kapha* corresponds to water and earth. Through analyzing the individual's body type and symptoms, Ayurvedic practitioners are able to diagnose illness or predisposition to illness.

See also DOSHAS.

U

urine therapy In Ayurvedic medicine, the practice of drinking, injecting, or externally applying one's own urine as a treatment for certain ailments or as a way of promoting health. Also called *amaroli*, urine therapy is part of the yoga and tantra tradition and is said to cleanse the body of impurities and encourage spiritual growth. Among the ailments some claim are treatable with urine therapy are asthma, flu, tuberculosis, toothache, allergies, heart disease, dysentery, edema, eye irritation, fatigue, fever, smallpox, infertility, hepatitis, Kaposi's sarcoma, morning sickness, depression, jaundice, tetanus, Parkinson's disease, diabetes, baldness, gonorrhea, leprosy, typhus, rheumatism, gastric ulcer, lymphatic disorder, bone fractures, chickenpox, pneumonia, hangover, common cold, sore throat, eczema, psoriasis, insect and snake bites, nettle sting, sea hedgehog sting, herpes simplex, sunburn, and skin cancer. A urine mask may be prepared for general skin care, and drinking urine is considered a spiritual practice that strengthens the immune system. Yogis, Ayurvedic practitioners, and others who espouse urine therapy say urine is sterile, has antiseptic properties, and contains harmless and nourishing components, as opposed to its being a toxic end or waste product of digestion. Its availability and lack of cost are also factors enthusiasts point out. Urine therapy has been practiced for thousands of years in the East, as evidenced by an approximately 5,000-year-old document describing Ayurvedic herbs and practices. Part of the document, called "Shivambu Kalpa Vidhi," which refers to "the method of drinking urine in order to rejuvenate," is named for Shiva (auspiciousness), the highest god in the Hindu pantheon. "Shivambu" means "the water of Shiva."

Urine therapy has also long been practiced in Western cultures including those of the ancient Romans and Greeks. Various uses of urine may be found in the following sources: the German encyclopedia *Johann Heinrich Zedler's Grossen Vollstandigen Universallexikon* of 1747; *The Water of Life*, by John W. Armstrong (Saffron Walden, England: Health Science Press, first edition 1944, 1990); *Auto-Urine Cure*, by R. V. Karlekar (Bombay, India: Shree Gajanan Book Depot Prakashan, 1969); *Miracles of Urine Therapy*, by Dr. C. P. Mithal (New Delhi, India: Pankaj Publications, 1978); *Urine Therapy; Self-Healing through Intrinsic Medicine*, by Dr. John F. O'Quinn (Fort Pierce, Fla.: Life Science Institute, 1982); *Your Own Perfect Medicine: The Incredible Proven Natural Miracle Cure That Medical Science Has Never Revealed!*, by Martha M. Christy (Scottsdale, Ariz.: Future Med, Inc., 1994); *The Golden Fountain: The Complete Guide to Urine Therapy*, by Coen van der Kroon (Swallcliffe, United Kingdom: Amethyst Books, 1996).

The examination of urine—urinalysis—is integral in Eastern and Western medical practices, particularly as a diagnostic test. Color, odor, amount, clarity, and other characteristics are observed while tests for acidity, alkalinity, toxins, microorganisms, proteins, and other measurements are performed by adding a sample of urine to certain chemicals or substances and obtaining results. In Ayurvedic medicine the oil drop test requires one drop of sesame oil per urine sample. Practitioners say that if the drop spreads immediately, the patient's ailment will be easy to treat, if it sinks to the middle of the sample, the ailment will be difficult to treat, and if it sinks to the bottom, the ailment will be more difficult. However, if the drop creates wavelike movements on the surface of the sample, a *vata* (one of the three *doshas*, or body types, set forth in Ayurveda) disorder is indicated. A *pitta* disorder is indicated if the drop disperses on the surface of the sample and creates rainbow-like colors; an oil drop that separates into "pearls" in the surface of the sample may indicate a *kapha* disorder.

Ayurveda also states that urine is a natural laxative and detoxifying agent and aids in nutrient absorption and fecal elimination in the large intestine. Practitioners recommend drinking one cup of one's own midstream urine every morning to benefit the large intestine. Urophiles, as urine-therapy enthusiasts are sometimes called, acknowledge that this therapy is repulsive to most people, especially because of the uremic smell and the idea that urine is a poisonous waste product. One report from the Xinhua news agency claims that more than 3 million Chinese drink their own urine to promote health.

vaginal pack, herbal   A pad or tampon with aci-dophilus powder, yogurt, or cottage cheese that may be applied to or inserted into the vagina as a home remedy for the treatment of yeast and other infections and vaginitis.

vata   One of the three body types designated in Ayurvedic medicine.

See also *DOSHA*.

vegetarianism   Generally the practice of eliminat-ing animal flesh from the diet for nutritional and/or philosophical or religious reasons. Vegetari-ans may be vegans, who do not eat any animal or animal-derived product; fruitarians, who eat only fruit and nuts; living foodists, who eat only germi-nated seeds, sprouts, vegetables, cereals, berries, nuts, and fruits; lactovegetarians, who do not eat eggs but do eat dairy products; or ovolactovegetar-ians, who eat eggs and dairy foods exclusively. Individuals in each subcategory have characteristic problems in acquiring the proper balance of nutri-ents to prevent deficiencies. Many proponents of vegetarianism, including Dean Ornish, M.D., believe vegetarianism is beneficial in the preven-tion, management, and treatment of cancer, car-diovascular and cerebrovascular disorders, obesity, rheumatoid arthritis, chronic renal failure, non-insulin-dependent diabetes, and macular degener-ation, among other diseases.

See also MACROBIOTICS; NUTRITION; ORNISH, DEAN.

veterinary alternative medicine   See PET THERAPY.

vibrational medicine   Any alternative treatment modality that focuses on using, manipulating, changing, or balancing electromagnetic frequencies of the body, or the energy field, such as bioener-getic therapies, homeopathy, and flower essence remedies.

See also ACUPUNCTURE; BACH FLOWER REMEDIES; BIOENERGETICS; CHAKRAS; COLOR THERAPY; HOMEOPA-THY; LAYING ON OF HANDS; LIGHT THERAPY; MAGNETIC THERAPY; MERIDIANS; RADIONICS; REIKI; SOUND THERAPY; THERAPEUTIC TOUCH.

visualization   See GUIDED IMAGERY.

vital force   Life, or primal, energy.

See also ENERGY MEDICINE; *QI*; YIN-YANG.

vitalism   Another term for the theory of "vital energy."

See also ENERGY MEDICINE; *QI*; YIN-YANG.

vitamin   An organic compound that is required in small amounts for normal health, growth, and well-being of the body. Vitamins are not utilized primar-ily as a source of energy or as a source of structural tissue components, but rather as catalysts. Vitamins are micronutrients that promote physiologic processes necessary for continued life. There are 13 vitamins. Only three of these, vitamin D, biotin, and pantothenic acid, are manufactured by the body, and even these may not be present in sufficient quantities for good health. Therefore vitamins must be supplied by exogenous, or outside, sources. Vita-min deficiency results in a well-defined disease that is prevented or cured by replacement of that vita-min. For example, vitamin A is anti-infective and essential for the normal function of epithelial cells and the formulation of visual purple. An antiberiberi and antineuritic vitamin is thiamine, or vitamin B1. Vitamin K significantly affects blood coagulation.

Vitamin C prevents scurvy and is considered a natural antibiotic and possibly an antiviral nutrient. Vitamin D is important as an antirachitic, that is, agent that prevents bone and tooth disorders. The B vitamins affect growth, metabolism, lactation, and the nervous, endocrine, and gastrointestinal systems.

See also NUTRITION.

Voodoo (Vodun)   A healing tradition, often mistakenly considered a type of witchcraft, involving herbalism, traditional wisdom, baths, rituals, spells, charms, necromancy, prayers, and other modalities derived from the polytheism and ancestor worship of African slaves taken to Haiti and practiced largely in Caribbean and Latin American countries and in the United States. The name *Voodoo* or *Voodu* most likely originated from the Louisiana Creole word *voudou*, meaning deity or demon. Haitian Voodoo priestesses, called *mambos*, minister as doctor, psychic, psychotherapist, spiritualist, and social worker to clients who are required to participate in their healing processes.

Weil, Andrew American medical researcher and physician. A graduate of Harvard Medical School, Weil teaches at the University of Arizona College of Medicine and is the author of *Chocolate to Morphine*, (Houghton Mifflin, 1983); *The Natural Mind: A New Way of Looking at Drugs and the Higher Consciousness,* (Houghton Mifflin, 1972), *Health and Healing,* (Boston: Houghton Mifflin Company, 1983), T*he Marriage of the Sun and Moon: A Quest for Unity in Consciousness* (Houghton Mifflin 1980); and *Eating Well for Optimum Health* (New York: Alfred A. Knopf, 2000).

Weiss, Brian L. American psychiatrist, proponent of mind-body medicine, and author of several books including *Many Minds, Many Masters; Only Love Is Real; Through Time Into Healing* (New York: Simon & Schuster, 1992); *Mirrors of Time: Using Regression for Physical, Emotional,* and *Spiritual Healing* and *Messages from the Masters* (New York: Warner Books, 2000).

See also PAST-LIFE REGRESSION THERAPY.

Western herbalism See HERBALISM.

White Light Reiki A school of Reiki founded by Dr. Mikao Usui, of Kyoto, Japan, in the latter half of the 19th century. Usui added to traditional Reiki methods what he believed to be the healing energy of various Reiki symbols taught during the Second Degree and in Master's training. The various symbols, similar to ancient hieroglyphs or characters, are meant to activate energy and are made with the hand over the Reiki recipient as the practitioner determines for that individual's needs.

See also BIOENERGETICS; REIKI; VIBRATIONAL MEDICINE.

xenobiotics Biologically active foreign substances, such as environmental toxins that enter the body and impair normal functioning. (By-products of metabolism, known as *aama* in Ayurvedic medicine, are not included because they are produced internally.) A certain form of yogic breathing, known as *kappalbhati*, is reported to use forceful exhalation to serve as a route of elimination of any foreign or waste substances "clogging" the body. Also in yoga, a breathing technique called a "pranic bath" involves stimulating the sweat glands to force off undesirable matter through the skin. Both Ayurvedic and homeopathic medicine acknowledge the need to eliminate xenobiotics through the lungs, colon, bladder, and skin.

See also *AAMA*; YOGA.

xian The Chinese word for the salty taste of herbs.

xin The Chinese word to describe an acidic taste of herbs.

X rays, chiropractic A diagnostic procedure used in chiropractic treatment to reveal the condition of the spine.

See also CHIROPRACTIC.

xu In traditional Chinese medicine, the word for deficiency, one of the basic diagnoses.

See also YIN-YANG.

yin-yang   The Chinese symbol, also called the t'ai ch'i symbol, for universal opposite forces, or mutually interdependent polar forces, such as light/dark, and male/female, within a circular form, used in Chinese medicine to illustrate the ideal goal of balance and harmony.

Yin means "the shady side of the mountain" and *yang* means "the sunny side of the mountain" in Chinese medicine. Yin, the symbol or manifestation of darkness, coldness, quietness, inertia, and death, includes reference to the tissues, blood, fluids, and internal secretions of the body. Yin organs (also known as *zang*) are the liver, heart, spleen, lungs, and kidneys and are considered the solid organs that contain what Chinese medicine calls the essences—tears, sweat, saliva, mucus, and sexual secretions. Yin phenomena refer to cold, wet, quiescent, deteriorating, chronic, slow, empty, and contracted, and lack of yin generates heat and dryness. When yin decreases, yang dominates.

Yang, which includes bodily functioning and the generation of metabolic heat, decreases when yin dominates. Yang organs (also known as *fu*) are the gallbladder, small and large intestines, stomach, and bladder and are considered the hollow organs that transform and transport matter throughout the body as well as carry it out of the body when it becomes waste. Yang manifests as birth, warmth, activity, noise, form, and light. Among the yang phenomena are heat, dryness, growth, fullness, suddenness, and acuteness. Lack of yang generates cold and dampness.

In Traditional Chinese Medicine (TCM), yin-yang constitutes one set of four diagnostic sets of polar categories known as the Eight Guiding Principles. These principles—Cold-Hot, Deficient-Excess, Internal-External, and Yin-Yang—help practitioners identify patterns of distress and locate disease processes. A yin syndrome is characterized as cold, deficient, and internal; a yang syndrome is hot, excess, and external. Combinations of yin and yang syndromes are most frequently diagnosed. Yin-yang also serve as general categories that sum up the interaction of all the others. Acupuncturists aim to balance the disturbed energy or the imbalance of yin and yang that causes illness.

Macrobiotics, based on the Chinese concept of yin and yang, is a branch of alternative medicine involving nutrition that balances yin and yang characteristics. Macrobiotic therapists believe that excessive yin qualities (essentially calm and peacefulness) may result in depression, fatigue syndromes, and sleep disorders, and excessive yang (essentially energy and activity) qualities may lead to tension, insomnia, hyperactivity, and irritability. Yin and yang characteristics are also recognized in foods. Fruits, leafy green vegetables, nuts and seeds, tofu, and some other foods are considered to be yin. Whole grains, root vegetables, seafood, legumes, salt, and cottage cheese are considered yang.

Yin-yang also symbolizes sexuality and the masculine/feminine, anima/animus, passive/aggressive aspects of energy. Traditional Oriental wisdom proclaims that within every yin there is an element of yang, and within every yang an element of yin. This refers to the ability of each force to take on characteristics of the other or of both to dip into each other to create harmony in functioning. A popular example of this concept is found in mainstream psychology that touts men who summon their "feminine (yin) side" and women their "masculine (yang) side" when appropriate and/or necessary.

See also MACROBIOTICS.

yoga A system of physical postures, stretching, meditation, and regulated ways of breathing according to the Hindu philosophy that an individual strive for unity with the Supreme Being, or Universal Self. Yogic breathing and exercises have been widely accepted into the Western mainstream culture as healthful and healing practices. Yoga has been shown to help lower blood pressure and heart rate and suppress other bodily functions in order to achieve a state of total relaxation. An instructor or practitioner of yoga is called a yogi.

History of Yoga

The language of yoga is Sanskrit, considered the oldest literary language of India and the basis of many modern Indian languages such as Hindi and Urdu. The name Sanskrit means refined or polished. Yoga means "yoke, union," or the verb to join. The combination of breathing techniques, exercise, meditation, and "right action" is taught to anyone seeking to promote or restore health and perhaps adopt the belief that this will help unite his or her soul with God. It is believed that cleansing and strengthening the body and focusing the mind enable the spirit to connect with the divine. This connection is the result of achieving full consciousness or self-realization, also known as *atman*, and unity with *brahman* (totality). However, yoga is not considered a creed; nor does it oppose any religion. It is universal.

Meditation was the earliest form of yoga, and Buddha is considered by some to be the first yogi. Raja yoga, which specifically relates to quieting and focusing the mind, was developed about 5,000 years ago by sages of India. Hatha is one of seven limbs of Raja yoga, all of which are thought to be necessary to unite the body, mind, and spirit.

Yoga is also associated with Eastern religions such as Hinduism, which is one of many that adopted the philosophy, but yoga predates Hinduism by many centuries. Ancient engraved seals of deities striking yogic poses have been discovered in the Indus Valley, one of the world's first urban civilizations, located in what is now Pakistan and western India. These artifacts suggest that yoga must have existed before 3000 B.C.

As Eastern philosophies have become integrated into Western popular culture, so has yoga become a common activity. It is likely that much of what

we know about athletics was derived from the ancient practice known as Hatha (physical) yoga. There is a wealth of information available about the history of yoga described in ancient texts by philosophers and the variety of styles of Hatha yoga developed over the decades. Much of what we know of yoga relies on Hatha to inspire a spiritual interest in the subject, although yoga may be practiced solely for physical purposes such as stress relief and relaxation. The relaxation pose, for example, involves closing the eyes, breathing deeply, and drawing the focus away from life's details. Perhaps this is why many believe yoga is best approached not as a mere workout routine, but as a journey to one's whole, best self.

Patanjali

There is much debate about who is responsible for the oldest documentation of yoga. According to native Indic tradition, it was a grammarian known as Patanjali. Other than his brief work, *The Yoga Sutras of Patanjali*, dating back approximately 2,000 years, little more is known about his life. The text does not credit Patanjali or anyone else as the author. The first person to attribute this classical work to him was Vacaspati Mishra, the 10th-century author of the Tattva-Vaisharadi commentary on the Sutra. Many consider the Sutra to be the most important outline of the yogic path.

In 196 aphorisms contained in four chapters written in Sanskrit, *Yoga-Sutra* describes Raja yoga, an eightfold path for overcoming the obstacles of humankind's spiritual evolution. There are eight concepts, or "limbs," as they are commonly known, of Raja yoga: *yama* (moral discipline), *niyama* (religious discipline), *asana* (posture), *pranayama* (breath), *pratyahara* (releasing the mind from the senses), *dharana* (concentration), *dhyana* (meditation), and *samadhi* (super-consciousness).

Patanjali believed that practicing these eight disciplines and sowing the seed of nonattachment in one's heart would allow a person to achieve the ultimate freedom of spirit. He said, "Nonattachment is that effect which comes to those who have given up their thirst after objects either seen or heard." Many translations and commentaries of Patanjali's theories have been written over the centuries and are available today.

Gorakhnath

The first treatise on Hatha Yoga was written by Gorakhnath, who lived sometime between A.D. 900 and 1225. Although there are no known copies of the work remaining, the information imparted remains.

The *Goraksa-sataka*, Hundred verses of Goraksa (*Goraksanatha* is a Sanskrit form of *Gorakhnath*), describes six aspects of yoga referred to as limbs. This does not include the *yama* (restraint) and *niyama* (disciplines), which precede *asana* in Patanjali's text. There are no reliable facts about Gorakhnath, only legends. According to Bengal literature, he was born of the matted hair of the god Mahadeva (Shiva). As the purest and strongest of yogis, he put the goddess Durga to shame with his purity and strength. Gorakhnath has been described as the most influential Indian since Shankara.

The Upanishads, Vedanta, and Shankara

Much detail and understanding of yogic theory come from The Upanishads (pronounced oo-PAN-ee-shadz), which literally means secret teaching. Much of it is written in the form of dialogues between kings and yogis. The book is known as the Vedanta, meaning the end or final goal of wisdom. As in the *Yoga-Sutra*, there is no mention of an author. Composed ca. 900 B.C., it forms the last section of the Vedas, a four-part collection of hymns, mantras, prayers, and psalms dealing with religious ceremony and ritual. The parts are called Rig-Veda, Sama-Veda, Yajur-Veda, and Artharva-Veda.

According to the introduction in the book's translation by Swami Paramananda, these scriptures arrived in the Western world in the form of a Persian translation made in the 17th century. The first English translation was that of Raja Ram Mohun Roy (1775–1833). Several European translations have been published since then. It is a doctrine of *brahman*, the universal reality of consciousness, and the identity of *brahman* with the inner essence (*atman*) of the human being. It is a prototype for the later philosophical schools of Vedanta, which is based primarily on the Upanishads.

Adi Shankara (also known as Samkara), one of India's greatest sages, wrote Advaita Vedanta, the Vedanta treatise, among other texts. He is believed to have come closest to depicting the true path of yoga. He also wrote commentaries of the Brahma Sutras, the Upanishads, and the Gita. Regarded as an incarnation of Lord Shiva, he was born in 509 B.C. and died at age 32. By the age of eight he had mastered the four Vedas, and by age 12 the Shastras. Legend has it that a crocodile grabbed young Shankara's foot while he bathed in a river. He shouted to his mother that to spare his life, she must permit him to renounce evil. When she agreed, he uttered a mantra. After the crocodile let him go, he left home to search for a guru. He met Govinda, a realized sage, and attained self-realization (*samadhi*). Later he established four monasteries called Mutts, which exist today throughout India.

For studies of logic and metaphysics Shankara's work is highly recommended. In S. Dasgupta's five-volume work, *A History of Indian Philosophy*, Shankara is synopsized as follows: "So great is the influence of the philosophy propounded by Shankara and elaborated by his illustrious followers, that whenever we speak of Vedanta philosophy we mean the philosophy that was propounded by Shankara" (vol. 1, p. 429).

Ramakrishna Paramhansa

Ramakrishna Paramhansa (1836–86) was a scholar of the Vedas, Upanishads, Sufism, the Bible, Sikhism, and Buddhism. He did not found any organization or claim to know a new path to salvation. He grew to realize that different religions lead to the same goal. He was known to say, "As many faiths, so many paths" and "Man's upliftment is the main goal in life." His main disciple, Swami Vivekananda, was once quoted as saying, "My master used to say that such names as Hindu, Christian, etc., stand as great barriers to all brotherly feeling between man and man. We must try to break them down first. They have all lost their good powers and now only stand as baneful influences under whose black magic even the best of us behave like demons. Well, we will have to work hard and we must succeed."

Swami Vivekananda

When Swami Vivekananda was born, January 12, 1863, in Calcutta, his parents named him

Narendra. He became a disciple of Sri Rama-krishna Paramhansa, who renamed him Swami Vivekananda. He went on to become one of India's leading social reformers. His lectures focused on humanitarianism and service to God through service to others rather than on dogma, as well as on Hinduism and its true meaning. In 1897 this pioneer of the Vedanta movement in the United States and England founded the Ramakrishna Mission, one of India's largest charitable institutions. Although he died at age 39, his contributions were so appreciated that he is known as the "patron saint" of modern India.

Swami Paramananda (1884–1940)

The author, poet, and teacher Swami Paramananda was the youngest monastic disciple of Swami Vivekananda, founder of the Ramakrishna Order, the most widely known religious and philanthropic organization in India. He was one of the first Eastern teachers to travel to the United States, in 1906. In 1909 he founded the Vedanta Centre in Boston. He wrote several books, including *Change Your Mind, A Practical Guide to Buddhist Meditation.*

Bhagavad-Gita

The title of this book-length Sanskrit poem, Bhagavad-Gita, means "song of the Lord." The Bhagavad Gita is the most widely read scripture in India. Also known as the Gita, it is part of the *Mahabharata* (Great India), a religious classic of Hinduism. The story spotlights Lord Krishna and Prince Arjuna on the eve of the battle of Kurukshetra. Krishna persuades Arjuna to fight his fear of the opposing army with the armor of spiritual wisdom attained through yoga (union with God).

In chapter 6 of the Gita, considered the most important authority of yoga philosophy, Krishna advises Arjuna, "When his mind, intellect and self (ahamkara) are under control, freed from restless desire, so that they rest in the spirit within, a man becomes a Yukta—one in communion with God. A lamp does not flicker in a place where no winds blow; so it is with a yogic, who controls his mind, intellect and self, being absorbed in the spirit within him. When the restlessness of the mind, intellect and self is stilled through the practice of Yoga, the yogic by the grace of the Spirit within himself finds fulfillment. Then he knows the joy eternal which is beyond the pale of the sense which his reason cannot grasp. He abides in this reality and moves not therefrom. He has found the treasure above all others. There is nothing higher than this. He who has achieved it, shall not be moved by the greatest sorrow. This is the real meaning of Yoga—a deliverance from contact with pain and sorrow."

Unlike the Upanishads, the Gita teaches that surrender to God is a more easily attainable spiritual path than pure knowledge. Various chapters of the Gita deal with renunciation and meditation. It says that the person who works according to his or her dharma (purpose in life) but cares not for the reward of those actions is a true yogi. Union with God can be achieved by following a divine set of guidelines that fall under the categories of *hatha* (physical practice), *jnana* (knowledge), *karma* (right action), *bhakti* (devotion), *raja* (control of the mind), and *mantra* (chant).

The Hatha Yoga Pradipika

Although the *Yoga-Sutra* is revered by all practitioners, Patanjali describes only a simple cross-legged posture used for meditation. A few more *asanas* (postures) are described in what is considered the bible of the physical component of yoga, *The Hatha Yoga Pradipika*. This 500-page text was written by Sri Yogindra Svatmarama in the 14th century and provided the first textual evidence of *asanas*. The *Pradipika* is divided into four parts. The first explains *yamas* (restraints on behavior), *niyamus* (observances), *asanas* (postures), and *nutrition*. The second discusses *pranoyama* (control or restraint of energy) and the *shatrurmas* (internal cleansing). The third part talks about *mudras* (hand gestures), *bandhas* (locks), the *nadis* (channels of energy through which prana flows), and the *kundalini* power. The fourth describes *pratyahara* (withdrawal of the senses), *dharana* (concentration), *dhyana* (meditation), and *samadhi* (absorption).

Krishnamacharya

Tirumalai Krishnamacharya (1888–1989) receives much credit for shedding new light on what is now considered the Hatha yoga of modern times. By age 12 he was already a serious student of the Vedas. In 1924 he opened a school of yoga in Mysore, India. In 1976 he and his son, T.K.V. Desikachar, founded the Krishnamacharya Yoga Mandiram, a center for alternative treatment, in Chennai, India. While teaching, he wrote his first book, *Yoga Makarandam* (*Secrets of Yoga*). One secret was that yoga can help control the heartbeat. He believed that yoga is most authentic and useful when adapted to suit the individual. He encouraged students to practice according to their own ability and needs rather than follow a course of idealized poses. He also stressed the importance of following the breath from the beginning of a practice to the end in order for the individual to realize his or her highest potential.

Jiddu Krishnamurti

Unlike many gurus, Jiddu Krishnamurti claimed not to want any followers during his more than 60 years of lecturing all over the world. His goal was to convince people that the possibility for peace throughout the world depended on change in each individual. Krishnamurti, who lived to be 90 years old, felt that to follow another person, no matter who it may be, is evil. That is why he did not create an organization or authorize anyone to interpret his work His only wish was that his written and recorded talks be made available to the public.

Indra Devi

Born in 1899, Indra Devi, a woman of Russian descent, was moved to visit India in 1927 after hearing Krishnamurti speak in Holland. Two years later she became a film actress and adopted her name after Indira Gandhi. At 31 she ended her film career, married a diplomat and took up yoga in Bombay. Eventually she studied with Sri Krishnamacharya in Mysore. She became a popular yoga teacher among Hollywood movie stars in the 1940s and 1950s and paved the way for other yoga instructors who migrated to America. She now lives and teaches in Argentina. She is known to have said, "The solution to a better and full life is in the practice of yoga, where you can find all the answers. You can also transmit peace through yoga. I do not belong to any religion. Everything is between God and myself."

Sri Aurobindo Ghose

Sri Aurobindo Ghose was considered a yogi, a revolutionary, a poet, and a visionary. As a leader of the struggle for India's independence from British rule, he was jailed in 1909 for terrorist activities. While in jail he had his first spiritual experiences. He said, "It was no longer by its [the jail's] high walls that I was imprisoned; no, it was Vasudeva [the father of the Vedic gods Krishna and Balarama] who surrounded me."

In 1926 he founded Aurobindo Ashram as well as his own philosophy on samadhi. To get there he prescribed a blend of ancient spirituality and integral yoga. He believed that striving for spiritual realization does not require a withdrawal from society.

Papa Ramdas (1884–1963)

Until the age of 36 Papa Ramdas lived an ordinary life. His focus shifted after exposure to the teachings of Sri Ramakrishna and Swami Vivekananda, among others, who inspired him to renounce his worldly possessions and follow God. He realized that his desire was attainable through God. He founded Anandashram. Swami Sivananda, founder of the Divine Life Society located in the Himalayas, characterized him as follows: "Ramdas is the living example of one that has realized Cosmic Consciousness. Thus he is permeated with bliss. All his actions, utterances and his writings bubble with this bliss."

Paramhansa Yogananda (1893–1952)

The author of the well-known *Autobiography of a Yogi* and founder of the Self-Realization Fellowship in 1920, Paramhansa Yogananda was the first yoga master of India to live and teach in the West. He arrived in America in 1920 and created a tremendous stir with what he called a "spiritual campaign." He said, "Self-Realization is the knowing in all parts of body, mind, and soul that you are now in possession of the kingdom of God; that you do not have to pray that it come to you; that God's omnipresence is your omnipresence; and that all that you need to do is improve your knowing."

He continued to lecture and write up to his passing in 1952.

Swami Sivananda (1887–1963)

The physician Swami Sivananda was forever changed when he happened to treat a wandering monk who offered information on yoga and Vedanta. He was moved to help people heal not only on a physical level, but on a spiritual level. He became a monk and founded the Divine Life Society. His teachings can be summarized as "Serve, Love, Give, Purify, Meditate, Realize."

B.K.S. Iyengar

Born in 1918, B.K.S. Iyengar is one of the world's most recognized yoga practitioners. He has written many books on the subject, including *Light on Yoga*, (New York: Schocken Books, 1995) and *Light on Pranayama*, (New York: Crossroad/Herder and Herder, 1995). He was a sick child, who survived bouts of malaria, tuberculosis, and typhoid. At 15 he was introduced to yoga by his brother-in-law, Sri T. Krishnamacharya, who offered him basic instruction to improve his health.

By 1937 he was ready to teach yoga himself. In 1952 he met the violinist Yehudi Menuhin, who arranged for him to teach in Europe. His popularity soared in 1966 when *Light on Yoga* became an international best-seller. The culmination of more than 60 years of dedication to yoga is his most recent book, *Yoga: The Path to Holistic Health*, published in 2001.

Branches of Yoga

The physical aspect of yoga called Hatha yoga has been incorporated into mainstream fitness and health programs. Sanskrit for Sun and Moon, *Hatha yoga* focuses on balancing yin and yang, or opposite universal forces, for the purpose of improving respiration, circulation, and digestion and boosting the immune and nervous systems. Although yoga instructors offer various types of Hatha, along with meditation and *pranayama* (breathing), all branches seek to unite the body, mind, and spirit through deep breathing. The following are types of Hatha yoga:

1. Ananda yoga: a system of "energization exercises" that incorporates the use of silent affirmations. The concept is that the affirmations consciously direct energy and raise the individual's level of awareness. Ananda (Sanskrit for bliss) was founded in the 1960s by Swami Kriyananda (J. Donald Walters), who became a disciple of Paramhansa Yogananda in 1948. The Ananda Sangha organization offers instruction in Kriya yoga and yoga techniques according to Yogananda. Currently there are five Ananda communities on the West Coast, retreat centers in northern California and Rhode Island, a retreat/community in Italy, and affiliated meditation groups throughout the world.

2. Anusara yoga: A blend of hatha yoga techniques and biomechanics; Anusara, meaning "to step into the current of divine will," was developed in 1997 by John Friend, who studied yoga with Sri K. Patabhi Jois, T.K.V. Desikachar, and B.K.S. Iyengar. Anusara yoga is based on the philosophy that all people are divine in body, mind, and spirit regardless of their individual limitations, and that it is best to see the good in all things. Friend cited attitude, alignment, and action as components of every *asana* (posture).

3. Ashtanga yoga: First described in an ancient hatha yoga text, the "Yoga Korunta," and later rediscovered by the sage Patanjali in the "Yoga Sutras," ashtanga is called the "eight-limbed yoga," which is based on stamina, strength, and flexibility. The goal is to cleanse and purify the internal organs with forward and backward bends.

4. Bikram yoga: Developed by the brother of Yogananda, Bishnu Ghosh, and Bikram Choudhury, Bikram yoga requires that the 26 postures and deep breathing exercises be done in a room heated to approximately 104–105°F and repeated twice.

5. Integral yoga: A meditative practice structured to lead from the physical body (*asana*) and the vital body (*pranayama*) to the mental, that is, a mindful balance of effort and relaxation; it is a scientific system developed in 1966 by the Reverend Sri Swami Satchidananda. Integral yoga has evolved into an international organization, with more than 40 institutes and centers throughout the United States and abroad that offer Hatha yoga, meditation, yoga philosophy and various branches of yoga practice, and vegetarian diet.

6. Integrative yoga therapy: The use of gentle postures, guided imagery, and breathing techniques for the treatment of heart disease, psychiatric disorders, and acquired immunodeficiency syndrome (AIDS), integrative yoga

therapy (IYT) was founded in 1993 by Joseph Le Page in San Francisco, California. Le Page designed a teacher-training program specifically for conventional and medical settings aimed at rehabilitation.

7. ISHTA yoga: ISHTA yoga is a blend of postures, breathing, and meditation geared to access human potential developed by Alan Finger, founder of Yoga Zone Studios and second-generation yoga master who has been practicing for more than 40 years. The Yoga Zone has four studios in New York for more than 1,700 students per week. Finger began his yoga studies as a teenager in his native South Africa under the instruction of his father, Kavi Yogiraj Mani Finger, who studied yoga in India. Alan Finger became a Western Yoga Master and in 1992 developed ISHTA yoga, which in Sanskrit refers to developing a personal yoga practice that meets individual needs. The acronym ISHTA refers to the Integrated Science of Hatha Tantra and Ayurveda, a physical and spiritual form of yoga. ISHTA combines Ashtanga, Viniyoga, Iyengar, and the practices of Paramahansa Yogananda. Finger's company has published a book, more than 50 videos, and the nationally televised *Yoga Zone* television show that aired on the Health Network.

8. Iyengar yoga: Founded by B.K.S. Iyengar, who adapted it from Patanjali's traditional yoga methods, Iyengar is one of the most commonly practiced forms of yoga in the United States. It involves the use of tools, such as belts, chairs, blocks, and walls to help make postures more attainable for beginners and individuals with physical limitations.

9. Jivamukti yoga: Created by David Life and Sharon Gannon in 1984, Jivamukti combines meditation and physical challenge with Sanskrit chanting, readings, references to scriptural texts, a diverse selection of music, poetry, postures, and breathing techniques.

10. Kali Ray TriYoga: Founded by Kali Ray (Kaliji) in 1980, the TriYoga Center in Santa Cruz, California, was established to offer a system of yoga based on a series of flowing, dancelike movements accompanied by music in a meditative environment.

11. Kripalu yoga: Kripalu yoga is the form of yoga practiced at its homebase, the Kripalu Center for Yoga and Health, a nearly 30-year-old nonprofit education fellowship located in Lenox, Massachusetts, and the largest retreat center for yoga and holistic health in North America. The organization was founded in 1966, when Yogi Amrit Desai created the Yoga Society of Pennsylvania, a nonprofit organization providing yoga classes and training for yoga teachers. The center was renamed to honor Yogi Desai's guru, Swami Kripalvananda. Swami Kripalu is better known as Bapuji, which means beloved grandfather. He was a master of kundalini yoga as well as a respected speaker, writer, and musician. Kripalu's philosophy consists of three conceptual stages. Willful practice focuses on body alignment, breath, and consciousness; willful surrender is the practice of holding postures to the level of tolerance and beyond to deepen concentration, and release tension.

12. Kriya yoga: A technique of pranayama (energy control) used during meditation to accelerate one's spiritual progress. *Kriya*, the Sanskrit word for action, is geared to divine union through a certain act or technique. It was introduced to the West by Paramahansa Yogananda and combines an esoteric meditation technique with other practices of raja and hatha yoga. It is considered to be one of the most effective techniques for achieving self-realization (*samadhi*). The Ananda Sangha organization offers Kriya preparation classes, including the year-long Ananda Course in Self-Realization.

13. Kundalini yoga: The source of all forms of yoga, Kundalini is a comprehensive science of breathwork, postures, sound, chanting, and meditation with the goal of merging with the universal Self. Known as the Yoga of Awareness, *Kundalini* means "coiled one," referring to the power of the Absolute or Consciousness that creates and sustains the universe. The idea is that the coiled and dormant form of this power is harbored by everyone and symbolizes the potential of consciousness. Yogi Bhajan introduced Kundalini to the West in 1969; he believed that it is everyone's birthright to be healthy, happy, and holy and that people of all

religions can realize their greatest potential. Kundalini combines *asanas*, *pranayama*, and other techniques to strengthen and focus the *prana*, a subsidiary power of Kundalini. Siddha yoga is a popular variation of Kundalini that relies on a guru to awaken the Kundalini through mantra, meditation, chanting, and seva, or selfless service.

14. Laya yoga: Laya yoga is a form of meditation focusing on the energy centers located in the spine and head, which are regarded as doorways to higher consciousness. Laya yoga is geared toward overcoming selfishness and self-centeredness and developing the ability to cope with any fear or issue that blocks "heart expansion."

15. Mantra yoga: Mantra, from the Sanskrit word *manas*, or mind, focuses on the meditative word or prayer repeated for a length of time. Although the most common mantra is Om, or Aum, the vibration of God, from which all other mantras are derived, one may choose from many mantras or obtain an individual mantra from a guru. The repetition of the word *Japa*, meaning "in the name of God," may be used as a mantra. Other common mantras are Om Namo Sivaya (to call upon the energy of Siva) and Om Nama Narayanaya (which calls upon the god Vishnu). Bija-mantras are used to address the seven charkas, or energy zones of the body. The major ones are Lam, Vam, Ram, Yam, Ham, Ksam, Bam (or Om).

16. Office yoga: Office yoga practice is also called Desktop yoga because the stretches do not require moving away from a chair or desk. Incorporating ergonomics and working conditions that promote the well-being of office workers, office yoga offers stress relief from the daily business world routine and confinement to the office.

17. Phoenix Rising yoga: Based at the Phoenix Rising Center in West Stockbridge, Massachusetts, Phoenix Rising yoga blends classical techniques with contemporary mind-body psychology in order to allow the release of physical and emotional tension. A Phoenix Rising session is a one-on-one, one-and-a-half-hour experience of assisted yoga postures, nondirective dialogue, and guided breathing. Much physical and emotional healing can be accomplished by this form of yoga for individuals who prefer privacy and personal attention.

18. PowerBreathing: PowerBreathing is a deep, slow breathing technique developed by the yoga teacher Yonah Offner. The goal is to allow the diaphragm to work properly by unblocking the three lower chakras. More information on PowerBreathing is available on Offner's website, www.powerbreathing.com.

19. Power yoga: Power yoga is the Western form of Ashtanga yoga developed by Beryl Bender Birch, author of *Power Yoga* and *Beyond Power Yoga* (New York: Simon & Schuster, 2000). A student of classical yoga since 1971 and graduate of Syracuse University, Birch addresses the positive mind-body therapeutic effects of yoga, to which she has added more challenging postures and a unique breathing technique called *ujjayi* that extend the Ashtanga yoga method. The initial goal of the practice is to create heat and energy flow in the body, to flush out mental and physical toxins and to stretch and strengthen muscles. As in all authentic yoga systems, the ultimate spiritual goal is the realization of the Self or the recognition of the true Self as divine consciousness.

20. Sivananda yoga: Sivananda yoga is a method geared toward balancing the intellect, heart, body, and mind that includes proper exercise (*asanas*), proper breathing (*pranayama*), proper relaxation (*savasana*), proper diet (vegetarian), positive thinking (*vedanta*), and meditation (*dhyana*). Introduced to the United States of America in 1957 by Swami Vishnu-devananda, founder of the International Sivananda Yoga Vedanta Centers, Sivananda yoga is based on the teachings of Swami Sivananda of Rishikesh, India, who taught students to "serve, love, give, purify, meditate, and realize."

21. Svaroopa yoga: Svaroopa yoga is a method that includes gentle poses directed toward "core opening," or unraveling tensions all along the spine, developed by Rama Berch, who founded and directs the Master Yoga Foundation in La Jolla, California, and who has also directed the yoga program for Dr. Deepak Chopra's Center for Well-Being. Berch discovered that many of

her students "impose the pose upon their body rather than unfolding it from within," and therefore adapted classical asanas to help students experience the deeper effects she realized from Kundalini yoga. With the goal of opening the body and experiencing the transcendent inner state called *svaroopa* by Patanjali in the "Yoga Sutras," Svaroopa focuses on alignment and support and makes frequent use of chair poses to help release deep-muscle tension. Each pose is based on integrated principles of asana, anatomy, and yoga philosophy.

22. Tantra yoga: *Tantra* means expansion in Sanskrit; a Tantra yogi teaches ways to expand all levels of consciousness to realize the Supreme Reality (samadhi). Although Tantra yoga may be confused with tantric sex, the goal is to awaken and balance male-female energy for the sake of inner peace and overcoming of personal limitations and subconscious blockages. According to Srinivasan of the Sivananda Yoga organization, Tantra yoga has been practiced for the spiritual regeneration of the Hindus. Often considered a secret doctrine, the Tantra is also known as Gupta Vidya. Srinivasan said one must acquire this knowledge not from books, but from the practical Tantrikas, the Tantric Acharyas, and Gurus. The tantric student must be "endowed with purity, faith, devotion, dedication to Guru, dispassion, humility, courage, cosmic love, truthfulness, non-covetousness, and contentment."

23. Tibetan yoga: A method of yoga little known in the West, Tibetan yoga is the name used by Buddhists to describe tantric meditation and breathwork. In 1939 Peter Kelder published *Ancient Secret of the Fountain of Youth* (New York: Doubleday, 1998), which contains a series of postures called "The Five Rites of Rejuvenation." The author Christopher Kilham produced a modern version: *The Five Tibetans: Five Dynamic Exercises for Health, Energy, and Personal Power* (Inner Traditions, 1994). Kilham's book explains five flowing movements that start with 10 to 12 repetitions and progress to 21, with the purpose of restoring the spin of the chakras to their youthful rate. It is believed that if the chakras are perfectly balanced, the body resists aging. Few classes are available on this method.

24. Viniyoga: Viniyoga is a method incorporating *asana, pranayama*, meditation, ritual, and prayer for the higher purpose of enhancing an individual's ability to adapt. The late Sri T. Krishnamacharya and his son, T.K.V. Desikachar, advocated treating each yoga student as an individual who wishes to reach particular goals in a way that is comfortable for him or her. Gary Kraftsow, a yoga teacher since 1976, wrote *Yoga for Wellness: Healing with the Timeless Teachings of Viniyoga* (New York: Viking Penguin, 1999) and *Yoga for Transformation: Ancient Practices and Teachings for Healing the Body, Mind, and Heart* (New York: Penguin, 2002). Kraftsow met Desikachar and T. Krishnamacharya and created a link with the Viniyoga tradition through his American Viniyoga Institute, which offers retreats, seminars, and Viniyoga Teacher and Therapist Training throughout the United States, Canada, and Europe.

25. White Lotus yoga: A nondogmatic approach developed by the husband-and-wife team Ganga White and Tracey Rich, White Lotus yoga is dedicated to the development of the whole human being. White and Rich produced five yoga videos that highlight the practice of partner yoga in 1978, and White is also the author of *Double Yoga* (New York: Penguin, 1981). The technique involves a flowing vinyasa approach that ranges from gentle to vigorous and consists of alignment, breath, and the basic yoga principles. White Lotus includes the Flow Series, or Flow Yoga, which uses proper body alignment, attunement with breath, focused attention, and the development of a balance of strength, flexibility, and endurance. It also includes moving sequences, standing poses, inversions, backbends, forward bends, twists, balances, *bandha, mudra* (hand gestures), and *pranayama*. White and Rich's 40-acre retreat in the Santa Ynez Mountains in Santa Barbara, California, offers weekend and week-long yoga-immersion experiences as well as 16-day teacher-training programs.

26. YogaDance: A combination of standing movements and yogic stretches developed by Jeff

Hoffman, a native New Jersey yogi for 27 years, the practice focuses on relaxation, breath, self-observation, and individual awareness, according to Hoffman, whose website is www.verycalm.com. Simple and common yoga *asanas* (postures) include *balasana* (the child's posture), *paschimottanasana* (posterior stretch), *bhujangasana* (cobra), *shalabhasana* (locust), *ardha matsyendrasana* (half-spinal twist), *shavasana* (corpse), *sarvangasana* (shoulder stand), and *ardha matsayana* (half-fish). Yoga therapy is known to be beneficial as a preventive health and exercise regimen and as complementary treatment for back pain, arthritis and rheumatism, anxiety, migraines, insomnia, nerve or muscle disease, menstrual problems and premenstrual syndrome, menopause symptoms, high blood pressure, heart disease, asthma, bronchitis, duodenal ulcer, hemorrhoids, diabetes, obesity, and substance addictions.

Z

zanfu zhi qi The energy, or *qi*, of the body's organs, according to traditional Chinese medicine.

zang fu The term for the internal organ systems in traditional Chinese medicine.
See also YIN-YANG.

zero balancing A hands-on mind-body system designed by Dr. Fritz Smith in 1973 to align body energy with the body's physical structure. It aims to help relieve physical and mental symptoms, improve the ability to deal with stress, and organize vibratory fields in order to promote a sense of wholeness and well-being. Founded in 1991, the Zero Balancing Association represents the integration of Eastern views of energy with Western views of science and teaches how to use energy as a working tool in relation to body structure. It is the integration of the client's body energy with his or her body structure to create clearer, stronger fields of energy in the mind-body and balance energy in the tissues and the skeletal system. More information is available by contacting www.zerobalancing.com.

zheng qi The traditional Chinese medicine term for normal energy, or *qi*, that flows through the meridians (channels) and organs of the body.
See also QI.

Zikr The Sufi practice of remembrance that includes chanting, drumming, meditating, releasing false impressions and delusions, and embracing new dimensions of inner reality.
See also ISLAMIC SUFI HEALING PRACTICES.

zone therapy Originally, European technique that involves the stimulation of the body's regional energetic zones for the treatment of a variety of disorders. After the laryngologist William Fitzgerald, of Saint Francis Hospital in Connecticut, found that zone therapy with finger pressure applied to certain points on the hands and mouth could induce numbness and relieve some symptoms, he introduced its benefits to the American public. Later, the physiotherapist Eunice Ingham further developed Dr. Fitzgerald's work by mapping out bodily reflexes (reflex points) and regions on the soles of the feet, which contain approximately 7,200 nerve endings. When finger pressure is applied to certain areas—the ball of the foot, representing the lungs and breast, for example—stimulation and a healing effect are directed to the lungs or breast. Ingham's techniques brought forth reflexology, as it is known today, as a form of bodywork.
See also ACUPRESSURE; CHAKRAS; REFLEXOLOGY; YIN-YANG.

zong qi In Chinese traditional medicine energy, or *qi* (*ch'i*), that is gathered in the thorax as other types of *qi* combine in that area.

Zukav, Gary The Harvard University graduate and winner of the 1979 American Book Award for *The Dancing Wu Li Masters* (New York: Bantam Books, 1979). Zukav, of California, became one of the New Age movement's intellectual explorers with his vision that goes beyond physics and science to the new mind-expanding theory of personal experience, that is, the power of our own thoughts and how this power can help in life transformations. Zukav is also the author of *The Seat of the Soul* (New York: Simon & Schuster, 1989).

173

APPENDIXES

I. Professional and Lay Organizations

II. The American Medical Association
   Report 12 of the Council on Scientific Affairs

III. New National Institutes of Health Study

IV. Herbs Used in Alternative Medicine Disciplines

V. National Center for Complementary and
   Alternative Medicine Five-Year Strategic Plan
   2001–2005

VI. Historic Timeline of Alternative and
   Complementary Therapies

APPENDIX I
PROFESSIONAL AND LAY ORGANIZATIONS

Academy for Guided Imagery
P.O. Box 2070
Mill Valley, CA 94942
(800) 726-2070
http://www.interactiveimagery.com

Accreditation Commission for Acupuncture and Oriental Medicine
(301) 608-9680

Acupressure Institute
1533 Shattuck Avenue
Berkeley, CA 94709
(800) 442-2232
http://www.acupressure.com

Acupuncture Foundation of Canada
7321 Victoria Park Avenue, Unit 18
Markham, ON
Canada L3R 2ZB

Advanced Health Research Institute
211 South State College Blvd., Suite 316
Anaheim, CA 92806
(888) 792-1102
http://www.ahrinstitute.com

Aidan Incorporated
621 South 48th Street
Tempe, AZ 85281
(800) 529-0269 or (480) 446-8181
http://www.aidan-az.com

AIDS Alternative Health Project
4753 N. Broadway, Suite 1110
Chicago, IL 60640
(773) 561-2800
http://www.danceforlife.org

American Academy of Anti-Aging Medicine (A4M)
2415 North Greenview
Chicago, IL 60614
(773) 528-4333
http://www.worldhealth.net

American Academy of Biological Dentistry (AABD)
P.O. Box 856
Carmel Valley, CA 93924
(831) 659-5385
http://www.biologicaldentistry.org

American Academy of Environmental Medicine
7701 East Kellogg Avenue, Suite 625
Wichita, KS 67207
(316) 684-5500
http://www.aaem.com

American Academy of Medical Acupuncture
4929 Wilshire Blvd., Suite 428
Los Angeles, CA 90010
(323) 937-5514 or (800) 521-2262
http://www.medicalacupuncture.org

American Academy of Neural Therapy
1200 112th Avenue N.E.
Bellevue, WA 98004
(425) 688-8818
http://www.neuraltherapy.com

American Academy of Osteopathy
3500 DePauw Blvd., Suite 1080
Indianapolis, IN 46268
(317) 879-1881
http://www.academyofosteopathy.org

American Alliance of Aromatherapy
P.O. Box 750428
Petaluma, CA 94975-0428
(707) 778-6762

**American and International Boards of
    Environmental Medicine (ABEM/IBEM)**
65 Wehrle Drive
Buffalo, NY14255
(716) 837-1380

American Alternative Medical Association
708 Madelaine Drive
Gilmer, TX 75644-3140

American Apitherapy Society, Inc.
P.O. Box 54
Hartland Four Corners, VT 05049
(800) 823-3460

American Aromatherapy Association
P.O. Box 3679
South Pasadena, CA 91031
(818) 457-1742

American Art Therapy Association
1202 Allanson Road
Mundelein, IL 60060

**American Association of Acupuncture
    and Oriental Medicine**
1424 16th Street N.W., Suite 501
Washington, DC 20036

**American Association of Acupuncture
    and Bioenergetic Medicine**
2512 Manoa Road

Honolulu, HI 96822
(808) 946-2069

**American Association of Drugless
    Practitioners**
(888) 764-AADP
(A division of American Alternative Medical
Association)

**American Association of
    Naturopathic Physicians**
601 Valley Street, Suite 105
Seattle, WA 98109
(206) 298-0126
http://www.naturopathic.org

American Association of Oriental Medicine
433 Front Street
Catasauqua, PA 18032
(888) 500-7999
http://www.aaom.org

**American Association of
    Orthopedic Medicine**
30897 C.R. 356-3
P.O. Box 4997
Buena Vista, CA 81211
(800) 992-2063
http://www.aaomed.org

**American Association of Professional
    Hypnotherapists**
4149-A El Camino Way
Palo Alto, CA 94306
(650) 323-3224
http://www.aaph.org

**American Association for
    Therapeutic Humor**
222 Meramec, Suite 303
St. Louis, MO 63105
(314) 863-6232

**American Board of Chelation Therapy
    Great Lakes College of Clinical Medicine**
1407-B North Wells Street
Chicago, IL 60610
(800) 286-6013 or (312) 266-7246
http://www.glccm.org

American Board of Hypnotherapy/American Institute of Hypnotherapy
2002 E. McFadden, Suite 100
Santa Ana, CA 92705
(714) 245-9340 or (800) 872-9996
http://www.aih.cc

American Bodywork and Massage Professionals
28677 Buffalo Park Road
Evergreen, CO 80349
(800) 458-2267
http://www.abmp.com

American Botanical Council
P.O. Box 144345
Austin, TX 78714-4345
(512) 926-4900
http://www.herbalgram.org

American Center for the Alexander Technique
129 West 67th Street
New York, NY 10023
(212) 799-0468

American Chiropractic Association
1701 Clarendon Boulevard
Arlington, VA 22209
(800) 986-4636
http://www.acatoday.com

American Chronic Pain Association
P.O. Box 850
Rocklin, CA 95677
(916) 632-0922

American College of Addictionology and Compulsive Disorders
975 Arthur Godfrey Road, Suite 500
Miami Beach, FL 33140
(305) 534-3635

American College of Advancement in Medicine (ACAM)
23121 Verdugo Drive, Suite 204
Laguna Hills, CA 92654
(800) 532-3688
http://www.acam.org

American College of Hyperbaric Medicine (ACHM)
P.O. Box 25914-130
Houston, TX 77265
(713) 528-0657

American College of Nutrition
722 Robert E. Lee Drive
Wilmington, DE 28480
(252) 452-1222
http://www.am-coll-nutr.org

American College of Osteopathic Pain Management and Sclerotherapy
5002 East Woodmill Drive
Wilmington, DE 19808
(800) 476-6114

American College of Traditional Chinese Medicine
455 Arkansas Street
San Francisco, CA 94107
(415) 282-7600
www.actcm.org

American Colon Therapy Association
17739 Washington Blvd.
Los Angeles, California 90066
(310) 572-6223

American Council of Hypnotist Examiners Hypnotism Training Institute of Los Angeles
700 south Central Avenue
Glendale, CA 91204

American Council on Science and Health
1995 Broadway, 2nd Floor
New York, NY 10023
(212) 362-7044
http://www.acsh.org

American CranioSacral Therapy Association Upledger Institute
11211 Prosperity Farms Road
Palm Beach Gardens, FL 33410
(407) 622-4706
http://www.upledger.com

American Dietetic Association
216 W. Jackson Boulevard, Suite 800
Chicago, IL 60606
(312) 899-0040 or (800) 366-1655 or
   fax (312) 899-1979

American Foundation for Homeopathy
1508 Glencoe Street, Suite 44
Denver, CO 80220-1338

American Health Institute
12381 Wilshire Blvd.
Los Angeles, CA 90025
(310) 820-6042
http://www.ahealth.com

American Herb Association
P.O. Box 1673
Nevada City, CA 95959

American Herbal Pharmacopoeia
P.O. Box 5159
Santa Cruz, CA 95063
(831) 461-6318
http://www.herbal-ahp.org

American Herbal Products Association
8484 Georgia Avenue, Suite 370
Silver Spring, MD 20910
(301) 588-1171
http://www.ahpa.org

American Herbalists Guild
1931 Gaddis Road
Canton, GA 30115
(770) 751-6021
http://www.americanherbalist.com

American Holistic Health Association
P.O. Box 17400
Anaheim, CA 92817
(714) 779-6152
http://mail@ahha.org

**American Holistic Medical Assocation
(AHMA)**
6728 Old McLean Village Drive
McLean, VA 22101

(703) 556-9245
http://www.holisticmedicine.org

American Holistic Nurses Association
P.O. Box 2130
2133 E. Lakin Drive, Suite 2
Flagstaff, AZ 86003-2130

**American Holistic Veterinary
   Medical Association**
2218 Old Emmorton Road
Bel Air, Maryland 21015
(410) 569-0795
http://www.ahvma.org

American Imagery Association
4016 Third Avenue
San Diego, CA 92103
(619) 794-8814

American Imagery Institute
P.O. Box 13453
Milwaukee, WI 53213
(414) 781-4045

American Institute of Hypnotherapy
16842 Von Karmen Avenue, Suite 475
Irvine, CA 92606

American Massage Therapy Association
820 Davis Street, Suite 100
Evanston, IL 60201
(847) 864-0123
http://www.amtamassage.org

American Medical Association
515 N. State Street
Chicago, IL 60610
(312) 464-5000

American Music Therapy Association (AMTA)
8455 Colesville Road, Suite 1000
Silver Spring, MD 20910
(301) 589-3300
http://www.musictherapy.org

**American Oriental Bodywork
   Therapy Association (AOBTA)**
Laurel Oak Corporate Center, Suite 408
1010 Haddonfield-Berlin Road

Voorhees, NJ 08043
(856) 782-1616
http://www.healthy.net/association/pa/body
    work/about1.htm

American Osteopathic Association
142 East Ontario Street
Chicago, IL 60611
(312) 202-8200 or (800) 621-1773

American Polarity Therapy Association
P.O. Box 19858
Boulder, CO 80308
(303) 545-2080
http://www.polaritytherapy.org
or
P.O. Box 44-154
West Sommerville, MA 02144

American Physical Therapy Association
1111 North Fairfax Street
Alexandria, VA 22314-1488
(703) 706-3248
http://www.apta.org

**American Psychotherapy and
    Medical Hypnosis Association**
280 Island Avenue, Suite 404
Reno, NV 89501
(775) 786-5650
http://www.apmha.com

**American Qigong Association and
    East-West Academy of the Healing Arts**
P.O. Box 31211
San Francisco, CA 94131
(415) 788-2227
http://www.eastwestqi.com

**American Reflexology Certification Board
    and Information Service**
P.O. Box 620607
Littleton, CO 80162
(303) 933-6921

American Shiatsu Association
P.O. Box 718
Jamaica Plain, MA 01230

**American Society of the
    Alexander Technique**
P.O. Box 517
Urbana, IL 61801
(800) 473-0620
http://www.alexandertech.org

**American Society of
    Bariatric Physicians**
5600 South Quebec Street, Suite 109A
Englewood, CO 80111
(303) 779-4833 or fax (303) 779-4834

American Society of Clinical Hypnosis
2200 E. Devon Avenue, Suite 301
Des Plaines, IL 60018

American Society for Clinical Nutrition
9650 Rockville Pike
Bethesda, MD 20814
(301) 530-7110

**American Speech-Language-Hearing
    Association**
10801 Rockville Pike
Rockville, MD 20852
(800) 638-8255
http://www.asha.org

American Vegan Society
P.O. Box H
Malaga, NJ 08328
(609) 694-2887

American Yoga Association
3130 Mayfield Road, W-301
Cleveland Heights, OH 44118
(216) 371-0078
or
513 South Orange Avenue
Sarasota, FL 34236
(813) 953-5859

Anchor Point Institute, L.L.C.
505 E. 200 South, Suite 250
Salt Lake City, UT 84102
(801) 534-1022
http://www.nlpanchorpoint.com

Aromatherapy Institute and Research
P.O. Box 1222
Fair Oaks, CA 95628

Aromatherapy Seminars
3379 South Robertson Blvd.
Los Angeles, CA 90034
(800) 677-2368

Arthritis Trust of America
7111 Sweetgum Road, Suite A
Fairview, TN 37062-9384

Association for Applied Psychophysiology and Biofeedback
10200 West 44th Avenue, Suite 304
Wheat Ridge, CO 80033
(303) 422-8436
http://www.aapb.org

Association of Vegetarian Dietitians & Nutrition Educators
3674 Cronk Road
Montour Falls, NY 14865
(607) 535-6089

Aston Training Center
P.O. Box 3568
Incline Village, NV 89450
(775) 831-8228
http://www.AstonEnterprises.com

Autism Research Institute
4182 Adams Avenue
San Diego, CA 92116
(619) 281-7165
http://www.autism.com/ari/contents.html

Autism Services Center
Prichard Building, 605 9th Street
P.O. Box 507
Huntington, WV 25710-0507
(304) 525-8014

Autism Society of America
7910 Woodmont Avenue, Suite 300
Bethesda, MD 20814-3067
(301) 657-0881 or (800) 3-AUTISM
http://www.autism-society.org

Ayurvedic & Naturopathic Medical Clinic
2115 112th Avenue N.E.
Bellevue, WA 98004
(425) 453-8022
http://www.ayurvedic science.com

The Ayurvedic Institute
11311 Menaul Blvd. N.E.
Albuquerque, NM 87112
(505) 291-9698
http://www.ayurveda.com

The Ayurveda Institute
P.O. Box 282
Fairfield, IA 52556

Bio-Electro-Magnetics Institute
2490 West Moana Lane
Reno, NV 89509-3936
(702) 827-9099

Bonnie Prudden Pain Erasure
P.O. Box 65240
Tucson, AZ 85719
(800) 221-4634
http://www.bonnieprudden.com

Bowen Research and Training Institute, Inc.
P.O. Box 627
Palm Harbor, FL 34682
(727) 937-9077

Canadian Association of Ayurvedic Medicine
P.O. Box 749 Station B
Ottawa, ON, Canada K1P 5P8
(613) 837-5737

Canadian Holistic Medical Association
42 Redpath Avenue
Toronto, ON, Canada M4S 2J6

Canadian Institute of Stress
Medcan Clinic Office Suite 1500
150 York Street
Toronto, ON, Canada
M5H 3S5
(416) 236-4218

Center for Applied Psychophysiology Menninger Clinic
P.O. Box 829
Topeka, KS 66601-0829
(800) 351-9058
http://www.menninger.edu

Center for Mind/Body Medicine
5225 Connecticut Avenue N.W., Suite 414
Washington, DC 20015
(202) 966-7338
http://www.cmbm.org

Community Nutrition Institute
2001 S Street N.W., Suite 530
Washington, DC 20009
(202) 462-4700

The Cranial Academy
8202 Clearvista Parkway, Suite 9-D
Indianapolis, IN 46256
(317) 594-0411

DAMS (Dental Amalgam Mercury Syndrome)
P.O. Box 7249
Minneapolis, MN 55407-0249
(800) 311-6265

Dr. Edward Bach Centre
Mount Vernon, Bakers Lane
Sotwell, Oxon OX10 0PZ, U.K.
(44-0)-1491-834678
http://www.bachcentre.com

Dr. Edward Bach Healing Society
644 Merrick Road
Lynbrook, NY 11563

Ellon (Bach U.S.A.), Inc.
P.O. Box 32
Woodmere, NY 11598

EMDR Institute
P.O. Box 51010
Pacific Grove, CA 93950
(408) 372-3900
http://www.emdr.com

Environmental Dental Association
9974 Scripps Ranch Boulevard, Suite 36
San Diego, CA 92131
(800) 388-8124

Environmental Health & Light Research Institute
16057 Tampa Palms Boulevard, Suite 227
Tampa, FL 33647
(800) 544-4878

Esalen Institute
Highway 1
Big Sur, CA 93020
(408) 667-3000
http://www.esalen.orh

Feldenkrais Guild of North America
3611 S.W. Hood Avenue, Suite 100
Portland, OR 97201
(800) 775-2118
http://www.feldenkrais.com

Flower Essence Society
P.O. Box 459
Nevada City, CA 95959
(530) 265-0258 or (800) 548-0075
http://www.flowersociety.org

Flower Healing
P.O. Box 33-0841
Miami, FL 33233
(888) 875-6753
http://www.flowerhealing.com

Georgiana Institute
P.O. Box 10
137 Davenport Road
Roxbury, CT 06783
(860) 355-1545
http://www.georgianainstitute.org

Gordon Research Institute
708 E. Highway 260
Payson, AZ 85541
(520) 474-3684
http://www.fordonresearch.com

The Hakomi Institute
P.O. Box 1873
Boulder, CO 80306
(888) 421-6699
http://www.hakomiinstitute.com

Healing Touch International
12477 W. Cedar Drive, Suite 202
Lakewood, CO 80228
(303) 989-7982
http://www.healingtouch.net

Hellerwork Internationl
3435 M Street
Eureka, CA 95503
(800) 392-3900
http://www.hellerwork.com

Herb Research Foundation
1007 Pearl Street, Suite 200
Boulder, CO 80302
(303) 449-2265
http://www.herbs.org

**Holistic Animal Therapy Association
of Australia (HATAA)**
International fax: 011+6189201 0282

Holistic Dental Association
P.O. Box 5007
Durango, CO 81301
(970) 259-1091
http://www.holisticdental.org

Homeopathic Educational Services
2124 Kittredge Street
Berkeley, CA 94704
(510) 649-0294 or (800) 359-9051
http://www.homeopathic.com

Inner Peace Music
P.O. Box 2644
San Anselmo, CA 94979
http://www.innerpeacemusic.com

Insight Meditation Society
1230 Pleasant Street
Barre, MA 01500

(978) 355-4378
http://www.dharma.org

**International Academy of Oral Medicine
and Toxicology**
P.O. Box 608531
Orlando, FL 32860-8531
(407) 298-2450
http://www.iaomt.org

**International Alliance of
Healthcare Education**
11211 Prosperity Farms Road, Suite D-325
Palm Beach Gardens, FL 33410
(800) 311-9204
http://www.iahe.org

**International Association for
Colon Therapy**
2051 Hilltop Drive, Suite A-11
Redding, CA 96002
(916) 222-1498

**International Association of
Professional Natural Hygienists**
Regency Health Resort and Spa
2000 South Ocean Drive
Hallandale, FL 33009
(305) 454-2220

International Center for Reiki Training
29209 Northwestern Highway, Suite 592
Southfield, MI 48034
(800) 332-8112
http://www.reiki.org

International Chiropractors Association
1110 North Glebe Road, Suite 1000
Arlington, VA 22201
(703) 528-5000
http://www.chiropractic.org

**International Clinical
Hyperthermia Society**
1502 East Country Line Road South
Indianapolis, IN 46227
(317) 887-7651
http://www.hyperthermia-ichs.org

**International College of Advanced
  Longevity Medicine**
1407-B N. Wells Street
Chicago, IL 60610
(888) 855-5050
http://www.healthy.net/icalm

**International College of
  Applied Kinesiology**
6405 Metcalf Avenue, Suite 503
Shawnee Mission, KS 66202-3929
(913) 384-5336
http://www.icak. com

**International Medical and Dental
  Hypnotherapy Association**
4110 Edgland, Suite 800
Royal Oak, MI 48073
(800) 257-5467 or (248) 549-5594
http://www.infinityinst.com

**International Integral Qigong and
  Tai Chi Training Institute**
Health Action
243 Pebble Beach
Santa Barbara, CA 93117
(805) 682-3230
http://www.qigong-chikung.com and
  http://www.healerwithin.com

International Institute of Reflexology
5650 First Avenue North
P.O. Box 12462
St. Petersburg, FL 33733
(727) 343-4811

International Rolf Institute
205 Canyon Road
Boulder, CO 80306
(303) 449-5903
http://www.rolf.org

**International Society for
  Orthomolecular Medicine**
16 Florence Avenue
Toronto, ON, Canada M2N 1E9
(416) 733-2117
http://www.orthomed.org

**Life Sciences Institute of
  Mind-Body Health**
4636 S.W. Wanamaker Road
Topeka, KS 66610
(785) 271-8686
http://www.cjnetworks.com/~lifesci

Light Therapy Institute
1055 W. College Avenue #107
Santa Rosa, CA 95401
(707) 525-4747

Matrix, Inc.
P.O. Box 49145
Colorado Springs, CO 80949
(866) 948-4638 or (719) 522-0566
http://www.hugnet.com

Milton H. Erickson Foundation
3606 North 24th Street
Phoenix, AZ 85016
(602) 956-6196

**Mind-Body Medical Institute
  Beth Israel Deaconess Medical Center**
185 Francis Street, Suite 1A
Boston, MA 02215
(617) 632-9530
http://www.mbmi.org

Mozart Effect Resource Center
3526 Washington Avenue
St. Louis, MO 63103
(800) 721-2177
http://www.mozarteffect.com

**The Naropa Institute
  Somatic Psychology Department**
2130 Arapahoe Avenue
Boulder, CO 80302
(303) 444-0202 or (303) 546-5284

**National Association for
  Holistic Aromatherapy**
2000 Second Avenue, Suite 206
Seattle, WA 98121
(888) ASK-NAHA
http://www.naha.org

**National Acupuncture
  Detoxification Association**
P.O. Box 1927
Vancouver, WA 98668
(888) 765-NADA
http://www.acudetox.com

National Center for Homeopathy
801 North Fairfax, Suite 306
Alexandria, VA 22314
(703) 548-7790
http://www.homeopathic.org

**National Commission for the
  Certification of Acupuncturists**
P.O. Box 97075
Washington, DC 20090
(202) 232-1404

The National Guild of Hypnotists
P.O. Box 308
Merrimack, NH 03054
(603) 429-9438
http://www.ngh.net

**National Council Against Health Fraud
  (NCAHF)**
119 Foster Street
Peabody, MA 01960
(978) 532-9383

National Institute of Endocrine Research
1817 S. Eastern Avenue
Las Vegas, NV 89104
(805) 496-0275
http://www.endocrineresearch.com

National Institute of Nutrition
2565 Carling Avenue, Suite 400
Ottawa, ON, Canada K1Z 8RI

National Qigong Association
P.O. Box 540
Ely, MA 55731
(218) 365-6330
http://www.nqa.org

Nelson Bach USA, Ltd.
Wilmington Technology Park
100 Research Drive
Wilmington, MA 01887-4406
(978) 988-3833 or (800) 319-9151
http://www.nelsonbach.com

The North American Vegetarian Society
P.O. Box 72
Dolgeville, NY 13329
(518) 568-7970

**Nurse Healers—Professional Associates
  International**
3760 South Highland Drive, Suite 429
Salt Lake City, UT 84106
(801) 273-3399
http://www.therapeutic-touch.org

Nurse Healers Professional Associates, Inc.
1211 Locust Street
Philadelphia, PA 19107
(215) 545-8079
http://www.therapeutic touch.org

Our NET Effect (ONE) Foundation
1991 Village Park Way, Suite 201-A
Encinitas, CA 92024
(800) 638-1411
http://www.onefoundation.org

The Pacific Institute of Aromatherapy
P.O. Box 6723
San Rafael, CA 94903
(415) 479-9121
http://www.pacificinstituteofaromatherapy.com

The Qigong Institute
561 Berkeley Avenue
Menlo Park, CA 94025
http://www.qigonginstitute.org

The Raj, Maharishi Ayur-Veda Health Center
1734 Jasmine Avenue
Fairfield, IA 52556
(641) 472-9580
http://www.theraj.com

The Rosen Method
http://www.rosenmethod.org

The Rubenfeld Synergy Center
(877) 776-2468
http://www.rubenfeldsynergy.com

**Sacro-Occipital Research
Society International**
P.O. Box 6067
Leawood, KS 66206
(888) 245-1011
http://www.sorsi.com

**Sharp Institute for Human Potential
and Mind-Body Medicine**
8010 Frost Street, Suite 300
San Diego, CA 92123
(800) 82-SHARP
http://www.sharp.com

Simonton Cancer Center
P.O. Box 890
Pacific Palisades, CA 90272
(800) 459-3424 or (310) 459-4434
http://www.simontoncenter.com

**Society for Light Treatment and
Biological Rhythms, Inc.**
P.O. Box 591687
174 Cook Street
San Francisco, CA 94159
(415) 876-0716
http://www.sltbr.org

**Society for Orthomolecular
Health Medicine**
2698 Pacific Avenue
San Francisco, CA 94115
(415) 922-6462
http://www.orthomed.org

Sound, Listening and Learning Center
2701 East Camelback, Suite 205
Phoenix, AZ 85016
(602) 381-0086
http://www.soundlistening.com

Sound Healers Association
P.O. Box 2240
Boulder, CO 80302
(303) 443-8181
http://www.healingsounds.com

Sound Health Research Institute, Inc.
P.O. Box 416
Athens, OH 45710
(740) 698-9119
http://www.soundhealthinc.com

**Stress Reduction and Relaxation Program
University of Massachusetts Medical Center**
55 Lake Avenue North
Worcester, MA 01655
(508) 856-2656
http://www.umassmed.edu/cfm

The Trager Institute
3800 Park East Drive, Suite 100, Room 1
Beachwood, OH 44122
(216) 896-9383
http://www.trager.com

Vegetarian Education Network
P.O. Box 3347
West Chester, PA 19381
(717) 529-8638

World Chiropractic Alliance
2950 N. Dobson Road, Suite 1
Chandler, AZ 85224
(800) 347-1011
http://www.worldchiropracticalliance.org

APPENDIX II
THE AMERICAN MEDICAL ASSOCIATION REPORT 12 OF THE COUNCIL ON SCIENTIFIC AFFAIRS

Alternative Medicine

NOTE: This report represents the medical/scientific literature on this subject as of June 1997.

The terms "alternative medicine," "complementary medicine," or "unconventional medicine" refer to diagnostic methods, treatments and therapies that appear not to conform to standard medical practice, or are not generally taught at accredited medical schools. The scope of alternative medicine is broad, with widespread use among the American public of a long list of treatments and practices, such as acupuncture, homeopathy, relaxation techniques, and herbal remedies. In an editorial about alternative practices in the *New England Journal of Medicine*, Murray and Rubel comment, "Many are well known, others are exotic and mysterious, and some are dangerous."[1] This report will help to clarify and categorize the alternative medical systems most often used, create a context to assess their utility (or lack thereof), and discuss how physicians and the medical profession might deal with the issues surrounding these unconventional measures in health and healing. . . .

At the turn of the last century, the effort led by the American Medical Association (AMA) to improve the quality of medical education and bring quality controls to curricula ultimately led to the landmark report by Flexner in 1910. Among other outcomes, the resulting changes in medical education led to the acceptance of the biological, disease-oriented models that dominate medicine in the United States today. State licensing boards, influenced by the AMA, limited the practice of medicine to graduates of accredited institutions, and research funding became the domain of the major teaching centers. All these factors put great pressure on smaller schools (and their graduates, many of whom were homeopaths) that could not meet the emerging requirements for medical education and practice. As a result, many schools that taught practices such as homeopathy were closed, homeopaths were shunned and stigmatized, and their therapies became the "alternatives" to the standards that evolved after acceptance of the Flexner reports. In contrast, Osteopathic schools like allopathic schools developed rigorous standards and practices.

I. Alternative Systems and Techniques

Most observers from outside the fields of alternative or unconventional medicine find no common or unifying theory or basis for its use; indeed, it may be that the variety of treatments in itself enhances their popularity. Many such therapies are characterized by a charismatic leader or proponent, and are driven by ideology; some spring from folk practices or quasi-religious groups, while others are recognized elements of religions such as those practiced by Native Americans.

Many alternative practitioners are unlicensed (except for chiropractic, and in some states, acupuncturists, naturopaths, and homeopathic therapists) and unregulated, particularly those dealing in alternative nutritional therapy.

The adherents of these fields, however, state that "most alternative systems of medicine hold some common beliefs."[2] Many theories of alternative medicine attempt to pose a single explanation for most human illness; the therapy is thought to correct the source of the problem, not merely treat its symptoms. The recuperative power of the human body and the potential for certain stimuli to enhance this natural healing are central to many therapies. Other unifying threads include:[2]

- Importance of spiritual values to health
- Integration of individuals in the "stream of life"
- Attribution of a causal, independent role to various "manifestations of consciousness"
- Use of whole (unsynthesized) substances
- Maintaining the injunction to "do no harm"
- The philosophy that achieving and maintaining health is very different from fighting disease
- A belief that personal experience and anecdote are as reliable as scientific study in determining whether something is effective.[3,4]

John Renner, MD, a board member of the National Council Against Health Fraud, has proposed a set of definitions[3] that are useful in discussing of alternative therapies, treatments, and devices.

1. "Proven" products and services are those that have been scientifically tested, optimally through controlled clinical trials and double-blind studies, and found to be both safe and effective for the specific condition for which their use is proposed.
2. "Experimental" therapies or products are those undergoing controlled trials to determine their proper application, dose, frequency of use, general safety, and efficacy. Such trials should be conducted under the supervision of recognized entities such as the Food and Drug Administration (FDA), the National Institutes of Health (NIH), or in academic medical centers, with proper human subjects review and full informed consent among any persons involved.
3. "Untested" methods are those that have never been subjected to rigorous clinical testing or evaluation under standard protocols and controlled conditions. Many of the herbal, homeopathic, and dietary products described in the previous narrative would fall in this category.

4. "Folklore" remedies have usually been passed down through cultural tradition and oral history, including many home remedies such as chicken soup for colds and honey and lemon tea for sore throat. Most folk medicine is not done for personal enrichment and is noncommercial.
5. "Quackery" or health fraud involves commercial marketing or use of therapies, products, or procedures with no proven effectiveness that could also cause physical harm; indirectly harms patients by delaying appropriate therapy or diverting care to unproven methods; and often involves financial fraud as well. Promises of cure for cancer, human immuno-deficiency virus (HIV), and other conditions for which little hope is present attract desperate patients willing to try anything. Anecdotal testimonials are the main basis for the "success" of these modalities.

The failure (real or perceived) of many physicians and medical specialities to understand and practice preventive medicine and to communicate effectively with patients, and conventional medicine's dependence on costly diagnostic and procedural interaction that ignores the human side of medicine may have helped spur public interest in alternative and unconventional therapy.

II. Theories of Alternative Medicine

Mind-Body Interventions

Much of alternative medicine deals with the relationship between the mind (as distinct from the brain and its biochemistry) and the body, with a chief goal of achieving a sense of psychological or spiritual well-being in persons and a feeling of wholeness even in the face of a disease process or condition. Patients with a wide range of conditions and disorders benefit from applications of techniques in this area; cancer, chronic pain and burns, chemical dependence, several neurological and psychiatric conditions, blood pressure and cholesterol reduction, home births, and other problems have been the subject of this set of treatments. Some of the therapy sounds very familiar to orthodox clinicians—stress management through meditation, music and art therapy, hypnosis, focused relaxation, and psychotherapy are all known to physicians as useful treatments. Biofeedback has been used for years in helping with anxiety and stress-related disorders, and for adjunctive therapy in blood pressure management. Some of the clinical applications of these techniques are, however, decidedly unconventional. Guided imagery to produce spontaneous remission of cancer, for example, or hypnotherapy for immune disorders and hemophilia fall into this category. Meditation is touted for its ability to increase intelligence and longevity, and yoga for better diabetic control. Advocates call for research into the "nonlocal effects of consciousness" as well as for more traditional kinds of review such as the effects of personal belief, values, and meaning on health and illness.

Diet/Nutrition

The knowledge that good nutrition and a balanced diet help maintain health is not new, or news. A cornerstone of belief in most alternative systems is the repudiation of the "modern, affluent diet" and its replacement with a diet rich in whole, "organic" products, often vegetarian in approach. Many healers maintain that certain diets promote anti-tumor immunity or cardiovascular health; other regimens advocate specific micronutrients or vitamins for particular conditions or overall longevity. There seems to be a continuum of beliefs ranging from promoting dietary supplements beyond the Recommended Dietary Allowances (RDAs), to elimination or addition of specific foods to "treat" specific conditions.

Much of the dietary intervention stressed by alternative healers is prudent and reasonable. The American diet is unarguably too rich in fat and empty calories. Dietitians and nutritionists are licensed in many states, and are an invaluable source of advice to physicians and patients alike regarding nutrition and dietary management of a host of conditions. But the approach taken by some alternative practitioners encourages what many consider the excessive use of health foods and dietary supplements, often of a proprietary nature and meant to enrich themselves while promoting several myths:[4]

1. it is difficult to get the nourishment one requires from ordinary foods

2. vitamin and mineral deficiencies are common
3. most diseases are caused by faulty diets and can be prevented by nutritional interventions
4. any use of food additives and pesticides is poisonous

Herbal Remedies

Herbal medicine is a booming industry in the United States. The American market for herbal remedies has doubled since 1985, to $1.13 billion in 1993 (excluding homeopathic remedies and teas). Growth is expected to continue at 10% to 15% per year through 1997. Four-fifths of all people, worldwide, still rely to a great extent on traditional medicines based on plants and their components.[5]

The use of herbs in medicine is ancient in its origins, and several examples are well known to both physicians and the public: foxglove as the treatment for "dropsy" and later, the source for digitalis, and quinine's origins in *Cinchona* bark. New therapies such as taxol continue to show the usefulness of plants as a source of our pharmacopoeia. The director of collaborative services in the Department of Pharmacology at the University of Illinois at Chicago, a national botanical authority, states that only 90 plant species account for most of the plant-derived drugs in common use by physicians, about 120 drugs in all. Three-fourths of this list was discovered by following up on traditional folk medicine claims.[5]

Basic to the use of herbs in alternative medicine is the belief that whole plant material is superior to synthesized or isolated chemicals derived from plant sources. The material may be flowers, bark, roots, or leaves, used singly or in combination, often taken in the form of teas, or ground and taken as tablets, or used in salves. These compounds are thought to produce fewer unintended or dangerous effects, and a "balanced" action as opposed to single drugs. There is little evidence for this belief, however, and no standardization of the dose in herbal healing. The safety of many of the compounds is unknown, or the potential toxicity ignored.[6,7]

Folk healers, herbalists, naturopaths, traditional Chinese healers, homeopaths, and a host of others in alternative practices commonly use herbal remedies. As with other nutrition therapies, herbs are prescribed to prevent or treat specific conditions, and are consumed by many persons to maintain health. For example, a recent meta-analysis study on St. John's wort (*Hypericium perforatum*) suggests that this herb shows promise in treating mild to moderately severe depression.[8] An accompanying editorial points out several limitations in these interesting data, including the need for trials longer than 8 weeks, better patient selection and categorization of diagnosis, and comparisons with therapeutic doses of standard antidepressants.[9]

The conclusion that St. John's wort needs more study is distinctly different, however, from the one expressed by the president of Bastyr University, a school of naturopathy in Seattle, Washington. In an article written in a popular consumer magazine,[10] he describes common drugs he "personally would never take," offering "natural alternatives that help correct the underlying problem" that he describes as "safer, more effective, and less expensive" than such treatments as estrogens for menopausal symptoms, non-steroidal anti-inflammatory drugs, and conventional antidepressants. He advocates the use of St. John's wort or other herbs for mild to moderate depression. He does caution readers to consult with their doctor before beginning his suggested treatments, or making changes in current medication regimens.

Regulation of herbal and plant products in Germany has been assigned to a special commission within the Federal Health Agency that has produced a series of monographs on the safety of these products. More than 200 such products have been approved, some of which seem to have salutary effects. As opposed to the FDA requirements of evidence from randomized studies, the German commission demands a less stringent standard for efficacy, allowing material such as case reports, historical data, and other data in the scientific literature.[11]

The Dietary Supplement Health and Education Act of 1994 regulates the claims that can be made about the effects of herbal and nutritional products. The Act gives the FDA some controls over herbal supplements, vitamins, and amino acid preparations and similar products, classifying them as dietary supplements. Manufacturers cannot make claims as to the health or therapeutic benefits of their products on package labels and labeling without receiving FDA prior approval. However, general claims related to well-being and to the effect of a substance on the structure or function of the body can be made without any evaluation or approval by the FDA. The Act also shifts the burden of proof to the FDA to prove that a product in this category is unsafe prior to taking regulatory action, rather than requiring the manufacturer to obtain FDA approval by showing that the product is safe before offering the product to the public. New labeling requirements and an Office on Dietary Supplements in the NIH also are called for by the Act.

Because this category of products can be marketed without FDA review or approval, standards for dosage and other manufacturing safeguards, or evidence of safety, some health fraud experts worry that this new law will make it easier for nutrition to be misused by hucksters, and will hamper the FDA's ability to effectively monitor safety among the growing number of herbal and nutritional remedies being offered to the public. The burden now rests with the consumer to interpret claims made by the manufacturers of these products. For example, persons with acquired immunodeficiency syndrome (AIDS) might believe a claim made by an herbal product of "boosting T-cells" is true and leads to an improvement in the course of the disease from using the product.

An example of FDA intervention in this area involves ephedrine alkaloid containing dietary supplements that have been promoted as euphoric agents that are safe alternatives to illegal drugs, as well as for purposes such as weight loss, energy or body building. [NB: FDA has recorded very few adverse events with products marketed as euphorics.] Containing "natural" sources of ephedrine such as ma huang, ephedra, Ephedra sinica, or extracts of these substances, these compounds have been shown to have adverse effects such as headache, dizziness, palpitations, and possibly, clinically significant effects such as heart attack, stroke, seizures, and psychosis. The FDA considers marketing of these products, often aimed at adolescents looking for a "high," to be in violation of the Act, and is currently considering regulatory steps to ensure the safety of ephedrine-containing dietary supplements and what further action should be taken in this area.

Our ability to increase our understanding of the role of herbal remedies in medicine is hampered by deforestation, and the loss of knowledge held about plant therapies by indigenous people as the Amazon and other remote areas are developed. Activity in biodiversity is being supported by the NIH, the National Institute of Mental Health, the National Science Foundation, and the US Agency for International Development.[2] Both the traditional medical community and the adherents of alternative therapy have called for increased research into this area.

Manual Healing Methods

The healer's touch has been considered a therapeutic instrument for the entire history of medicine, dating back to instructions by Hippocrates about therapeutic massage. Ancient Chinese medicine has strong roots in this system, and several areas of alternative medicine are associated with manual healing methods. The major fields of manual healing include (1) methods that use physical touch, manipulation, and pressure—chiropractic and osteopathic manipulation are primary examples; (2) therapies that use an "energy field" that can influence healing; and (3) mixed interventions that use both physical touch and energy field therapy.

Osteopathy

Osteopathic physicians derive their theories from the work of Andrew Taylor Still (1828–1917), a physician's son who was trained as an apprentice to his father. After the Civil War, he began an empirical study of healing by manipulating bones and soft tissues to allow the free circulation of blood and lymph, and to restore the nervous system to what he considered a more normal function. Known as the "lightning bone-setter," he disdained the common practices of physicians in the last century such as venesection, emesis, and sedation with narcotics, preferring to use manipulation to enhance the body's innate ability to heal itself. Instead of using drugs, he believed that the solution to illness lay in treating the underlying condition, allowing the body's natural forces to return

the patient to health. He proposed that much more than headache and back pain could be treated with manipulation, and set forth a regimen of therapy that included treatment for serious conditions such as pneumonia, dysentery, and typhoid fever.

The first school of osteopathy was opened in Missouri in 1892, teaching a variety of methods: manipulation of soft tissue, isometric and isotonic muscle techniques, manipulation with varying "velocity," the use of the percussion hammer to strike the body to alleviate "restrictions" in the joints and muscles that allowed internal processes to function normally, and other unorthodox therapies. Since that time, osteopathic education and its practitioners have become nearly indistinguishable from their allopathic cousins, with the exception of manipulation techniques that continue to be integral parts of osteopathic diagnostic and treatment modalities. Modern osteopathic physicians are considered to be in the mainstream of medical practice, with rigorous standards for education and specialty training. Osteopathic physicians commonly complete allopathic postgraduate specialty training, and are licensed to practice the full scope of medicine in all states, without restrictions. Some advocates of alternative medicine criticize modern osteopaths for abandoning the original scope and breadth of manipulation therapy.

Chiropractic

As with many systems in alternative medicine, chiropractic holds that the innate ability of the body to heal itself can be optimized by achieving a "balance"; that proper function of the nervous system is key to this homeostasis; that "subluxations" of the spine and misalignment of joints impinge on nerves, causing imbalance in internal systems; and that manual release of these structural and functional joint pathologies can heal a number of conditions, and prevent illness as well.[12]

The theories behind chiropractic have been widely criticized. A 1968 study by the US Department of Health, Education, and Welfare concluded that chiropractic schools did not prepare students to adequately diagnose and treat patients, and recommended that their services not be covered under Medicare.[2,12] In 1972, Congress added Medicare benefits for "manual manipulation of the spine to correct a subluxation demonstrated to exist on x-ray." In 1974 the Council on Chiropractic Education was recognized to accredit schools of chiropractic, despite the absence of clear evidence of efficacy of chiropractic therapy.[12] Over the years, both political pressure and consumer acceptance has won licensure for chiropractic in all 50 states. Most of the nation's 45,000 chiropractors bill Medicare for services rendered, amounting to $181 million in 1990.[12] Most third-party payors accept claims from chiropractors.

Manipulation has been shown to have a reasonably good degree of efficacy in ameliorating back pain, headache, and similar musculoskeletal complaints,[13] and some chiropractors limit their practices to these conditions. While precise statistics are not available, a majority of chiropractors adhere to the method's original theories, and continue to claim that chiropractic manipulation cures disease rather than simply relieving symptoms. (Personal communication, Denny Futch DC, Vice President, National Association of Chiropractic Medicine.) They promote manipulation as useful in a host of conditions, ranging from infectious diseases to immune therapy, even claiming to prevent future conditions from occurring (even if years away) including menstrual irregularity, difficulty giving birth, and cancer.[12] Chiropractors commonly provide advice in nutrition and other preventive practices, and maintain that a regular series of "adjustments" is needed by most persons to maintain optimal health.

Energy Healing

Biofield, or energy healing, is described by its proponents as "one of the oldest forms of healing known to humankind."[14] Theories related to this practice involve transfer of energy from healer to patient in unknown ways, either from a supernatural entity or by manipulating the body's own "energy fields." Over 25 terms are used in various cultures to describe this life force. Biofield practitioners incorporate a holistic focus into therapy, and promote their methods as useful for stress and general improvement of health; relief of pain, edema, and acceleration of wound and fracture healing; improvement in digestion, appetite, and various emotional states; and treatment of conditions such as eating disorders, irritable bowel syndrome, and pre-menstrual syndrome.

Some unique conditions are "diagnosed" by biofield practitioners, such as "accumulated tension" and "congested energy" that, when released, supposedly lead to improved health. A common form of this therapy is used by nurses, and is called "therapeutic touch." It involves moving the hands over (but not in direct contact with) the patient's body either to create a general state of well-being by enhancing "energy flow" in the subject, or to release "accumulated tension" and induce balance and harmony. At least one school of nursing has demanded that its faculty cease teaching these modalities as part of their curriculum (personal communication, John Renner, MD).

Therapies that combine manipulation and biofield therapy include "network chiropractic spinal analysis," which combines soft-tissue chiropractic and applications of the biofield, followed by conventional chiropractic treatment; "craniosacral therapy," an offshoot of osteopathic medicine involving manipulation of cranial and/or sacral bones to relieve "restrictions" in motion of these bones that are thought to help persons with seizures, immune disorders, learning disabilities, and assorted other conditions; and "polarity therapy," in which touch, energy field manipulation, and other modalities correct distortions in one's "energy anatomy."[15]

Pharmacologic Methods

The area of pharmacologic treatment is rife with both opportunity and peril, since many of the modalities in unconventional medicine that use pharmacologic and biologic treatment may truly be deserving of clinical trials and well-funded investigation. At the same time, many therapies in this area represent true health fraud. Some areas under investigation include immunotherapies, including the use of antitumor antibodies; alternative strategies to treat menopausal conditions; the use of local anesthetic injection into autonomic ganglia and other sites, such as acupuncture points for chronic pain; and several cancer and HIV treatments. Some methods proposed for study and further dissemination have been associated with proponents using questionable methods and possibly fraudulent research. Several of these are cancer therapies, including "antineoplastons," popularized by a physician named Burzynski who claims he can "normalize" tumor cells by shutting off their undifferentiated growth using peptides extracted from urine. A review of this method in JAMA[16] concludes that no objective evidence exists to support the experimental claims.

Chelation with EDTA for heart disease and other cardiovascular conditions is another questionable practice in this category. Described by proponents as a nontoxic way to flush "toxins" and fatty deposits from the arterial system, it has also been touted for emphysema, kidney and endocrine disease, and arthritis. Ozone therapy has been advocated by alternative healers, as has intravenous hydrogen peroxide. Therapies involving bee pollen (and other products from bees) are in widespread use, with no scientific evidence for efficacy—but a Senator who attributed improvement in his health to bee pollen spurred the creation of the NIH Office of Alternative Medicine (OAM).

Investigators worry that the Internet has become a bazaar for alternative therapies, whose purveyors can use overseas addresses for distributing products that are not subject to any sort of scrutiny. There are now more than 100 commercial outlets for shark cartilage, a substance that is promoted for cancer treatment and prevention, arthritis, and a host of other ailments. Hormones such as DHEA (dihydroepiandosterone) get Internet claims for extending life, normalizing blood sugar and cholesterol, and sexual enhancement. Colloidal silver is said to be a "safe natural antibiotic" that "kills 650 disease causing organisms." Asparagus extract is said to "restrain and prevent metastasis of middle as well as late stage tumors," and the list goes on, with hundreds of alternative medicine home pages and links to mail order firms.[17]

Proponents of alternative pharmacotherapy argue that proper funding, well-organized trials, and modifications in FDA regulations for experimental therapy will help these therapies get a "fair hearing" by the traditional medical community. On the other hand, they have requested immunity from the FDA and other regulatory oversight, protecting investigators from fraud and licensing actions, raids, seizure of materials, import alerts,

and other interventions for all clinical trials endorsed by the OAM.[18]

III. Alternative Systems of Practice

Several distinct systems of alternative practice encompass many of the theories and methods described above.

Acupuncture

Acupuncture is an ancient technique with its origins in traditional Chinese medicine. The internal study of the body was forbidden in China, so structural anatomy as defined by dissection was unknown. Twelve organs, or "spheres of function," were thought present, having minimal equivalency to anatomic definitions used in Western medicine. Body function was described in theories of energy flow, or ch'i, from one organ to another. Each of these organs is described as having a superficial "meridian" with many numbered points, originally derived from Chinese astrologic calculations. By inserting needles into these points, acupuncturists believe energy flows can be manipulated or imbalance corrected, resulting in therapeutic effects on corresponding internal systems.

Western practitioners have increasingly begun to use acupuncture, but many may not be using techniques that correspond to traditional Chinese teaching. The American Academy of Medical Acupuncture is a group of more than 700 physicians who offer training and continuing medical education, and set "standards of practice" regarding use of these techniques in medical practice. Most often, acupuncture is used for acute or chronic pain relief, but some proponents also use it for smoking cessation and substance abuse treatment, asthma, arthritis, and other conditions. Endorphin release, stimulation of the peripheral nervous system, and pain mediation through the effects of other neuropeptides are currently thought to be the most likely conventional explanations for the effects of acupuncture.

Several variations on the general theme exist, including the use of heated needles, passing low-voltage current into the acupuncture point, and applying lasers to acupuncture points. Proponents from different traditions (i.e., Korean vs. Chinese) often disagree as to the "correct" location of acupuncture points for treating a given condition. Recently, the FDA reclassified acupuncture needles as devices that do not require clinical studies, thus easing requirements for marketing. Critics contend that acupuncturists, including many traditionally trained physicians, merely stick needles in patients as a way to offer another form of treatment for which they can be reimbursed, since many insurance companies will do so. Critical reviews of acupuncture summarized by Hafner[4] and others[19] conclude that no evidence exists that acupuncture affects the course of any disease.

Homeopathy

Homeopathy was begun in the early 1800s by Samuel Hahnemann (1755–1843), a traditionally trained German physician who renounced the practices of the day, such as bleeding and purging, taking an approach based in not inflicting harm. He studied the effect of drugs of the day on the body, and devised a new series of rules for their testing and later, their application. His primary theory is the "Law of Similars"—"like cures like." Coining the term homeopathy, he proposed that small amounts of a substance that could induce a set of symptoms in a patient could cure a disease with similar symptoms. This evolved into a highly structured, complex set of pharmacologic interventions or "provings" with formulation and administration of extremely dilute concentrations of substances and drugs, based in the "Law of Infinitesimals." Homeopaths believe that even extreme dilutions of a drug will have a salutary effect, and that the molecular structure of the diluent is somehow changed in the process of preparation, by vigorous shaking and striking the side of the flask containing the preparation. Then, the "memory" of the original drug is carried on even when, after multiple dilutions, none of the original substance could be theoretically present. Careful attention to the total history of the patient was emphasized, and the use of a single homeopathic remedy for a given condition or set of complaints was taught, based on detailed observations of the effects of these preparations.

Introduced into the United States in 1828, homeopathy spread and competed with traditional medicine, with results that were at least as favorable as bleeding and other customs of the day. By the turn of the century more than 14,000 homeopaths had been trained, and 22 schools taught the theory in the United States. As mentioned previously, advances in medical education, scientific theory, and pressure from organized medicine led to the decline of homeopathy. In 1938, a homeopath in the US Senate, Royal Copeland (D-NY), succeeded in giving homeopathic remedies legal status, adding the drugs found in the *Homeopathic Pharmacopeia of the United States* to the list of articles that the FDA recognizes as drugs. This automatically designated these drugs as "safe," although their efficacy was never proven.

Today, homeopathy is practiced mostly by persons licensed as physicians or holding another license allowing the prescription of drugs. Some lay healers use homeopathy, and homeopathic remedies abound in health food stores and many supermarkets that feature "organic" products. Some homeopathic healers continue the tradition of extensive patient interviews and the use of a single substance as instructed by Hahnemann's original treatises; others use several compounds simultaneously, and add other modalities to their range of treatments, such as massage and skeletal manipulation, acupuncture, and aromatherapy.

While most homeopathic remedies are not known to have harmed anyone (probably because of the extreme dilutions involved), the efficacy of most homeopathic remedies has not been proven. Some think it a placebo effect, augmented by the concern expressed by the healer; others propose new theories based on quantum mechanics and electromagnetic energy.

A randomized clinical trial of homeopathic remedies has been touted as showing the effectiveness of homeopathic treatments in childhood diarrhea.[20] However, it has been criticized for inconsistent/incorrect data analysis; use of different diagnostic and treatment categories but combining them in the conclusions of efficacy; and lack of chemical analysis of different treatments. The clinical significance of the results, given the self-limiting condition being studied, has been called into question.[21]

Homeopathy's adherents propose new trials of these therapies, systematic review of standard pharmacologic agents subjected to homeopathic dilutions and therapeutic application, and investigation into clinical outcomes following homeopathic treatment.

Naturopathy

Naturopathy is a term coined by John Scheel in 1895 to describe his methods of healing. A poorly developed set of principles and theories, naturopathy may have its roots in the spas of Europe that flourished at the turn of the century. About 20 schools of naturopathy were present in the United States in the early 1900s. The Flexner report and other pressures led to its decline. It never had the political and professional stature of other alternative methods, and until recently, education in naturopathy was available only through schools of chiropractic.

Currently, three naturopathic colleges have been accredited by the profession, led by Bastyr University in Seattle. Naturopathy is a four-year course of study that involves two years of anatomy, physiology, and basic sciences, and two years of applied courses. Naturopaths practice various treatments such as manipulation and massage, and use herbs, acupuncture, and traditional Oriental medicine. Its practitioners treat underlying causes of illness by facilitating the body's response to disease through its "life force." Questionable therapy such as prescriptions of colonic irrigation, and chelation therapy to "remove toxins" presumed present in the body are commonly used by naturopaths. Some naturopaths use "diagnostic" techniques such as iridology hair shaft analysis. Naturopaths are licensed in 11 states, but most third-party payors, including Medicare, do not cover their services. Recently, the King County, WA, governing council voted to subsidize a naturopathic clinic operated by Bastyr.

Ayurveda

Ayurveda is a mind-body set of beliefs and principles that has its roots in ancient India, and has been practiced for over 5,000 years. Disease is thought to arise from imbalance or stress in an individual's consciousness, and is exacerbated by unhealthy lifestyles. Three *doshas* determine one's unique "body type," and combined with diagnostic readings of the radial pulse, guides the healer to determinations of dysfunction and corresponding treatment.

Specific lifestyle and dietary interventions are prescribed, as well as measures to rid the body of certain toxins and metabolic byproducts that are thought to accumulate, to the detriment of the body. Meditation, exercise, herbal oil massage, and other therapy are promoted, much of which is proprietary and marketed commercially.

Folk Therapies

Besides traditional Oriental medicine, other cultural systems within the United States use folk treatment and rely to at least some extent on self-care remedies. Some of the healers are shamanistic and blend religion with their efforts to heal, such as in Native American healing ceremonies or in Latin American and Caribbean culture. For physicians practicing in areas with significant ethnic populations, knowledge of these folk beliefs and cultural sensitivity in history-taking, physical examination, and instruction may enhance clinical interactions. Practitioners of traditional Chinese medicine use acupuncture, a host of herbal remedies, and sometimes include substances derived from sources such as the gallbladder of bears, tiger teeth and bones, and rhinoceros horn, increasing the hazards facing these endangered species.

The Office of Alternative Medicine (OAM)

Because of the high prevalence of use of alternative medicine in the United States, Congress passed legislation in 1991 that created the OAM at the NIH, with a directive to begin a program of research on alternative therapies. Its purpose is to "coordinate and support evaluations and investigations that assess the scientific validity, clinical usefulness, and theoretical implications of health care practices that prevent or alleviate suffering or promote healing."

An initial budget of $2 million has grown to $5.4 million for FY 1995 and $11.1 million for FY 1997. The OAM is funding a wide variety of investigator-initiated grant projects and creating a clearinghouse for information on alternative medical practices. Ten centers for research in complementary and alternative medicine have been funded with grants of about $1 million each, to study specific health conditions, including cancer and women's health issues. Each center will develop a program infrastructure, establish research priorities, conduct small "collaborative research projects" within the first year or two, propose larger research projects for future funding, and create systematic reviews of specified areas of alternative medicine using rigorous standards.

The OAM is also re-evaluating its database and its methods for research development, including controlled trials of alternative therapies. As its evaluation director Carole Hudgings, PhD, states in the OAM's October 1996 newsletter, ". . . it is important that the scientific rigor applied in conventional medicine also be applied to complementary and alternative practices."

Critics of the OAM wonder why the NIH is putting its imprimatur on some of the more questionable alternative techniques, pointing out that doing so allows practitioners of such therapy to cloak themselves in legitimacy by such an association, claiming (often correctly) that their methods are "under study" at OAM. Initially, no rules were set up to guard against conflicts of interest by panel members, or to prevent them from using their panel membership in self-promotion.[22] As previously mentioned, proponents of alternative therapy make no secret of their desire to use OAM sanction to obtain freedom from regulatory oversight.

In an essay in the *New York Times*, two university scientists who discuss the OAM conclude, "Should there be an Office of Alternative Medicine to evaluate unconventional practices? Not one that elevates magical notions to matters of serious scientific debate. . . . It is important to distinguish these experiences [such as kindness or sunsets] from claims that ignore natural law."[23] Under its new director, it may be that the OAM will address these areas to the satisfaction of its critics.

The Context of Alternative Medicine

In a national survey, at least one-third of persons claimed to have used at least one alternative therapy in the past year, and one-third of these persons saw a provider of alternative medical therapy. Among those using an unconventional healer, 83% also saw a medical doctor for the same condition, but nearly 75% of them did not report the use of alternative care to their traditional physician. The survey data estimated that in 1990 the out-of-pocket cost of unconventional therapy in the United States, including the cost of herbal medicines and health food/nutrition therapy, exceeded $10 billion. Another $3 billion of these costs were borne by third-party payors. The total estimated cost, $13.7 billion, exceeds the cost of hospital care in the United States in 1990 ($12.8 billion) and is about half of all the out-of-pocket expenses to physician services ($23.5 billion). The authors suggest that the total number of annual visits to alternative practitioners may exceed those to primary care physicians.[25]

The Oxford Health Plan, based in Norwalk, CT, is currently adding a network of about 1,000 holistic providers from which plan participants will be able to obtain chiropractic, acupuncture, and naturopathic treatment *without* prior approval of a "gatekeeper" at a cost of 2% to 3% added to the premium. Plan managers may believe that alternative therapies can decrease costs by decreasing utilization of conventional services. However, the Eisenberg study showed that the cost of alternative therapies averaged $27 per provider visit, and totaled over $500/year among those who used alternative methods, who usually sought simultaneous care from conventional physicians.[25] The Oxford group has instituted several advisory committees to determine the "highest quality" of alternative practitioners, and plans to obtain feedback from patient encounters to monitor the type of treatments offered for different complaints. Quality-control committees will gauge appropriateness of care and whether the modality used lies within the scope of practice of the alternative therapist. They also hope to conduct outcomes research on this project. This new venture may have the effect of shifting the burden of seeking effective diagnosis and treatment to the consumer, since the plan has no clear idea whether most of the alternative treatments have any credibility besides that being claimed by proponents.

In an editorial, Campion[24] cites several reasons for the public's "expensive romance with unconventional medicine." People have easy access to many options in medical care; disaffection with traditional care is widespread, fueled by media accounts of medical misadventures and uncaring managed care institutions; alternative practitioners often give people more time and attention than traditional providers; people want to feel in control of their bodies; and most of all, they want to feel well.

Americans seek alternative care for a wide variety of conditions. In one national study, the most common complaints presented to unconventional practitioners were back complaints (36%), anxiety (28%), headache (27%), chronic pain (26%), and cancer or tumors (24%). About one-third of patients in the same survey reported using alternative healers for health promotion and disease prevention advice, or for nonserious conditions not related to their chief complaint.[25] A Canadian survey found that about 11% of children also attending a pediatric outpatient clinic in Quebec had been taken to chiropractic, homeopathic, naturopathic, and acupuncture practitioners, mostly for respiratory and ear-nose-throat problems. Parents assumed these treatments to be more "natural," and to have fewer side effects, but did not seek alternative therapy to receive more "personalized" care.[26]

Alternative therapy for cancer treatment has attracted much attention. Recent surveys show that from 3%[25] to 9%[27] of patients with cancer sought alternative methods of treatment for cancer. Older surveys with smaller data bases found higher usage rates, showing that 13%[28] to about 50% of patients with cancer sought alternative treatments.[29] That nearly half of all cancer patients have sought or seriously considered unconventional cancer therapy has been reported widely in the lay press as well, and adds to the perception that such practices are quite common and might be useful. Many cancer patients change diet, use multivitamin therapy, take shark cartilage, Chinese herbs, homeopathic pellets, and such therapies as mistletoe or mushroom extract with the expectation that their disease will be mitigated. The whole gamut of unconventional therapists is utilized by cancer patients, ranging from acupuncturists to Gestalt therapists.

Buckman and Sabbagh[30] point out that reports of success for many of the therapies being embraced by the public may be explained in several ways. The "cures" may have come from misdiagnosis, and when the anecdotes of healing are traced to the original sources, no data can be found. Patients may not have had the diagnosis for which they were "cured" or the data may have been falsified or misinterpreted by the healer. They may have experienced self-limiting or fluctuating illnesses, remission of which was wrongly attributed to the alternative treatment. After therapy, patients may not have been followed long enough to accurately assess cure or observe relapses. Concurrent conventional therapy is often being taken by patients who undergo alternative treatments, with inappropriate credit given to the unconventional method. Finally, misinterpretation of information by patients who believe themselves miraculously cured is often at the core of their success story. However, he points out that some of the clinical trials examining different areas of alternative therapy have raised enough questions to make further investigation of these methods desirable, in order to help answer the essential question in this debate: do these methods merely make one *feel* better, or do they really help one *get* better?

It is also interesting that in one survey of patients with cancer,[27] patients claimed little opposition by their physicians in seeking such care, but their physicians reported these encounters differently. Patients reported that their physicians recommended or approved their use of unconventional therapy 50% of the time, and 31% cited the physician as the source of information about alternative methods. Forty percent of patients in this group reportedly abandoned traditional therapy after finding alternative care. In the same study, 52% of physicians who treated this group of patients reportedly objected to unorthodox treatments, and only 2% said they had recommended such treatment, although 37% said they "went along with" the patients. Patients did not tell physicians about their alternative cancer care 35% of the time.

Other surveys report that for all uses of alternative medicine, up to 70% of patients may not reveal their use of unconventional treatment to their physician.[25] The former director of the OAM, Joseph Jacobs, MD, states that this lack of communication between doctor and patient about the use of alternative therapies "creates a very real challenge to the medical community, because not being able to understand what many [patients] are using outside of the medical mainstream presents a real barrier to good clinical care."[31]

On the other hand, many patients in the AIDS community, for example, have become quite vocal about the need for research in alternative medicine because they think many patients are being deceived by proponents of untested therapy, and have appealed to the OAM and others for definitive answers about unconventional AIDS treatments being offered.[31]

What do physicians think about alternative medicine? It is likely that most physicians are unaware of the scope, breadth, and extent of use of unconventional therapies in the United States.[1] The level of interest among physicians in learning more about alternative therapy, however, seems to be high. A regional survey of family physicians in the Chesapeake Bay area showed that more than 70% were interested in training in such practices as herbal medicine, prayer therapy, acupressure, vegetarian and megavitamin diet therapy, acupuncture, and biofeedback.[32] The results of this study, however, are curious in that 26% of respondents claim to have had training in chiropractic methods, 22% in acupuncture, and nearly 10% report training in traditional Oriental or Native American medicine. While informal training courses in these areas may be available, the scientific basis for such instruction is weak to nonexistent, and not usually accredited by specialty societies or traditional organized medical associations that govern continuing medical education. It would be most unusual if over 20% of family physicians in this area actually use chiropractic in their practice.

In a national survey of referral patterns by board-certified family physicians and internists, 94% indicated willingness to refer for at least one alternative therapy, 90% for at least two, 85% at least three, 77% at least four, and 66% at least five such modalities. The list of therapies for which these physicians expressed a willingness to refer patients included: relaxation techniques—86%, biofeedback—85%, therapeutic massage—66%, hypnosis—63%, acupuncture—56%, and meditation—54%. By contrast, 47% said they would refer for chiropractic, 24% for "spiritual" healing, 15% for homeopathy, 14% for energy healing, and 6% would refer for megavitamin or herbal therapy. In

the same survey, 22% of respondents reported personally providing relaxation therapy, 17% "lifestyle diet (vegetarian, macrobiotic, etc.)," 5% hypnosis, 3% massage or chiropractic therapy, and 1% homeopathic or acupuncture therapies.[33]

The authors of the Chesapeake Bay study[32] cite surveys of physicians in Great Britain, Israel, and New Zealand that show "similar interest" in studying alternative medicine. A more recent meta-analysis of European physicians and their attitudes about alternative medicine shows that on average, physicians view complementary medicine to have an "effectiveness rating" of 46 ± 18 on a scale of 0–100. There was no trend among these data to suggest increasing endorsement of alternative medicine by conventional practitioners, but the authors conclude that European physicians give these therapies a "considerable degree of acceptance."[34] They caution, however, that the perceived usefulness of such therapies by physicians or the public should not be equated with proven efficacy.

Many persons who are proponents of alternative medicine understand and acknowledge the role of traditional Western medicine for such problems as surgical intervention for appendicitis and fractures, or antibiotic therapy for specific infectious diseases. However, many in the alternative medical community spend a good deal of energy denigrating the role of allopathic intervention as dangerous, expensive, and impersonal. In the "deconstructionist" mode, they often change the vocabulary to make their methods seem rational and reasonable. In a critique of alternative medicine, Wallace Sampson, MD, points out that an editorial in *Alternative Therapies* poses:

"a non sequitur: present knowledge is adequate to dismiss the utility of most alternative methods; but [the editorial claims] there are ineffable qualities that [conventional] methods cannot detect and alternatives cannot define; therefore, alternative methods must be accepted, their practitioners licensed, and their services paid for by public funds and health insurance."[35]

In an unpublished survey of all 125 US medical schools, Sampson has found that just over 50 schools offer elective, for-credit courses on alternative therapy, and 18 other schools offer lecture series or seminars on the subject. His survey reveals that most are being given by "supporters or proponents of alternative methods," and that the "scientific view" is offered in only 7 courses.

In an editorial,[36] Alpert argues that alternative medicine should not be "condemned out of hand," but suggests that traditional medicine approach alternative therapy based on five principles. Convinced that many unconventional treatments will eventually become mainstream, he proposes that physicians:

1. Maintain an open-minded attitude about all potentially new therapeutic interventions that include those commonly referred to as alternative.
2. Encourage carefully performed and appropriately controlled studies of these new therapies.
3. Do not ignore or ridicule the potential of the placebo effect to produce marked therapeutic benefit.
4. Do not accept all new therapies as efficacious on first acquaintance. Practitioners of quack medicine continue to abound as in all earlier times. Claims of therapeutic efficacy should be rationally examined and tested.
5. Avoid hubristic and arrogant attitudes toward alternative medical practices because one might be embarrassed by the subsequent demonstrations of their clinical efficacy.

Alpert says that these statements are guiding the University of Arizona as it sets up a program to "integrate and evaluate valuable alternative medical practices into routine allopathic care." Andrew Weil, MD, who has written several books on alternative medicine, is heading the new program.

It is clear that in the quest for wellness, the public is seeking new approaches to medical care. Some of the reasons may be understandable, such as the desire to find a healer with time to listen, to receive compassionate care, and to establish a partnership with a provider in seeking health.

In "Turning from Science and Reason," an address at the 1996 AMA National Leadership Conference, Jeremiah Barondess, MD, stated that many physicians may not deal effectively enough with illness, elements he identifies as those symptoms, anxieties, and concerns that make people

feel sick, as opposed to our emphasis on disease, defined too often in biochemical and molecular terms that are far removed from the person being examined. Patients, he says, are increasingly taking more responsibility for their own health. Many are disaffected with medicine in general, as part of a trend of public suspicion of authoritarian, insular sections of society.

Some of the interest in alternative medicine may be due to an "outbreak of irrationalism" that includes New Age interest in "channeling" and astrology.[37] Television talk shows and the proliferation of books and tapes on alternative therapies are gobbled up by an uncritical public that does not understand how to sort quack theories from what might be reasonable. Carl Sagan has recently lamented the phenomenon of our increasing scientific illiteracy and the rise of pseudoscience and superstition, noting that "baloney, bamboozles, careless thinking, and wishes disguised as fact. . . ripple through mainstream political, social, religious, and economic issues in every nation."[39]

Political decisions allow licensing of alternative practitioners without any scientific basis for accreditation of their schools or the methods used by their practitioners. Congress has recently dismantled its own scientific oversight section, the Office of Technology Assessment. Political pressure from the health food and vitamin supplement industry has hampered the FDA's ability to monitor their products, and legislative proposals have been advanced to allow such products to be covered by food stamps—in effect, paying for pills instead of food.[38] There is, indeed, reason for concern.

Given the growing interest in alternative medicine by the public, accurate, even-handed education about alternative medicine is vital for both the public as well as for physicians, who should be familiar with unconventional therapies and be able to advise patients on their use. Sound, good quality research is needed to determine the potential benefits and avoid the risks inherent in unconventional therapy.

Recommendations

The following statements, recommended by the Council on Scientific Affairs, were adopted as AMA Policy at the 1997 AMA Annual Meeting.

1. There is little evidence to confirm the safety or efficacy of most alternative therapies. Much of the information currently known about these therapies makes it clear that many have not been shown to be efficacious. Well-designed, stringently controlled research should be done to evaluate the efficacy of alternative therapies.
2. Physicians should routinely inquire about the use of alternative or unconventional therapy by their patients, and educate themselves and their patients about the state of scientific knowledge with regard to alternative therapy that may be used or contemplated.
3. Patients who choose alternative therapies should be educated as to the hazards that might result from postponing or stopping conventional medical treatment.
4. Courses offered by medical schools on alternative medicine should present the scientific view of unconventional theories, treatments, and practice as well as the potential therapeutic utility, safety, and efficacy of these modalities.

References

1. Murray RH, Rubel AJ. Physicians and healers—unwitting partners in healthcare. *N Engl J Med* 1992;326:61–645.
2. Dossey L, Sawyers JP. *Introduction to Alternative Medicine: Expanding Medical Horizons.* Washington, DC: US Government Printing Office; 1994. NIH 94-066.
3. Renner JH. *Health Smarts.* Kansas City, Missouri: HealthFacts Publishing; 1990.
4. Hafner AW. *Reader's Guide to Alternative Health Methods.* Chicago: American Medical Association; 1992.
5. Coleman C. Herbal healing. Associated Press. *Daily Herald,* Chicago, Illinois. February 1, 1996: Section 4, p.1–2.
6. Tyler VE. The overselling of herbs. In: Barrett S, Jarvis WT, eds. *The Health Robbers.* Buffalo, NY: Prometheus Books; 1993.
7. Vautier G, Spiller RC. Safety of complementary medicines should be monitored. *BMJ* 1995;311:633.
8. Linde K, Ramirez G, Mulrow CD, et al. St. John's wort for depression—an overview and meta-analysis of randomized controlled trials. *BMJ* 1996;313: 352–358.
9. DeSmet P, Nolen WA. St. John's wort as an antidepressant. *BMJ* 1996;313:241–242.
10. Pizzorno JE. Ten drugs I would never take. *Natural Health.* September–October 1996; 84–85, 142–148.
11. Tyler V. Herbal remedies. *J Pharm Technol* 1995;11:214–220.
12. Barrett S. The spine salesmen. In: Barrett S, Jarvis WT, eds. *The Health Robbers.* Buffalo, NY: Prometheus Books; 1993.
13. Bigos S, Bowyer O, Braen G, et al. Acute low back problems in adults. *Clinical Practice Guideline.* Quick Reference Guide Number 14. Rockville, MD: US Department of Health and Human Services, Public Health Service, Agency for Health Care Policy and Research AHCPR Pub. No.95-0643. December 1994.
14. Brennan B, Rosner A, Demmerle A, et al. Manual healing methods. In: *Alternative Medicine: Expanding Medical Horizons.* Washington, DC: US Government Printing Office; 1994. NIH 94-066.
15. Brennan B, Rosner R, et al. Manual healing methods. In: *Alternative Medicine: Expanding Medical Horizons.* Washington, DC: US Government Printing Office; 1994. NIH 94-066.
16. Green S. "Antineoplastons": An unproven cancer therapy. *JAMA* 1992;267:2924–2928.
17. Bower H. Internet sees growth of unverified health claims. *BMJ* 1996;313:381.
18. Moss RW, Wiebel FD, et al. Pharmacologic and biological treatments. In: *Alternative Medicine: Expanding Medical Horizons.* Washington, DC: US Government Printing Office; 1994. NIH 94-066.
19. Taub A. Acupuncture: nonsense with needles. In: Barrett S, Jarvis WT, eds. *The Health Robbers.* Buffalo, NY: Prometheus Books; 1993.
20. Jacobs J, Jimenez LM, Gloyd SS, et al. Treatment of acute childhood diarrhea with homeopathic medicine: a randomized clinical trial in Nicaragua. *Pediatrics* 1994;93:719–725.
21. Sampson W, London W. Analysis of homeopathic treatment of childhood diarrhea. *Pediatrics* 1995;96:961–964.
22. Skolnick A. Science reporters hear wide range of data at 12th annual conference. *JAMA* 1993;270:2416.
23. Park RL, Goodenough U. Buying snake oil with tax dollars. *New York Times;* January 3, 1996, P. A-15.
24. Campion EW. Why unconventional medicine? *N Engl J Med* 1993;328:282–283.
25. Eisenberg DM, Kessler RC, Foster C, et al. Unconventional medicine in the United States. *N Engl J Med* 1993;328:246–52.
26. Spigelblatt L, Laine-Ammara G, Pless IB, Guyver A. The use of alternative medicine by children. *Pediatrics* 1994;94:811–814.

27. Lerner IJ, Kennedy BJ. The prevalence of questionable methods of cancer treatment in the United States. *CA-Cancer J Clin* 1992;42:181–190.

28. Cassileth BR, Lusk EJ, Strouse TB, et al. Contemporary unorthodox treatment in cancer medicine: A study of patients, treatments, and practitioners. *Ann Intern Med* 1984;101:105–112.

29. Cassileth BR. Unorthodox cancer medicine. *Cancer Invest* 1986;4:591–598.

30. Buckman R, Sabbagh K. *Magic or Medicine? An Investigation of Healing and Healers.* New York, NY: Prometheus Books; 1995.

31. Jacobs J. Presentation to AMA Council on Scientific Affairs. September 8, 1996.

32. Berman BM, Singh BK, Lao L, et al. Physicians' attitudes toward complementary or alternative medicine: A regional survey. *J Am Board Fam Pract* 1995; 8:361–366.

33. Blumberg DL, Grant WD, Hendricks SR, Kamps CA, Dewan MJ. The physician and unconventional medicine. *Altern Ther* 1996;1:31–35.

34. Ernst E, Resch KL, White AR. Complementary medicine. what physicians think of it: A meta-analysis. *Arch Intern Med* 1995;155:2405–2408.

35. Sampson W. Antiscience trends in the rise of the "alternative medicine" movement. *Ann N Y Acad Sci* 1996;775:188–197.

36. Alpert JS. The relativity of alternative medicine. *Arch Intern Med* 1995;155:2385.

37. Krauthammer C. The return of the primitive. *Time*; January 20, 1996;P.82. Essay.

38. Skolnick A. Experts debate food stamp revision. *JAMA* 1995;274:781–783.

39. Sagan C. *The Demon-Haunted World: Science as a Candle in the Dark.* New York: Random House; 1995.

APPENDIX III
NEW NATIONAL INSTITUTES OF HEALTH STUDY

The National Center for Complementary and Alternative Medicine (NCCAM) and 16 federal cosponsors announce the launch of an Institute of Medicine (IOM) study of the scientific and policy implications of the use of complementary and alternative medicine (CAM) by the American public. The $1 million, nearly two-year study, will be conducted by the IOM, a component of the National Academies.

The National Academies is a private, nonprofit, nongovernmental institution created by a congressional charter to be an advisory body for the nation on scientific and technological matters. The IOM draws upon volunteer panels of experts to examine policy matters regarding the public's health. NCCAM, the primary sponsor of the study, is the federal government's lead agency for scientific research on CAM.

The IOM will assemble a panel of approximately 16 experts from a broad range of CAM and conventional disciplines, such as behavioral medicine, internal medicine, nursing, epidemiology, pharmacology, health care research and administration, and education. During the course of the study, the IOM panel will assess research findings, hold workshops, and invite speakers to address the panel, among other activities, in order to

- Provide a comprehensive overview of the use of CAM therapies by the American public
- Identify significant scientific and policy issues related to CAM research, regulation, integration, training, and certification
- Develop a conceptual framework to help guide decision making on these issues and questions

The value of undertaking this study emerged from discussions among members of the Trans-Agency CAM Coordinating Committee, chaired by Stephen E. Straus, M.D., NCCAM Director. The Committee felt that the IOM had the expertise to consider questions of CAM research and policy critically

"Americans use CAM therapies in record numbers," said Dr. Straus. "The IOM's report will give us a clearer understanding of the scope of CAM use by Americans, as well as CAM's public health impact, and scientific and policy issues that will better inform our research decisions."

The IOM study, led by Senior Program Officer Lyla M. Hernandez, MPH, of the Board on Health Promotion and Disease Prevention, will not conduct new surveys of the public regarding CAM use. Rather, the IOM panel will gather and analyze existing data. In addition, the IOM study, which will recruit panel members after October 1, 2003 plans to address many key questions, such as the following:

- What are the methodological difficulties in evaluating some CAM therapies?
- How are the different CAM professions regulated in the United States?
- What is the current situation for coverage of CAM by insurers and other third parties?
- What are the policy and regulatory issues regarding licensing and certifying of CAM practitioners?

The answers to these questions and the information generated by the IOM panel of leading scholars drawn from both conventional medicine and CAM, and from education, should serve to complement the recommendations of the White House Commission on Complementary and Alternative Medicine Policy released earlier this year.

The agencies cosponsoring the IOM study include the following:

Agency for Health Care Research and Quality
John E. Fogarty International Center
National Cancer Institute
National Center for Complementary and
    Alternative Medicine
National Center for Research Resources
National Institute on Aging
National Institute on Alcohol Abuse and
    Alcoholism
National Institute of Allergy and Infectious Diseases
National Institute of Arthritis and Musculoskeletal
    and Skin Diseases
National Institute of Child Health and Human
    Development
National Institute of Dental and Craniofacial
    Research
National Institute of Diabetes and Digestive and
    Kidney Diseases
National Institute on Drug Abuse
National Institute of Mental Health
National Library of Medicine
NIH Office of Behavioral and Social Sciences
    Research
NIH Office of Dietary Supplements

For information on the National Academies, visit www.nationalacademies.org. For information on the Institute of Medicine, visit www.iom.edu.

The National Center for Complementary and Alternative Medicine (NCCAM) is dedicated to exploring complementary and alternative medical (CAM) practices in the context of rigorous science, training CAM researchers, and disseminating authoritative information to the public and professionals. For additional information, call NCCAM's Clearinghouse toll free at 1-888-644-6226, or visit the NCCAM Web site at nccam.nih.gov.

APPENDIX IV
HERBS USED IN ALTERNATIVE MEDICINE DISCIPLINES

Achillea millefolium	yarrow
Achyranthes bidentata	achyranthes root
Acorus calamus	sweet flag
Actaea racemosa ([L] Nutt)	black cohosh
L. (formerly Cimicifuga racemosa)	black cohosh
Aesculus hippocastanum	horse chestnut
Agastache rugosa	agastache
Agrimonia pilosa	agrimony
Akebia trifoliate	akebia
Alchemilla vulgaris	lady's mantle
Alisma plantago	alisma
Allium sativa	garlic
Aloe vera	aloe
Althea officinalis	marshmallow
Amomum villosum	cardamom
Amygdalus communis	sweet almond seed
Anemarrhena asphodeloides	anemarrhena
Angelica archangelica	angelica
Angelica sinensis	dong quai, danggui
Angelica sp	angelica
Apium graveolens	celery
Aquilaria agallocha	aquilaria wood
Aralia sp.	spikenard
Arctium lappa	burdock, gobo
Arctostaphylos uva-ursi	bearberry (uva ursi leaves)
Areca catechu	areca peel
Aristolochia sp.	snakeroot, guaco
Arnica montana	arnica
Artemesia spp.	southernwood, wormwood, absinthe, sage brush, lad's love, mugwort, tarragon, sweet annie
Asafoetida	asafoetida
Asarum sieboli	asaram
Asparagus spp	asparagus
Astragalus sp.	vetch, rattlepod, locoweed
Astragalus membranaceus	huang-qi
Atractylodes sppn	atractylodes
Baking soda	
Bamboo shavings	*Phyllostachys nigra*
Benincasa hispida	benincasa
Berberis sp.	barberry
Betula sp.	birch
Biota orientalis	biota
Borago officinalis	borage
Boswellia serrata	frankincense
Brassica alba	mustard seed
Bryonia sp.	bryony
Bupleurum chinense	bupleurum
Calamus draco	calamus gum
Calendula officinalis	marigold
Calophyllum sp.	punna, kamani
Capsicum frutescens	cayenne, red pepper
Carthamus tinctorius	carthamus

Castor oil	
Caulophyllum thalictroides	blue cohosh
Capsicum minimum	cayenne pepper
Centaurea sp.	cornflower, knap weed
Centaurium erythraea	century, feverwort
Centella asiatica	gotu kola, hydrocotyle
Chamomilla recutita	chamomile
Chrysanthemum morifolium	chrysanthemum
Cimicifuga (now known as Actaea racemosa) (NUTT.)	black cohosh
Cinnamomum zeylanicum	cinnamon
Citrus aurantium	aurantium
Citrus grandis	tangerine
Citrus reticulata	citrus
Clematis spp.	clematis
Codonopsis spp.	codonopsis, dang shen
Coix lachryma-jobi	coix
Colchicum autumnale	autumn crocus, meadow saffron
Commiphora mukul	guggul
Commiphora myrrh	myrrh resin
Coptis chinensis	coptis
Coriander	
Cornus florida & C. officinalis	dogwood
Corydalis yanhusuo	corydalis
Crataegus oxyacantha	hawthorn
Cumin	
Curculigo orchioides	curculigo
Curcuma longa	turmeric
Cuscuta chinensis	cuscuta
Cynara cardunculus	cardoon
Cynara scolymus	artichoke
Cyperus rotundus	cyperus
Dendrobium nobile	dendrobium
Dianthus chinensis	dianthus
Dioscorea opposita	dioscorea
Dioscorea villosa	wild yams
Dipsacus asper	dipsacus
Dryopteris	male fern
Echinacea purpurea, E. angustifolia and E. pallida	echinacea
Eclipta spp	eclipta, han lian cao
Eleutherococcus (Acanthopanax) senticosus	eleuthero, Siberian Ginseng
Ephedra sinica	ephedra, ma huang
Epimedium spp	epimedium, yin yang huo
Equisetum arvense	horsetail
Equus asinus	donkey gelatin
Eriobotrya japonica	loquat leaf
Eriodictyon californicum	yerba santa
Eschscholzia californica Cham	California poppy
Eucalyptus globulus Labill	eucalyptus
Eucommia ulmoides	eucommia
Eugenia sp.	clove
Eugenia caryophyllata	clove bud
Eupatorium fortunei	eupatorium
Euphoria longan	longan
Eurale ferox	euryales
Evodia rutaecarpa	evodia
Flax seeds	
Filipendula ulmaria	meadowsweet
Foeniculum vulgare	fennel
Forsythia suspensa (Thunb.) Vahl	forsythia, lian qiao
Fritillaria cirrhosa	fritillary bulb
Fucus vesiculosus L.	bladderwrack
Ganoderma lucidum	ganoderma
Garcinia cambogia	citrin, gambooge
Garcinia kola	bitter kola
Garcinia mangostana	mangosteen
Garcinia sp.	garcinia
Gardenia jasminoides	gardenia
Gastrodia elata	gastrodia
Gentiana spp	gentian
Ginkgo biloba	ginkgo
Glauber's salt	sodium sulfate
Glehnia littoralis	glehnia
Glycyrrhiza glabra	licorice
Glycyrrhiza uralensis	licorice
Gotu kola	

Gossypium herbaceum L. *or hirsutum L*	cotton	*Loranthus parasiticus*	mulberry
Guatteria gaumeri *Greenman*	guatteria	*Luffa sp.*	luffa
		Lycium spp	lycium, wolfberry, matrimony vine
Gymnema sylvestre	gurmar	*Lycopus lucidus*	bugleweed
Gypsum mineral	calcium sulfate	*Lygodium japonicum*	lygodium spores
Haliotis divericolor	haliotis shell	*Magnetitum*	magnetite
Hamamelis virginiana L.	witch hazel	*Magnolia officinalis*	magnolia
Harpagophytum *procumbens*	devil's claw	*Mahonia aquifolium*	mahonia, Oregon grape
Hibiscus sp.	hibiscus, roselle	*Matricaria chamomilla*	chamomile
Humulus lupulus	hops	*Melaleuca alternifolia*	tea tree oil
Hydrastis canadensis	goldenseal, yellow root, eye root, eye balm, jaundice root, ground raspberry, Indian dye	*Melia toosendan*	melia
		Mentha haplocalyx	peppermint leaf
		Mentha pulegium/ *Hedeoma pulegioides*	European pennyroyal/ American pennyroyal
Hypericum perforatum	St. John's wort	*Millettia reticulata*	millettia
Ilex pubescens	ilex	*Momordica charantia*	bitter gourd, karela
Illicium verum	star anise	*Morinda sp.*	Noni, Nonu
Isiatis tinctoria	isiatis	*Morus alba*	morus
Juniperus sp	juniper	*Musa sp.*	plantain, banana
Kadsura sp.	kadsura	*Myristica fragrans*	nutmeg
Kochia scoparia	summer cypress, fireweed	*Nelumbo nucifera*	lotus seed
		Ocimum basilicum	basil, albahaca
Laminaria japonica	laminaria	*Onion*	
Larrea tridentata *(DC) Coville*	creosote bush or chaparral	*Ophiopogon japonicus*	ophiopogon
		Origanum vulgare	oregano
Lavandula sp.	lavender	*Paeonia suffruticosa*	Moutan peony
Lentinus edodes	shiitake, black mushroom	*Panax quinquefolium*	American ginseng
		Panax ginseng C. A. Mey. *P. quinquefolius*	Chinese ginseng, or American ginseng
Leonorus cardiaca	motherwort		
Leonorus heterophyllus	motherwort	*Passiflora alata*	passion flower
Lepidium meyenii Walp.	maca	*Perilla frutescens*	perilla
Lepidium sp.	cress	*Phaseolus mungo*	mung bean
Ligusticumwallichii auct. *Non. Franch*	Sichuan lovage, sin. chuan xiong	*Phytolacca dodecandra*	poke root, endod
		Pimpinella anisum	anise
Lilium brownii	lily bulb	*Piper longum*	long pepper
Lindera strychnifolia	lindera	*Pinellia seed*	*Pinellia ternata*
Litchi chinensis	litchi	*Piper methysticum*	kava
Lobelia inflata	lobelia	*Piper nigrum*	black pepper
Lonicera japonica	honeysuckle	*Plantago major/lanceolate*	plantain
Lonicera japonica Thunb.	honeysuckle, jin yin hua, ren dong teng	*Plantago psyllium/ovata*	psyllium, ispaghula
		Platycodon grandiflorum	platycodon root

Podophyllum peltatum,	mayapple,
P. hexandrum, P. emodi	mandrake, Indian
	apple, wild
	lemon, duck's
	foot
Polygala tenuifolia	polygala root
Polygonatum odoratum	polygonatum
Polyporus umbellatus	polyporus
Poria cocos	poria fungus
Polygonum aviculare	knotgrass
Potentilla sp.	cinquefoil,
	silverweed
Prunella vulgaris	self-heal
Prunus armeniaca	apricot or bitter
	almond seed
Prunus persica	peach seed
Pseudoginseng roo	panax
	pseudoginseng
Pseudostellaria	heterophyllapseu
	dostellaria root
Psoralia corylifolia	psoralea seed
Pueraria lobata	kudzu
Pygeum africanum	African prune
Raphanus sativus	radish seed
Red dates	*Zizyphus jujuba*
Red pepper	*Capsicum anuum*
Rehmannia glutinosa	rehmannia
Rheum officinale	rhubarb
Ribes nigrum L.	black currant
Rosa laevigata	rose hips
Rosmarinus officinalis L.	rosemary
Rubia	cordyfoliarubia
Rubus chingii	rubus
Rubus idaeus	aspberry leaves
Ruta graveolensrue	
Salix alba	white willow bark
Salvia officinalissage	leaves
Sambucus nigra L.	black elderberry
Sanguinaria canadensis L.	bloodroot
Sargassum fusiformsargassum	
Sassafras albidum (Nuttall)	sassafras
Saussurea lappa	saussurea
Schisandra chinensis	wu wei zi,
	wu ren chun
Scutellaria baicalensis Georgi	Baical skullcap

Serenoa serrulata &	saw palmetto
S. repens (Arecaceae)	
Siler divaricatumsileris	
Silybum marianum Gaertn.	milk thistle
Smilax glabra Roxb.	sarsaparilla
Stephania tetrandra	stephania root
Stevia rebaudiana Bertoni	sweetleaf,
	candyleaf
Swertia sp.	swertia
Symphytum officinale L.	comfrey
Syzygium sp.	clove, jamun
Tabebuia avellanedae	pau d'arco
Tabernanthe iboga	iboga
Tamarindus indica	tamarind
Tanacetum parthenium.	feverfew
Schultz-Bip	
Tanacetum vulgare (L.)	tansy
Taraxacum mongolicum	dandelion root
Taraxacum officinale	dandelion
(Dhudhal)	
Terminalia arjuna	myrobalan
Terminalia chebula	hirda
Thuja occidentalis	arborvitae
Thuja plicata	western red cedar
Thymus vulgaris	thyme
Tilia europea	linden
Tribulus terrestris L.	puncture vine,
	goathead
Trichosanthes sp.	snake gourd,
	gualou
Trigonella foenum	fenugreek
graecum L.	
Turmeric	Curcuma longae
turnera	diffusadamiana
Tussilago farfara	coltsfoot
Uncaria rynchophyllauncaria	stem
Uncaria tomentosa	cat's claw,
(Willd.) D.C.	uno de gato
Urtica dioica	stinging nettles
Vaccinium macrocarpon	cranberry
Vaccinium myrtillus	bilberry
Valeriana officinalis	valerian
Verbascum thapsus. L.	mullein
Viburnum sp.	cramp bark, high
	bush cranberry

Viscum album	mistletoe, European	*Yellow dock root*	*Rumex crispus*
(Phoradendron	(American)	*Zanthoxylum sp.*	prickly ash
leucarpum, P. flavescens,		*Zea mays*	corn silk
P. serotinum)		*Zingiber officinale Roscoe*	ginger
Vitex agnus-castus	chaste tree	*Zingiber officinalis*	dry ginger
White peony root	*Paeonia lactiflora*	*Ziziphus sp.*	jujube
Withania somnifera	ashwagandha	*Zizyphus jujuba*	black date
Yarrow Achillea	millefolium		

APPENDIX V
NATIONAL CENTER FOR COMPLEMENTARY AND ALTERNATIVE MEDICINE FIVE-YEAR STRATEGIC PLAN 2001–2005

Reproduced here is the complete text of the National Center for
Complementary Medicine and Alternative Medicine report
Expanding Horizons of Healthcare: Five Year Strategic Plan, 2001–2005.
Photographs included in the original report have not been included.

National Center for Complementary and Alternative Medicine wishes to extend its sincerest gratitude to the many organizations and individuals who contributed to the development of this plan.

A special note of thanks goes to those who helped shape the draft strategic plan of NCCAM 's predecessor, the Office of Alternative Medicine. Through their efforts, NCCAM was provided a well-developed foundation upon which to build. We thank NCCAM staff and members of the National Advisory Council on Complementary and Alternative Medicine, who subsequently crafted and provided input to multiple iterations of the document as it evolved to its final form. We are also grateful to the directors and other senior officials at the National Institutes of Health (NIH) and the Department of Health and Human Services, whose broad perspectives have been incorporated to enrich the document substantially.

Finally, we acknowledge the efforts of over 200 individuals and organizations that reviewed the draft plan on NCCAM's Web site during the six-week period it was posted for public comment. It is their thoughtful responses that guided us in our attempts to create a document that is meaningful to multiple audiences and better accommodates the divergent sensibilities of our many stakeholders.

We look forward to collaborating further as we implement our first strategic plan.

Table of Contents

Acknowledgments
Preface
Part I The Case for Action
Part II Future Directions
Part III NCCAM Strategic Plan 2001–2005
  Our Mission
  Our Vision
  Our Stakeholders
  Strategic Areas
    Strategic Area 1: Investing in Research
    Strategic Area 2: Training CAM Investigators
    Strategic Area 3: Expanding Outreach
    Strategic Area 4: Facilitating Integration
  Practicing Responsible Stewardship
  Endnotes
Part IV Appendices
    Appendix I Major Domains of Complementary
      and Alternative Medicine
    Appendix II Important Events in NCCAM
      History
    Appendix III Biographical Sketch, Stephen
      E.Straus, MD
    Appendix IV NCCAM Research and Research
      Training Portfolio
    Appendix V NCCAM Outreach Activities
    Appendix VI Evidence-Based Reviews
    Appendix VII NCCAM Cancer Advisory
      Panel for Complementary and Alternative
      Medicine

Appendix VIII Strategic Planning Process
Appendix IX National Advisory Council for
    Complementary and Alternative Medicine

Preface

The growing appeal of complementary and alternative medicine (CAM) at the dawn of the 21st century creates both an opportunity and the obligation for scientific study and evaluation. As Americans become increasingly activist in their pursuit of sustained and improved health and well-being by exploring unconventional healthcare practices, so too, have we in the research community now joined in that exploration. We bring to that endeavor a curiosity and open-mindedness, motivated by the prospect of enhancing the healthcare repertoire, while at the same time mindful of the need to help protect the public from harm.

In establishing the National Center for Complementary and Alternative Medicine (NCCAM) at the National Institutes of Health (NIH) in 1998, Congress crafted legislation empowering us to conduct basic and clinical research, train researchers, and educate and communicate our findings to the public and professionals. I am honored to have been appointed the first Director of NCCAM; I am committed to bring to this position the evidence-based standards of science that have guided me though 23 years of research on important human infectious and immunologic diseases at the NIH.

I come to NCCAM cognizant of the formidable challenges that lie ahead, but with an optimistic vision of the value that scientific scrutiny can bring to the CAM field. Already there is mounting evidence—the result of initial rigorous investigations—that several therapeutic and preventative CAM modalities will be proven effective. We are also hopeful that advances in neuroscience will yield greater understanding of what happens in acupuncture and meditation and what lies behind the placebo effect. Similarly, we expect that the basis for the effectiveness of selected herbal and nutritional supplements will be clarified and lead to their standardization and routine use, just as, a century ago, we learned what were the effective ingredients of willow and cinchona bark. Other modalities currently considered CAM will be found unsafe or ineffective, and an informed public will reject them.

As CAM interventions are incorporated into conventional medical education and practice, the exclusionary terms, "complementary and alternative medicine," will be superseded by the more inclusive, "integrative medicine." Integrative medicine will be seen as providing novel insights and tools for human health, practiced by healthcare providers skilled and knowledgeable in the multiple traditions and disciplines that contribute to the healing arts.

To achieve these goals and to ensure that our actions are commensurate with the public trust that has been given to NCCAM, we have developed our first strategic plan, *Expanding Horizons of Healthcare*. I am deeply grateful to my colleagues and the many organizations and individuals who have contributed to its development. Like the field of medicine itself, the Plan is a work in progress, and I look forward to our continued collaboration as our initiatives evolve. Together, we can strive to make NCCAM a recognized leader in the field within a vibrant, global research community.

Stephen E. Straus, MD, Director
*National Center for Complementary
and Alternative Medicine*

PART I The Case for Action

Advances in medical science in the 20th century, coupled with improvements in sanitation and public health, resulted in dramatic gains in the health and well-being of Americans and a remarkable increase in average life expectancy from 47 years in 1900 to 76 years today. This stunning success was largely the result of declines in deaths from acute infectious disease—for example, tuberculosis, diphtheria, influenza, pneumonia—made possible by the development of vaccines and the advent of antibiotic drugs. To be sure, new and re-emerging infectious diseases remain serious, both locally and globally, as the AIDS epidemic has taught us, but the challenges for conventional Western mainstream medicine[1] (also known as allopathy and biomedicine) come increasingly from chronic diseases prevalent among the growing ranks of mature and older Americans. These adults, more informed and more demanding than their forebears, have high hopes of living long and well, free of disease and disability. Yet many will experience chronic and degenerative diseases that can drain their energies and incomes, increase their pain and suffering, and diminish their quality of life. Despite impressive new treatments and technologies, chronic diseases often resist cure and even symptom relief. Moreover, the increased reliance on technology as well as the economic imperatives and time constraints of managed care mitigate against the expressions of care and concern that should characterize the physician-patient relationship, a dialogue that enhances the healing process beyond the immediate effects of drugs and other treatments.

These issues are emerging at a time when the triumphs of reductionist biology are a daily fact of life, climaxed by the stunning announcement of the sequencing of the human genome in June 2000. Indeed, the cumulative advances in cell and molecular biology over the past few decades have helped medicine evolve from art toward science. Now the very increase in knowledge, the wealth of databases and analytic tools and techniques, are pointing to the need for synthesis, for a way to put the information together to understand how living organisms work as a whole. For the research scientist, this means the need to balance reductionism with integrative biology. For the healthcare provider, it means the need to balance medicine as the science of genes and molecules with medicine as the artful interaction of genes, cells, organ systems, and the whole person with the social and physical environment, which together determine the state of health and well-being of the individual.

The Appeal of Nontraditional Approaches

Frustrated by the inability of mainstream medicine to meet all their expectations and needs, many people have turned to complementary and alternative medicine (CAM) approaches. These developments have been facilitated by the revolution in information technology, which is enabling easy access to sources of CAM information on the Internet and in print and electronic media. The advertising and marketing of alternative and complementary medicine have also grown apace, assuring increased public awareness and exposure to new products and approaches. Not surprisingly, more and more Americans—as many as 42 percent of the public according to one recent estimate—are adopting CAM approaches to satisfy their personal healthcare needs. Between 1990 and 1997, the number of Americans using CAM increased by 38 percent from 60 million to 83 million. Figure 1 indicates that visits to CAM practitioners between 1990 and 1997 increased from an estimated 427 million to 629 million, almost half again as many. Conservative estimates put expenditures for alternative medicine professional services at $21.2 billion in 1997, with at least $12.2 billion paid out-of-pocket. Indeed, Americans spent more out-of-pocket for CAM than they paid out-of-pocket for all hospitalizations—an amount comparable to the projected 1997 out-of-pocket expenditures for all U.S. physician services.[2]

CAM Described

Complementary and alternative medicine practices are best described as those not presently considered an integral part of conventional medicine.[3] Implicit in this definition is the acknowledgment that as CAM practices are proven safe and effective, they may become adopted into mainstream healthcare practice. Generally, patients who choose CAM approaches are seeking ways to

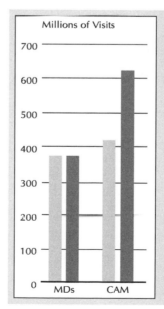

Figure 1
Growth of CAM Visits
From 1990 to 1997 the number of adults reporting use of CAM interventions increased from 60 million to 83 million. While the estimated number of visits to primary care physicians over the same time period remained stable, visits to CAM practitioners increased by 47 percent, exceeding visits to MDs by 243 million.

The five leading reasons for CAM visits were back problems, allergies, fatigue, arthritis, and headaches.
(Eisenberg et al 1998).

improve their health and well-being and to relieve symptoms associated with chronic or terminal illnesses or the side effects of conventional treatments. Interestingly, the overwhelming majority of patients adopting CAM approaches use them to complement conventional care, rather than as an alternative.[4]

As diverse and abundant as the peoples and cultures of the world, CAM practices may be grouped in five major domains: alternative medical systems; mind-body interventions; biologically based treatments; manipulative and body-based methods; and energy therapies[5], with some overlap across categories. For example, discrete practices such as meditation are considered mind-body interactions, but they are also included as part of some alternative systems of medicine. In addition to the examples below, Appendix I provides further information.

Alternative Medical Systems. Ayurvedic medicine, India's traditional medical system, is an example of an alternative system based on the principle that health is achieved by restoring the innate harmony of the individual. It emphasizes the equal importance of body, mind, and spirit. Many other non-Western societies embrace similar beliefs. Moreover, the dominant medical system in Europe from ancient Greece to the modern era was based on the belief that ill health resulted from an imbalance of the body's four humors (blood, phlegm, yellow bile, and black bile).

Mind-Body Interventions. The practice of meditation, certain uses of hypnosis, prayer, and forms of art, music, and dance therapy are considered CAM mind-body interventions. Biochemical evidence of connections and interactions between the nervous system and endocrine and immune systems and evidence of benefit have led to the entry of certain mind-body interventions, for example, cognitive-behavioral therapies and various means of stress reduction, into mainstream medicine.

Biologically Based Therapies. Herbal remedies, special diets, and food products used therapeutically are considered biologically based CAM practices. Herbs are defined as plants or plant products that produce or contain chemicals that act upon the body.

Manipulative and Body-Based Methods. Chiropractic approaches in which the spine (primarily) is manipulated to restore health and function to the body is an example of a body-based method. Various forms of massage that involve manipulation of soft tissues and/or the musculoskeletal system are other examples.

Energy Therapies. Therapies based on the activation or generation of energy fields either originating in the body or acting externally on the body are examples of energy therapies. Qi gong (pronounced'chee gung') is a component of traditional Chinese medicine that combines movement, meditation, and regulation of breathing to enhance the flow of vital energy (qi) in the body to improve circulation and enhance immune function.

CAM Yesterday; Mainstream Healthcare Today

As noted, CAM practices once considered unorthodox in the United States can become part of the mainstream healthcare repertoire following demonstration of safety and efficacy by rigorous scientific investigation. For example, before Nixon went to China in 1971 and James Reston's compelling memoir that same year[6], acupuncture was considered arcane. Today acupuncture is often prescribed to manage pain and sometimes to control the nausea associated with chemotherapy. More recently, investigators have reported positive results in the use of acupuncture to treat cocaine addiction.[7] (See the textbox.) Among the first drugs for treatment of high blood pressure was reserpine from the herb *Rauwolfia serpentina*, described many centuries ago in Indian Ayruvedic monographs. Indeed, some of our most important drugs, while not originating as CAM therapies, are derivatives of the active ingredients identified in herbal remedies. Such drugs of botanical origin include digitalis for the treatment of congestive heart failure and vincristine, and more recently, taxol, for treatment of cancers. There are indications that other herbal remedies and CAM practices may prove effective in preventing and treating chronic diseases, possibly reducing the costs of healthcare, as well as advancing our understanding of how healing works. At present, however, few of these practices have been tested for safety and effectiveness. Still others await discovery and validation of their worth.

Acupuncture for Addiction

53.8 percent of cocaine addicts treated five times a week with acupuncture at sites in the ear tested free of the drug at the end of an eight-week study. In comparison, researchers reported that only 23.5 percent of addicts given sham acupuncture and 9.1 percent of subjects who watched relaxation videos were drug-free when tested in the final week.Further studies are needed to confirm these encouraging results.

Resolving the Issues

Despite their potential, untested CAM therapies may have unintended negative consequences.[8] They may interfere with or displace effective treatments (see Figures 2 and 3); they may expose patients to potentially toxic substances; and they may absorb resources that might be better invested in more appropriate treatment. Thus, it is critical to evaluate widely used CAM treatments for both safety and efficacy, as determined experimentally in rigorously conducted clinical trials. As appropriate, CAM therapies should also be evaluated for effectiveness (the measured outcome of routine use within the general population).

Beyond testing prevalent CAM interventions, it is also important to identify promising CAM approaches that merit more intensive study. To pursue these investigations, we must train, encourage, and support skilled investigators in both CAM and conventional medical academic communities. Furthermore, we must present credible, rather than anecdotal, data to a curious public. Finally, we must broaden the knowledge base of CAM and conventional healthcare practitioners to encompass the full repertoire of safe and effective healthcare practices—truly expanding the horizons of healthcare. These practices can then be integrated into optimal interdisciplinary treatment plans developed in cooperation with patients. These imperatives dictate serious efforts in research, training, education, and communication, along with strategies to facilitate their interdisciplinary integration.

Responding to Public Demand

In 1993,Congress formally established the Office of Alternative Medicine (OAM) at the National Institutes of Health.[11] In 1998 Congress expanded the status, mandate, and authority of the Office by enacting legislation to create the National Center for Complementary and Alternative Medicine (NCCAM).[12] NCCAM is charged to "conduct basic and applied research (intramural and extramural[13]), research training, and disseminate health information and other programs with respect to identifying, investigating, and validating CAM treatments, diag-

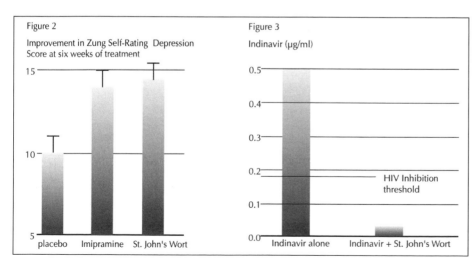

Figure 2

Improvement in Zung Self-Rating Depression Score at six weeks of treatment

(placebo, Imipramine, St. John's Wort)

Figure 3

Indinavir (μg/ml)

HIV Inhibition threshold

(Indinavir alone, Indinavir + St. John's Wort)

A Cautionary Tale
Figure 2 indicates the promise of St. John's wort as an antidepressant in a study showing that it compares favorably with a standard antidepressant, imipramine, and that both are significantly better than placebo.[9]

However, **Figure 3** indicates that if St. John's wort is taken by subjects who are also taking indinavir, an HIV protease inhibitor, levels of indinavir in the blood are reduced below the level required to block HIV multiplication.[10]

nostic and prevention modalities, disciplines and systems." Congress has expressed growing support for NCCAM's mission by providing progressive budget increases for the Center. (See Figure 4.)

Succinctly, NCCAM is dedicated to exploring complementary and alternative healing practices in the context of rigorous science, training researchers, and disseminating authoritative information. NCCAM's legislative history and milestones are summarized in Appendix II.

PART II Future Directions

NCCAM presently supports a broad portfolio of research[14], research training and educational grants and contracts, which are summarized in Appendix IV. In addition, the Center conducts outreach activities, including the dissemination of information through the NCCAM Clearinghouse and the NCCAM Web site *(http://nccam.nih.gov)*, which receives close to half a million hits a month. (See Appendix V for a more complete description of NCCAM outreach activities.) Programs to

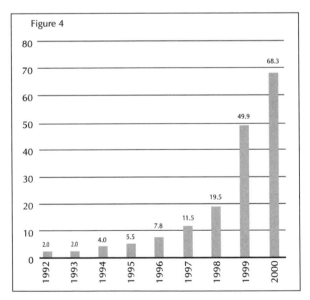

Figure 4

NCCAM funding.
Appropriations increased dramatically following the establishment of grant-making authority to NCCAM in 1998, totaling $68.3 million in FY 2000. The additional investment in CAM research by other Institutes and Centers brings the total investment in CAM research at NIH in FY 2000 to approximately $161 million.

expand basic and clinical research, train investigators to conduct CAM research, disseminate information, and facilitate integration of CAM and conventional healthcare delivery are essential in moving the CAM field forward. Our priorities in each of the four areas of research, research training, information dissemination, and integration are outlined below.

Research

The Clinical Imperative. The extensive use of untested CAM practices by the public dictates that NCCAM make clinical research[15] its highest priority and the centerpiece of its research portfolio. In this regard, the Center's approach differs significantly from that of the other NIH Institutes and Centers where the emphasis is on the discovery of new knowledge through basic research. In contrast CAM consumers and healthcare practitioners want to know now whether available options are safe and effective. Thus, while essential basic information will be sought in parallel, NCCAM is committed to the clinical study of promising CAM substances and modalities before knowledge becomes available about their active ingredients, mechanisms of action, stability, and bioavailability.

To help identify fertile areas for clinical investigation and the appropriate level of investment in these areas, the Center relies on evidence-based reviews (described in Appendix VI). These analyses indicate that information regarding the efficacy and safety of CAM therapies spans a continuum ranging from anecdotes and case studies through encouraging data derived from small, well-developed Phase I and II clinical trials (Table 1).

Several additional factors, such as the extent of utilization by consumers, the potential for public impact, the opportunity to expand the science base, feasibility, and cost are also considered, in no priority order, in selecting which treatments should be studied and at what depth.

Accordingly, NCCAM will support large (Phase III) clinical trials of CAM substances and modalities that appear from evidence-based reviews to be the most promising and important. A number of such trials are already underway, such as those to evaluate the use of St. John's wort for depres-

SYSTEMATIC REVIEWS

- Large randomized clinical trials
- Small randomized clinical trials
- Uncontrolled trials
- Observational studies
- Case Studies
- Anecdotes

Table 1 Hierarchy of Evidence
The weight of evidence supporting the safety and efficacy of any clinical modality ranges from the strongest—derived from large randomized controlled clinical trials (considered the gold standard)—through successively weaker levels of support, with case studies and anecdotes providing the weakest evidence. Systematic reviews may be conducted at and across all levels.

sion, research conducted in collaboration with the National Institute of Mental Health and the Office of Dietary Supplements; *Ginkgo biloba* to prevent dementia, in collaboration with the National Institute on Aging, the National Heart, Lung, and Blood Institute, and the National Institute of Neurologic Disorders and Stroke; glucosamine and chondroitin sulfate for osteoarthritis, in collaboration with the National Institute of Arthritis and Musculoskeletal and Skin Diseases; and acupuncture in the treatment of osteoarthritis of the knee. Many more widely used, promising therapies are deserving of definitive study, including milk thistle for chronic liver disease, Echinacea for respiratory virus infections, and melatonin and valerian for sleep disorders. For other, less well-studied, but still promising approaches, NCCAM will fund initial Phase I or Phase II trials to establish the scientific rationale and methodological feasibility needed to justify large, randomized clinical trials. NCCAM will also seek to determine the potential for toxic or adverse reactions and for interactions with prescription and over-the-counter medications. Finally, NCCAM will invest as well in careful studies of popular interventions for which reports of efficacy are only anecdotal and no rational biomedical explanation for the mechanism of action has been proposed, such as magnet therapy. NCCAM also plans to pursue studies of placebo

effects and how interactions between practitioners and patients may influence healing.

In addition to investigating individual therapies, NCCAM also aims to study entire systems of traditional and indigenous medicine that have been practiced over the centuries. Such studies may identify additional health tools of potential use to the American public and may present opportunities to address health disparities and the needs of special populations. This is an area highlighted for attention across the NIH and reflects the changing demographics of America. By 2050 it is estimated that the numbers of Latino, black, and Asian and Pacific Islander racial and ethnic groups will exceed the white non-Hispanic population. Many of these individuals will have absorbed traditions of healthcare and specific modalities practiced in their families and their countries of origin for generations.

Appropriate evaluation of CAM techniques and products will require that experts in the use of a given CAM modality are intimately involved in the design, conduct, and oversight of these studies. Also, diverse research designs will be needed to assess the spectrum of CAM techniques and products. For example, it is not possible to examine some CAM modalities (for example, massage) through double-blind trials, while others involve combinations of therapies that are custom-tailored to each patient's needs. In this regard, it is helpful that recent studies suggest that observational studies can be sufficiently well designed to yield data comparable to those of some randomized, controlled trials.[16][17][18] Notwithstanding the difficulties in designing some CAM studies, NCCAM will demand the same high standard of scientific excellence that is required throughout the NIH.

Basic Science Research. While clinical research is the centerpiece of NCCAM's research portfolio, NCCAM will pursue basic studies in parallel. The realization that herbals are not single agents but mixtures of many compounds makes our understanding of their underlying mechanisms of action all the more critical. Moreover, research projects such as those designed to understand the neurobiological basis for acupuncture-mediated analgesia and the essential components of St. John's wort that ameliorate depression may contribute to the knowledge base of conventional biomedical researchers and inspire novel treatment approaches and rational drug discovery. To take full advantage of the opportunities to build a base of CAM-related basic science discoveries, randomized clinical trials will be designed not only to test treatments, but also, to the extent possible, to determine underlying mechanisms of action, discover biomarkers, define pharmacokinetics, identify the active components in natural products, and collect data on the natural presentation and progression of the diseases under study. For example, NCCAM's current trial of *Ginkgo biloba* not only will test whether this ancient natural product delays the onset and progression of dementia, but the trial also represents the single largest prospective study of intellectual decline in aging Americans to date.

NIH Areas of Emphasis.   NCCAM shares the NIH-wide imperative to address pressing public health concerns, and our research aims are closely aligned with the NIH-designated areas of emphasis. Toward this end, the Center will contribute to the collective effort in three specified areas: the biology of brain disorders; new preventive strategies against disease; and new avenues for the development of therapeutics. The potential contribution of NCCAM with respect to this latter area is substantial. NCCAM also will participate in the trans-NIH effort to understand and eliminate the health disparities observed between minority and majority populations. To this end, NCCAM is developing a strategic plan to address health disparities to be incorporated into the overall NIH plan.

Collaboration.   The efficiency with which we advance our research agenda will be enhanced by leveraging the resources and expertise of our colleagues in other NIH Institutes and Centers, other government agencies,[19] research institutions, the academic and international communities, and industry. The opportunities for such collaborations are abundant and it is gratifying that we have already found many partners at NIH and other agencies, and that centers of excellence throughout the world have expressed interest in working with us.

Training

Our ability to achieve our research goals is dependent on the availability of a critical mass of skilled investigators in both CAM and conventional communities. Thus, NCCAM must encourage skilled researchers to investigate CAM approaches and train CAM and conventional practitioners to conduct or participate in rigorous studies. To this end, NCCAM will fully exploit the range of options within NIH's purview to promote the training and professional development of researchers. Specifically, we will make awards to both individuals and institutions, for both mentored and independent research, ranging from basic through clinical research projects. NCCAM also will work to promote collaborations between CAM and conventional practitioners and researchers, which are essential to moving the field forward.

Information Dissemination

We regard as one of our highest priorities the need to inform the public, which today is immersed in media reports and Internet claims regarding CAM approaches, towards the safest and most effective practices and away from those that are risky or unsafe. Using all forms of communication, we must disseminate credible, not anecdotal data to a curious public that deserves complete and accurate information. Thus, we will aim to make available an abundance of timely and relevant materials for distribution, not only through the interactive capabilities of the Internet, but also as hard copy. Critical materials will be translated for non-English readers, as appropriate. We will hold open forums to engage the public in dialogue and interact with the scientific community at professional meetings.

Integration

Finally, NCCAM must work to overcome the reluctance of conventional healthcare providers to consider CAM therapies for their patients. If we are to capitalize on the opportunities to achieve changes in both the CAM and conventional healthcare communities, we must increase opportunities for training medical and post-graduate professional students to become educated about

CAM. With this information, they may knowledgeably guide and refer patients toward safe and effective CAM applications and practitioners experienced in delivering them.

While many agree in principle regarding the merits of an integrated healthcare delivery system, there are numerous policy issues that await resolution before such a system can be fully implemented. These matters, including development and enhancement of clinical training programs, insurance reimbursement, licensing of CAM practitioners, and the relative roles of CAM and conventional providers, are not within the purview of

NIH. Rather, their resolution falls to NIH's sister agencies in the Department of Health and Human Services, actions based on the findings of the White House Commission on Complementary and Alternative Medicine Policy, and concerned organizations.

As a component of NIH, NCCAM's role is to provide the scientific evidence to inform policy makers

Ginkgo Biloba to Prevent Dementia in Aging Americans

For centuries, extracts from the leaves of the *Ginkgo biloba* tree have been used as Chinese herbal medicine to treat a variety of medical conditions. In Europe and Asia, standardized extracts from ginkgo leaves are routinely taken to treat a wide range of neuro-cognitive symptoms, including those of Alzheimer's disease. Little is known, however, about the safe dosage levels of *Ginkgo biloba* extract, let alone its actual effectiveness in preventing Alzheimer's disease. A newly funded NCCAM study, in collaboration with NIA, may help resolve these questions. In FY 1999, the University of Pittsburgh School of Medicine was awarded a six-year, $15 million cooperative agreement to coordinate a multicenter effort to study the efficacy of *Ginkgo biloba* extract in preventing dementia, a cognitive decline in memory and other intellectual functions, in older individuals. This study, the largest of its kind ever conducted on *Ginkgo biloba*, will include four clinical centers and enroll almost 3,000 people. Participants who take *Ginkgo biloba* will be compared to a second group of individuals who will take a placebo.

adequately. It is by holding CAM therapies to the highest standards of evidence, that we believe we will best facilitate the creation of an integrated healthcare delivery system in which conventional physicians and CAM practitioners work as an interdisciplinary team.

Part III NCCAM Strategic Plan, 2001–2005

The confidence of Congress in authorizing NCCAM to fund grants and contracts and providing increasing budgets to support them has served as the impetus for a review of Center activities with an eye to targeting its efforts toward expanding options of healthcare. For these reasons, we modified and expanded the 1998 Draft Strategic Plan developed by the then Office of Alternative Medicine to create this first NCCAM Five-Year Strategic Plan. The Plan embodies the principles discussed in Part II, articulates our mission and vision, identifies principal stakeholders, proposes strategic initiatives and goals, and specifies the management principles under which NCCAM will operate in carrying out its mission. We are indebted to our staff and NIH colleagues, advisory councils, workshop attendees, numerous healthcare providers, and the public at large for the cumulative wisdom that has informed the Plan. It represents the first step in an ongoing planning process that will be used periodically to ensure that our priorities match developments in the field as it matures, and that they reflect an appropriate balance between pursuing scientific opportunity and addressing the healthcare needs of the public in promoting health and in preventing and treating disease. The ongoing planning process (described in Appendix VIII) will continue to solicit and consider input from the public and our many other stakeholders, facilitated by our Office of Public Liaison.

Our Mission

We are dedicated to exploring complementary and alternative healing practices in the context of rigorous science, educating and training CAM researchers, and disseminating authoritative information to the public and professionals.

Our Vision

NCCAM will advance research to yield insights and tools derived from complementary and alternative medicine to benefit the health and well-being of the public, while enabling an informed public to reject ineffective or unsafe practices.

The role of the National Center for Complementary and Alternative Medicine is to apply the uncompromising standard of excellence in research to healthcare practices and products derived from many rich traditions. We will employ best-in-the-world practices for the conduct of science and the management of research, training, and related activities. We are committed to the timely dissemination of research findings to the communities we serve, and in so doing regard it as of the highest importance to facilitate the merger of valuable CAM and conventional approaches into a practice of "integrative medicine." Such a practice will involve multiple healthcare professionals working as an interdisciplinary team, thus expanding the repertoire of ways to achieve and maintain health.

NCCAM's vision will be realized only by creating and sustaining close partnerships across the spectrum of CAM consumers, investigators, and healthcare providers, and by reaching out to diverse stakeholder groups for advice and exchange of information.

Our Stakeholders

- Patients and the General Public
- Patient Advocacy Groups
- CAM Healthcare Researchers, Educators, and Practitioners
- Conventional Healthcare Researchers, Educators, and Practitioners
- Academic and Professional Associations
- NIH and other Government Agencies
- Research and Educational Institutions and Foundations
- International Research Organizations
- The Pharmaceutical, Nutriceutical, Dietary Supplement, and Biotechnology Industries
- The Media
- Congress
- Health Insurers

Strategic Areas

To achieve our vision, we have identified four strategic areas: Investing in Research, Training CAM Researchers, Expanding Outreach, and Facilitating Integration. Each of these strategic areas has evolved and will mature through an ongoing process of planning and evaluation, with substantial input from the National Advisory Council for Complementary and Alternative Medicine (Appendix IX lists members), and our stakeholders.

Strategic Area 1: Investing in Research

NCCAM will advance research by encouraging and supporting CAM research projects according to the philosophies and priorities outlined in Part II.[20] The Center's highest priority is clinical research, both with respect to individual therapies and entire systems of medicine. While NCCAM will pursue investigations at all levels of the hierarchy of evidence outlined in Table 1, our largest investment will be in Phase III clinical trials, with proportionately smaller investments in areas for which less evidence is available. NCCAM will also support basic science research, not only through studies whose primary aim is to elucidate basic mechanisms, but also by exploiting opportunities afforded by clinical trials.

The Center is also committed to building research capacity and infrastructure, both intramurally and extramurally, in the United States and abroad. Throughout these endeavors, the Center will pursue the many advantages afforded by collaborations nationally and internationally, as well as with fellow NIH Institutes and Centers, other government agencies, and industry.

Goal 1

Stimulate submission of high-quality applications in CAM priority areas by both CAM and conventional investigators

Objectives:

- Exhibit NCCAM information at professional meetings and conduct grant-writing workshops.

- Sponsor interdisciplinary conferences to stimulate broad-based research.
- Assist extramural CAM researchers and practitioners to develop and participate in high-quality research applications.

Goal 2

Expand the scope of the NCCAM extramural research portfolio and participation by research subjects

Objectives:

- Emphasize investigator-initiated research as the time-proven vehicle for advancing science on broad fronts.
- Support a broad base of rigorous CAM research, including, but not limited to, studies of basic biology and disease pathogenesis, elucidating mechanisms of action, outcomes research, pharmacologic investigations, epidemiology, and all phases of intervention trials (I–III).
- Support research to address health disparities among women, minorities, children, and other underrepresented populations.
- Solicit applications and proposals in areas for which the opportunities for impact are great and there is a paucity of investigator-initiated research.

Goal 3

Create an NCCAM intramural research program

Objectives:

- Design, conduct, analyze, and report rigorous CAM research, including, but not limited to, studies elucidating basic biology and pathogenesis mechanisms of action, outcomes research, pharmacologic investigations, epidemiology, and all phases of intervention trials (I–III).
- Conduct clinical and laboratory-based CAM research studies in close collaboration with extramural CAM scientists and with intramural staff of the other NIH Institutes and Centers.
- Provide an environment for training scientists and clinicians from diverse backgrounds in the healthcare professions in the conduct and analysis of CAM research studies, employing the highest standards of trial design and ethics.

Goal 4

Establish a global NCCAM research enterprise

Objectives:

- Establish programs of research on traditional and indigenous health practices in the United States and in those countries in which the most promising opportunities for CAM research are identified, in coordination with international organizations, and with all due respect to the heritage and practices of indigenous peoples.
- Align these programs with existing NIH-funded international research programs to ensure the immediate availability of research expertise in the field and the infrastructure to support them.

Strategic Area 2: Training CAM Investigators

NCCAM will develop a cadre of investigators in CAM research by providing appropriate career development opportunities; by increasing the knowledge, experience, and capacity of CAM practitioners to conduct rigorous research; and by enhancing conventional practitioners' and researchers' knowledge and experience in specific CAM areas.

Goal 1

Increase the number, quality, and diversity of CAM investigators

Objectives:

- Stimulate collaborations between CAM practitioners and investigators in the conventional academic medical community.
- Develop programs to train individuals in CAM-related laboratory and epidemiological research.
- Train doctors of medicine, osteopathy, chiropractic, and naturopathy, and others with advanced degrees in relevant clinical disciplines,[21] to conduct CAM-related clinical research.

- Initiate quality research training programs.
- Increase the number of trainees from under-represented populations.
- Establish an interdisciplinary, intramural NIH research training program.

Strategic Area 3: Expanding Outreach

NCCAM will strive to create a public image that conveys our dedication to exploring complementary and alternative healing practices and pursuing rigorous science, providing extensive, accurate information to consumers with sensitivity and compassion, and involving our broad range of stakeholders in shaping the Center's agenda. To this end, NCCAM will use a variety of methods, media, and technologies to provide a timely source of evidence-based, CAM information, and actively seek input from its stakeholders.

Goal 1

Enhance NCCAM's capacity to provide information to consumers, practitioners, and investigators

Objectives:

- Develop and disseminate reliable scientific information that is culturally sensitive, engaging to the reader, and updated frequently to reflect the pace of change in the field.
- Respond with compassion and understanding to inquiries from consumers, directing them as appropriate, to a network of resources.
- Collaborate on information dissemination with other NIH entities and government agencies, international organizations, and foreign government and nongovernment agencies.

Goal 2

Establish an effective dialogue with CAM stakeholders

Objectives:

- Sponsor regional Town Hall Meetings to provide a forum for the public to contribute input and for NCCAM to share information regarding important research efforts and findings with the community.

- Seek ongoing, substantive input from leaders of CAM practice communities, CAM training institutions, advocacy groups, the mainstream academic and scientific communities, industry, partners in other NIH Institutes and Centers, and Federal agencies.
- Exhibit NCCAM-funded discoveries and opportunities at conventional scientific meetings and those of our CAM constituents.
- Develop media opportunities and strategies to disseminate research information and increase public understanding of NCCAM's mission.

Strategic Area 4: Facilitating Integration

NCCAM will work to facilitate a more integrated practice of medicine. Within this paradigm, CAM and conventional healthcare professionals would function as interdisciplinary teams to deliver an expanded repertoire of safe and effective treatments that include a focus on the whole person. This goal is consistent with the increasing interdisciplinary nature of health-related research and the renewed focus on integrative biology. Only by holding CAM therapies to the highest standards of evidence will we best accomplish this broad aim.

Goal 1

Facilitate development of health education curricula that respect and incorporate insights and opportunities afforded by safe and effective CAM and conventional practices

Objectives:

- Fund educational grants to develop model curricula regarding CAM practices for schools of medicine and allied disciplines.
- Fund educational grants to develop model curricula regarding conventional medical practices and research methods for schools of complementary and alternative medicine disciplines.

Goal 2

Facilitate coupling of effective CAM and conventional practices within a coordinated, interdisciplinary healthcare delivery system

Objectives:

- Sponsor national meetings, consensus conferences, and workshops on validated CAM therapies to enable practitioners and all other concerned parties to identify effective interventions for use in treating patients.

- Disseminate CAM research findings to healthcare providers.

- Identify and develop methods to overcome barriers to the integration of safe and effective CAM practices.

- Support demonstration projects focusing on how most effectively to translate CAM research findings into practice. These projects will emphasize the development of partnerships between researchers and healthcare systems and organizations that have incorporated CAM practices into the delivery of clinical care.

- Facilitate integration of effective CAM practices into routine healthcare delivery for NIH Clinical Center patients.

- Support enhanced communication and partnership-building between conventional and CAM healthcare institutions.

Practicing Responsible Stewardship

NCCAM will enhance customer service and continue to develop its valuable human resources, effective leadership, sound management practices, and efficient business systems in ways that reflect the trust placed in it by the American public.

Goal 1

Develop NCCAM's human resources

Objectives:

- Exploit all available strategies to recruit and retain a motivated, highly qualified, well-trained, versatile, and flexible workforce that is committed to NCCAM's vision.

- Define roles and responsibilities of each staff member clearly.

- Vest staff with authority, accountability, and autonomy.

- Provide the resources staff needs to be successful in performing their respective roles.

- Foster diversity among NCCAM employees and enhance understanding and appreciation of cultural differences.

- Promote a work culture characterized by integrity, mutual respect, teamwork, and open communication.

- Reward excellence.

- Foster staff career development through practical experience, training, and other methods.

- Emphasize quality of work life.

Goal 2

Establish effective leadership, management, and administrative practices

Objectives:

- Elevate standards of performance.

- Emphasize customer service.

- Enhance administrative infrastructure.

- Evaluate major NCCAM functions.

Goal 3

Engineer for efficiency

Objectives:

- Streamline and automate business activities based on benchmarking best practices.

- Provide training for staff to enhance core competencies to maximize use of systems, technology, and equipment.

- Develop exacting management systems.

ENDNOTES

1   Conventional medicine refers to medicine as practiced by holders of MD (medical doctor) or DO (doctor of osteopathy) degrees and their allied health professionals, some of whom may also practice complementary and alternative medicine.

2   Eisenberg, D.M. et al. "Trends in Alternative Medicine Use in the United States," 1990–1997. *JAMA.* 1998; 280:1569–1575.

3   This is the definition that NCCAM chooses to employ. There are others as well. For example, the definition

assigned by Ernst,E. et al. (Complementary medicine—a definition. Br J Gen Pract. 1995;45:506), and adopted in a slightly altered form by the Cochrane Collaboration (see Appendix VI) is "diagnosis, treatment and/or prevention which complements mainstream medicine by contributing to a common whole, by satisfying a demand not met by orthodoxy or by diversifying the conceptual frameworks of medicine."

4   Astin, J.A."Why Patients Use Alternative Medicine—Results of a National Study." *JAMA*. 1998;279:1548–1553.

5   These are the categories within which NCCAM has chosen to group the numerous CAM practices; others employ different, broad groupings. Note also that only limited examples are provided within each category, and that no attempt was made to be exhaustive. Thus, the absence of any one CAM modality does not in any way imply its intentional omission.

6   *The New York Times*. July 26,1971:1,6.

7   Avants,S.K., Margolin, A., Holford, T.R., Thomas R. Kosten, T.R. "A Randomized Controlled Trial of Auricular Acupuncture for Cocaine Dependence." *Arch Intern Med*. 2000;160(15):2305–2312.

8   Nortier, J.L., Martinez, M.M., Schmeiser, H.H., Volker, M.A., Bieler, C.A., Petein, M., Depierreux, M.F., DePauw, L., Abramowicz, D.,Vereerstraeten, P., Vanherweghem, J.L. Urothelial Carcinoma Associated with the Use of a Chinese Herb *(Aristolochia fangchi), New England Journal of Medicine*. 2000; 342(23):1686–1692.

9   Philipp, M., Kohnen, R., Hiller, KO. "Hypericum Extract Versus Imipramine or Placebo in Patients with Moderate Depression: Randomised Multicentre Study of Treatment for Eight Weeks." *BMJ*. 1999;319:1534–1539.

10   Piscitelli, S. C., Burstein, A. H., Chaitt, D., Alfaro, R. M., Falloon, J."Indinavir Concentrations and St. John's Wort." *Lancet*. 2000; 355(9203):547–548.

11   Previous legislation provided $2 million in Fiscal Year 1992 to establish the Office of Alternative Medicine.

12   The legislation also established the White House Commission for Complementary and Alternative Medicine Policy to study and report to the President and the Congress on public policy issues related to CAM.

13   Approximately 82 percent of NIH's overall investment is made through approximately 35,000 grants and contracts supporting research and training in more than 2,000 research institutions throughout the U.S. and abroad. These grants and contracts comprise the NIH Extramural Research Program. Approximately 10 percent of the budget goes to NIH's Intramural Research Programs, the more than 2,000 projects conducted mainly in its own laboratories. About 8 percent of the budget is expended to administer the extramural and intramural research programs.

14   NCCAM's portfolio does not yet reflect the desired balance across all potential CAM practices. This is in part due to the lack of a research tradition in some fields of practice. To redress this situation, NCCAM will work with CAM communities to develop the requisite expertise. NCCAM also will seek to enlist experienced investigators with the expertise needed to undertake research across all CAM domains. These include areas such as neuroscience, bioimaging, and molecular biology.

15   For an overview of the concepts and practices involved in clinical trials, see http://clinicaltrials.gov.

16   Concato,J.,Shah,N.,Horwitz,R.I."Randomized, Controlled Trials, Observational Studies, and the Hierarchy of Research Designs." *New England Journal of Medicine*. 2000;342:1887–1892.

17   Benson,K.,Hartz,A. "A Comparison of Observational Studies and Randomized, Controlled Clinical Trials." *New England Journal of Medicine*. 2000;342:1878–1886.

18   Pocock,S.J.,Elbourne,D.R."Randomized Trials or Observational Tribulations?"2000;342:1907–1909.

19   To foster NCCAM's collaboration within the Department of Health and Human Services and with other Federal agencies, NCCAM has organized the NCCAM Trans-agency CAM Coordinating Committee (NTACCC),which carries forward the work of the Trans-agency CAM Coordinating Committee established in 1997 by the NIH Director. The Committee comprises representatives of 22 of the NIH Institutes and Centers and the NIH Offices of AIDS Research, Behavioral and Social Sciences Research, Dietary Supplements, Extramural Research, Rare Diseases, Medical Applications of Research, Research on Minority Health, and Research on Women's Health. The Departments of Agriculture, Education, and Defense also are represented, and the Department of Health and Human Services sends representatives from multiple components (the Agency for Healthcare Research and Quality, Centers for Disease Control and Prevention, Food and Drug Administration, Health Resources and Services Administration, Indian Health Service, Substance Abuse and Mental Health Services Administration). The White House Commission on Complementary and Alternative Medicine Policy is also represented.

20   Information for those interested in applying for grants may be found at http://nccam.nih.gov.

21   Note: The appropriate advanced degree varies by discipline.

PART IV APPENDIX I

MAJOR DOMAINS OF COMPLEMENTARY AND ALTERNATIVE MEDICINE

Complementary and alternative healthcare and medical practices are those healthcare practices that are not currently an integral part of conventional medicine.[1] The list of practices that are considered CAM changes over time as CAM practices and therapies that are proven safe and effective become accepted as mainstream healthcare practices. NCCAM groups CAM practices within five major domains, acknowledging that other groupings are possible: native medical systems,(2)mind-body interventions, (3)biologically based treatments,(4)manipulative and body-based methods, and (5)energy therapies. The individual systems and treatments comprising these categories are too numerous to list in this document. Instead, we are providing examples within each domain. The absence of any one CAM modality in no way implies its intentional omission. Note also that there is some overlap across domains so that a CAM practice chosen as an example within one domain might also be classified within one or another of the five domains.[2]

I. Alternative Medical Systems—Alternative medical systems involve complete systems of theory and practice that have evolved independently of, and often prior to, the conventional biomedical approach. Many are traditional systems of medicine that are practiced by individual cultures throughout the world, including a number of venerable Asian systems.

Traditional oriental medicine emphasizes the proper balance or disturbances of qi (pronounced chee),or vital energy, in health and disease, respectively. Traditional oriental medicine consists of a group of techniques and methods, including acupuncture, herbal medicine, oriental massage, and qi gong (a form of energy therapy described more fully below). Acupuncture involves stimulating specific anatomic points in the body for therapeutic purposes, usually by puncturing the skin with a needle.

Ayurveda is India's traditional system of medicine. Ayurvedic medicine (meaning "science of life") is a comprehensive system of medicine that places equal emphasis on body, mind, and spirit, and strives to restore the innate harmony of the individual. Some of the primary Ayurvedic treatments include diet, exercise, meditation, herbs, massage, exposure to sunlight, and controlled breathing.

Other traditional medical systems have been developed by Native American, African, Middle-Eastern, Tibetan, and Central and South American cultures.

Homeopathy and naturopathy are also examples of complete alternative medical systems. Homeopathy is an unconventional Western system developed in Germany that is based on the principle that "like cures like," i.e., that the same substance that in large doses produces the symptoms of an illness, in very minute doses cures it. Homeopathic physicians believe that even dilute remedies have great potency, provided that they are precisely selected based on detailed evaluations of symptoms to determine a patient's sensitivity. Therefore, homeopaths use small doses of specially prepared plant extracts and minerals to stimulate the body's defense mechanisms and healing processes in order to treat illness.

Naturopathy views disease as a manifestation of alterations in the processes by which the body naturally heals itself and emphasizes health restoration as well as disease treatment. Naturopathic physicians employ an array of healing practices, including diet and clinical nutrition; homeopathy; acupuncture; herbal medicine; hydrotherapy (the use of water in a range of temperatures and methods of applications); spinal and soft-tissue manipulation; physical therapies involving electric currents, ultrasound, and light; therapeutic counseling; and pharmacology.

II. Mind-Body Interventions—Mind-body interventions employ a variety of techniques designed to facilitate the mind's capacity to affect bodily function and symptoms. Only a subset of mind-body interventions are considered CAM. Many that have a well documented theoretical basis and for which there is supporting scientific evidence, for example, cognitive-behavioral approaches, are now considered "mainstream." On the other hand, meditation, certain uses of hypnosis, dance, music, and art therapy, and prayer and mental healing are categorized as complementary and alternative.

III. Biologically Based Therapies—This category of CAM includes natural and biologically based practices, interventions, and products, many of which overlap with conventional medicine's use of dietary supplements. Included are herbal, special dietary, orthomolecular, and individual biological therapies.

Herbal therapies employ individual herbs or mixtures of herbs for therapeutic purposes. Herbs are plants or plant parts that produce and contain chemical substances that act upon the body. Special diet therapies, such as those proposed by Drs. Atkins, Ornish, Pritikin, and Weil, are believed to prevent and/or control illness as well as promote health. Orthomolecular therapies aim to treat disease with varying concentrations of chemicals, such as, magnesium, melatonin, and megadoses of vitamins. Biological therapies include, for example, the use of laetrile and shark cartilage to treat cancer and bee pollen to treat autoimmune and inflammatory diseases.

IV. Manipulative and Body-Based Methods—This category includes methods that are based on manipulation and/or movement of the body. For example, chiropractors focus on the relationship between structure (primarily the spine) and function, and how that relationship affects the preservation and restoration of health, using manipulative therapy as an integral treatment tool. Some osteopathic physicians practice osteopathic manipulation, a full-body system of hands-on techniques to alleviate pain, restore function, and promote health and well-being. Massage therapists manipulate muscle and connective tissue to promote optimal function of those tissues and promote relaxation and well-being.

V. Energy Therapies—Energy therapies focus either on fields believed to originate within the body (biofields)or those from other sources (electromagnetic fields).

Biofield therapies are intended to affect energy fields that purportedly surround and penetrate the human body. The existence of such fields is not yet experimentally proven. Some forms of energy therapy manipulate biofields by applying pressure and/or manipulating the body by placing the hands in, or through, these fields. Examples include Qi gong, Reiki, and Therapeutic Touch. Qi gong is a component of traditional oriental medicine that combines movement, meditation, and regulation of breathing to enhance the flow of vital energy (qi) in the body, to improve blood circulation, and to enhance immune function. Reiki, the Japanese word representing Universal Life Energy, is based on the belief that by channeling spiritual energy through the practitioner the spirit is healed, and it in turn heals the physical body. Therapeutic Touch is derived from the ancient technique of "laying-on of hands "and is based on the premise that it is the healing force of the therapist that affects the patient's recovery and that healing is promoted when the body's energies are in balance. By passing their hands over the patient, these healers identify energy imbalances.

Bioelectromagnetic-based therapies involve the unconventional use of electromagnetic fields, such as pulsed fields, magnetic fields, or alternating current or direct current fields. These therapies have been used to treat asthma or cancer or manage pain and migraine headaches, among other conditions.

APPENDIX II
Important Events in NCCAM History

October 1991

Legislative action (P.L.102–170) provides $2 million in funding for FY to establish an office within the NIH to investigate and evaluate promising unconventional medical practices.

Stephen C.Groft, PharmD, appointed Acting Director of the new Office of Alternative Medicine (OAM).

September 1992

Workshop on Alternative Medicine convened in Chantilly, Virginia, to discuss the state of the art of the major areas of alternative medicine and to direct attention to priority areas for future research activities.

October 1992

Joseph J. Jacobs, MD, MBA, appointed first Director, OAM.

June 1993

OAM formally established under the National Institutes of Health Revitalization Act of 1993 (P.L.103–43) to facilitate study and evaluation of complementary and alternative medical practices and to disseminate the resulting information to the public.

September 1993

First OAM research project grants funded through the National Center for Research Resources.

December 1993

Alternative Medicine Program Advisory Council established.

September 1994

Alan I. Trachtenberg, MD, MPH, appointed Acting Director, OAM.

January 1995

Wayne B. Jonas, MD, appointed second Director, OAM.

October 1995

Research Centers Program established to provide a nationwide focus for interdisciplinary CAM research in academic institutions.

October 1996

Public Information Clearinghouse established.

November 1996

OAM designated as a World Health Organization Collaborating Center in Traditional Medicine.

September 1997

First Phase III clinical trial funded to test the efficacy of *Hypericum perforatum* for treatment of depression.

October 1998

National Center for Complementary and Alternative Medicine established, by Congressional mandate, under provisions of the Omnibus Appropriations Bill (P.L.105–277). This bill amended Title IV of the Public Health Service Act and elevated the OAM to an NIH Center.

January 1999

William R. Harlan, MD, named Acting Director, NCCAM.

February 1999

Charter creating NCCAM, making it the 25th independent component of the National Institutes of Health signed. The law gave the NCCAM Director control of the Center's day-to-day financial and administrative management, as well as broad decision-making authority and fiscal responsibility for grants and contracts. Dr. Donna E. Shalala, Secretary, Department of Health and Human Services (DHHS), approved the charter of the Center on February 1, 1999, its first official business day.

May 1999

First independently awarded NCCAM research project grant made.

NCCAM Trans-Agency CAM Coordinating Committee (TCAMCC) established by the NCCAM Director to foster NCCAM's collaboration across the Department of Health and Human Services and other Federal agencies. This committee superseded a transagency committee established by the NIH Director in 1997.

June 1999

Special Emphasis Panel chartered to enable NCCAM to conduct peer review of CAM research project grant applications.

July 1999

Cancer Advisory Panel for Complementary and Alternative Medicine (CAPCAM) created to assess preliminary clinical data related to treatment of cancer submitted by CAM practitioners.

August 1999

National Advisory Council on Complementary and Alternative Medicine chartered.

October 1999

Stephen E. Straus, MD, appointed first Director, NCCAM.

APPENDIX III

STEPHEN E.STRAUS, MD, NCCAM DIRECTOR
Biographical Sketch

Dr. Stephen E. Straus was appointed the first director of the National Center for Complementary Alternative Medicine (NCCAM) on October 6, 1999. Born on November 23,1946, in New York City, Dr. Straus received his BS in life sciences from the Massachusetts Institute of Technology in 1968 and MD from the Columbia University College of Physicians and Surgeons in 1972.His postgraduate included an internship and residency in medicine at Barnes Hospital, St. Louis, Missouri, and a fellowship in infectious disease at Washington University, St. Louis. Dr. Straus is board certified in internal medicine and infectious diseases.

Dr. Straus began his NIH career in 1973 as a research associate in the National Institute on Allergy Infectious Diseases (NIAID),and he returned to NIAID in 1979 upon completion of his training in St.Louis. In pursuit of his research interests in molecular biology, pathophysiology, and treatment and prevention of human viral and immunological diseases, Dr. Straus has conducted both basic and research. Dr. Straus has published over 300 research articles and edited several books. Since joining NIAID, he has assumed progressively higher levels of leadership, serving first as senior investigator and as Head of the Medical Virology Section in the Institute's Laboratory of Clinical Investigation and then Chief of the Laboratory, a position he continues to hold concurrently with the Directorship of NCCAM.

Among Dr. Straus's accomplishments is his demonstration that acyclovir suppresses recurrent genital and herpes, and the characterization of a previously unrecognized genetically determined disease, the lymphoproliferative syndrome. The recipient in 1999 of the Dutch National ME Fund Award (the national prize from the Netherlands for research in myalgic encephelomyelitis/chronic fatigue syndrome), Dr. Straus's professional achievements have been recognized by his election to the Infectious Diseases of America, the Association of American Physicians, and the American Society for Clinical Investigation. He is a recipient of five medals and other commendations from the U.S. Public Health Service, including the Distinguished Service Medal for innovative clinical research, and the DHHS Secretary's Distinguished Award for drafting the blueprint to reinvigorate clinical research at the NIH. He serves on the boards of several scientific journals, including the *Journal of Virology* and *Virology*.

APPENDIX IV

NCCAM RESEARCH AND RESEARCH TRAINING PORTFOLIO[3]

NCCAM supports a diverse portfolio of research and research training activities, many cofunded with other NIH Institutes. Research activities include the conduct of clinical trials to test the safety and efficacy of CAM modalities that are currently in wide use, the establishment of Centers to develop the infrastructure and capacity for CAM research and research training, and research programs initiated by individual investigators.

RESEARCH PROJECTS

NCCAM has made awards to study a number of health conditions and populations. Included are a large number of Phase I (to evaluate safety), Phase II (to assess clinical activity) and Phase III clinical trials (to determine clinical efficacy) of a range of CAM therapies.

ARTHRITIS

RCT—Acupuncture Safety/Efficacy in Knee Osteoarthritis (Brian Berman, MD, University of Maryland, Baltimore)—This multisite, Phase III trial is designed to determine the short-and long-term safety and efficacy of acupuncture in the treatment of elderly patients with osteoarthritis of the knee using three randomly assigned participant groups for comparison: (1)true acupuncture group, (2)sham acupuncture group, and (3)education and attention control group.

Study of the Efficacy of Glucosamine and Glucosamine/Chondroitin Sulfate in Knee Osteoarthritis (Daniel Clegg, MD, University of Utah) *Cofunded with the National Institute of Arthritis and Musculoskeletal and Skin Diseases*—This four-year, multisite, Phase III study will determine whether glucosamine, chondroitin sulfate and/or the combination of glucosamine and chondroitin sulfate are more effective than placebo and whether the combination is more effective than glucosamine or chondroitin sulfate alone in the treatment of knee pain associated with osteoarthritis of the knee.

CANCER

RCT—Gonzalez Regimen (Karen Antman, MD, Columbia University, supplement to Cancer Center Support Grant) *Cosponsored with the National Cancer Institute*—This is a randomized, controlled, Phase III trial comparing the efficacy of the Gonzalez Regimen versus standard care in the treatment of inoperable pancreatic adenocarcinoma. The Gonzalez Regimen consists of intensive pancreatic proteolytic enzyme therapy with ancillary nutritional support and detoxification procedures.

Self-transcendence in Breast Cancer Support Groups (Doris Coward, PhD, University of Texas, Austin) *Cofunded with the National Institute of Nursing Research*—This randomized, Phase II open trial proposes to expand the traditional role of breast cancer support groups by conscious promotion of self-transcendence views and behaviors, and to document, over time, changes in measures of self-transcendence, well-being and immune function in support group participants.

Shark Cartilage Trial (Charles Loprinzi, MD, North Central Cancer Treatment Group, Mayo Clinic)—The intent of this multisite, Phase III, randomized, blinded, controlled trial is to test the efficacy and safety of a powder preparation of shark cartilage for the treatment of patients with breast or colo-rectal cancer.

Shark Cartilage Trial (Roy Herbst, PhD, MD, University of Texas/M.D. Anderson Cooperative Research Base)—This is a multisite, randomized, controlled, double-blind Phase III trial comparing the efficacy of purified shark cartilage and placebo in 500 individuals with inoperable, nonsmall cell lung cancer. All individuals will also receive standard chemotherapy and radiotherapy with survival as the primary outcome measure.

CARDIOVASCULAR DISEASES

Acupuncture and Hypertension: Efficacy and Mechanisms (Norman M. Kaplan, MD University of Texas Southwestern Medical Center)—Acupuncture has been advocated as safe and effective treatment of essential hypertension and other cardiovascular disorders (for example, heart failure, myocardial ischemia) that have sympathetic neural components. Using a randomized, double-blind placebo-controlled design for their Phase II trial, the investigators will test two major hypotheses: (1)electroacupuncture produces a long-lasting reduction in sympathetic nerve activity, thereby providing a safe and effective complementary treatment of human hypertension; (2)a major mechanism mediating the blood pressure lowering effect of acupuncture is the activation of somatic afferents, which trigger a naloxone-sensitive reflex suppression of central sympathetic outflow.

Effect of High-Dose Vitamin E on Carotid Atherosclerosis (Ishwarlal Jialal, MD, University of Texas Southwestern Medical Center)—The primary aim of study is to test the effect of high-dose alpha tocopherol (AT) supplementation on the progression of carotid atherosclerosis in patients with coronary artery disease (stable angina pectoris or previous myocardial infarction) in a two-year, placebo-controlled, Phase II randomized trial. Since AT supplementation decreases low-density lipoprotein oxidation and certain proatherogenic properties of activated monocytes, these parameters will also be studied and correlated with carotid atherosclerosis. While the patients will be monitored for clinical events during the study, this will not constitute a major aim since the study is not powered to adequately assess this. Thus, this study will determine if high-dose AT supplementation is beneficial in retarding carotid atherosclerosis.

Effects of Meditation on Mechanisms of Coronary Heart Disease (C. Bairey Merz, MD, Cedars-Sinai Medical Center)—This project is a randomized controlled, single-blinded, Phase II trial investigating whether transcendental meditation will reduce cardiac events in patients with coronary heart disease. The control groups will participate in a cardiology education program. The primary outcome is arterial vasomotor dysfunction (brachial artery reactivity) and the secondary outcome is autonomic nervous system imbalances (heart rate variability).

DENTAL DISORDERS

Acupuncture for Dental Pain: Testing a Model (Lixing Lao, DDS, PhD, University of Maryland)— This double-blind, randomized controlled trial tests the hypothesis that acupuncture can produce better analgesic effects than control procedures on postoperative dental pain caused by extraction of a partially impacted third molar model. The first pilot phase will develop and validate two sham procedures to test the efficacy of acupuncture. The Phase II trial will test the efficacy and safety of real acupuncture compared to the sham model developed in the Phase I study.

DIGESTIVE DISORDERS

Acupuncture and Moxa For Chronic Diarrhea in HIV Patients (Joyce K. Anastasi, RN, PhD, LAc, Columbia University Health Sciences)—This study is designed to assess the efficacy of two alternative medicine treatments for chronic diarrhea associated with HIV. It is a randomized, controlled, blinded Phase III clinical trial in which parallel groups are studied under the intent-to-treat principle. True acupuncture, moxibustion, and combination therapy, in which specific meridian points are stimulated according to protocol, will be compared to each other and with the control group. Endpoints will include diarrhea frequency and stool consistency.

GENERAL MEDICAL SCIENCES

Biomechanical Effect of Acupuncture Needling (Helene M. Langevin, MD, University of Vermont)— This investigation will lead to quantification of needle grasp by measuring the peak force required to pull out acupuncture needles inserted at acupuncture points and control points in 80 normal human volunteers. Needling operations will be carried out by a computer-controlled device, eliminating potential investigator bias. All needling parameters will be consistent with clinical practice. The investigators will also study varying dwell times after insertion and different types of needle manipulation. They will correlate the force required to withdraw the needle with the depth of its insertion into muscle and subcutaneous tissue, which will allow determination of which tissue is most responsible for needle grasp.

Complementary and Alternative Medicine Data Archive (Eric L. Lang, PhD, Sociometrics Corporation)—The goal of this project is to facilitate access to, and statistical analysis of, outstanding scientific data sets and documentation on CAM through the creation of an international CAM Data Archive.

Melatonin and Cerebral Blood Flow Autoregulation (Mohan Viswanathan, PhD, Children's Research Institute)—The present project will attempt to define the physiological role of melatonin receptors in cerebral blood flow. The study will focus on functional studies and signal transduction mechanisms of melatonin receptors in the cerebral arteries and pharmacological characterization of melatonin binding sites.

Nonpharmacologic Analgesia for Invasive Procedures (Elvira Lang, MD, Beth Israel Deaconess Medical Center)—It is proposed that the use of nonpharmacologic analgesia (a combination of relaxation training, hypnosis and guided imagery) during invasive radiologic procedures will reduce the need for intravenous drugs, improve patient safety, and prove cost effective. To test these hypotheses, the relative performance of nonpharmacologic analgesia will be compared to standard care in a randomized, Phase III trial.

LIVER DISEASE

Herbal Remedies and the Treatment of Liver Disease (Mark Zern, MD, Thomas Jefferson University)—The objective of this study is to investigate the effectiveness of a number of herbal remedies, employing a rigorous scientific approach, to determine the relative effectiveness of these agents and the mechanisms by which they may be inhibiting liver injury and fibrosis. Both in vitro models of liver cell injury and rat models of liver injury and fibrosis will be employed.

MENTAL HEALTH

A Placebo-Controlled Clinical Trial of a Standardized Extract of Hypericum perforatum in Major Depressive Disorder (Jonathan Davidson, MD, Duke University) *Cofunded with the National Institute of Mental Health and the Office of Dietary Supplements*—The purpose of this multisite, Phase III trial is to study the acute efficacy and safety of a standardized extract of *Hypericum perforatum* in the treatment of patients with major depression. This three-arm, double-blind clinical efficacy study will compare a standardized extract of Hypericum to placebo over an eight-week period. Subjects responding to treatment will be followed for an additional four months. A third treatment group, using a selective serotonin reuptake inhibitor, will be included to ensure the validity of the trial.

Acupuncture in the Treatment of Depression (John Allen, PhD, University of Arizona)—This randomized, double-blind, placebo-controlled Phase III trial is testing the efficacy of acupuncture to treat major depression. The study is unique in that treatment effects will be assessed from the perspectives of both western psychiatry and Chinese medicine.

Method for Making an Improved St. John's Wort Product (Trevor P. Castor, PhD, Aphios Corp.)—The project seeks to develop an improved St. John's wort product that can be manufactured in a standardized and reproducible manner and in strict accordance with current Good Manufacturing Practices of the Food and Drug Administration.

Omega-3 Fatty Acids in Bipolar Disorder Prophylaxis (Andrew Stoll, MD, McLean Hospital) *Cofunded with the National Institute of Mental Health*—The purpose of this Phase III clinical trial is to assess the efficacy of omega-3 fatty acids in preventing recurrence in patients with bipolar disorder, type I. One hundred and twenty outpatients with bipolar disorder, type I, will be randomly assigned to receive add on treatment with omega-3 fatty acids or placebo, for one year. The primary goal is to assess the prophylactic effects of omega-3 fatty acids in a cohort of bipolar patients with a relatively high risk of recurrence.

Oxidative Cell Injury in First Episode Psychotic Patients (Sahebarao Mahadik, PhD, Medical College of Georgia)—This project seeks to establish that increased oxidative cell injury exists at the onset of psychosis and that probably continued injury contributes to deteriorating course of illness in some patients. Results from this study could provide a mechanism by which dietary antioxidants might reduce some abnormal pathologies leading to psychosis.

MUSCULOSKELETAL DISORDERS

Efficacy of Acupuncture in the Treatment of Fibromyalgia (Dedra A. Buchwald, MD, University of Washington)—Ninety-six patients with fibromyalgia will be recruited for a 12-week, 24-treatment, 3-arm, randomized, controlled Phase II clinical trial. The active treatment group will receive true acupuncture. Control groups will be treated with acupuncture for an unrelated condition. These patients will receive needle insertion at nonchannel, nonpoint locations, or a true placebo. Short-and long-term efficacy and side effects will be measured using both subjective and objective measures of overall health and pain, to determine the optimal duration of treatment and examine the concordance of allopathic and acupuncture-based measures of outcome.

Evaluating the Efficacy of Acupuncture for Back Pain (Daniel Cherkin, DrPH, Center for Health Studies, Seattle, Washington) *Cofunded with the Agency for Healthcare Research and Quality*—The goals of this Phase II study are (1) to develop and evaluate methods for improving randomized trials to assess the efficacy of acupuncture, and (2) to use this information to design and pilot-test a randomized clinical trial of acupuncture for persistent low back pain. The trial will compare acupuncture to standard medical care, and standardized to individualized acupuncture treatment.

Pilot Study of Acupuncture in Fibromyalgia (Daniel J. Claw, MD, Georgetown University Medical Center)—A randomized, blinded, sham-controlled, 2-by-2 factorial Phase II trial will be conducted to examine the individual and synergistic effects of needle placement and stimulation on the efficacy of acupuncture as a therapeutic modality in fibromyalgia. The design allows determination of dose-effect for the analgesic effect of acupuncture.

Trial of Acupuncture for Carpal Tunnel Syndrome (Arthur Weinstein, MD, George

Washington University Medical Center)-The major specific aim of this pilot study is to demonstrate that using a "single blind-mute "methodology, true and sham acupuncture can be administered in a standardized and unbiased fashion. The condition to be studied is carpal tunnel syndrome (CTS), a common,well-delineated syndrome causing hand pain with characteristic clinical and objective elec-trodiagnostic findings. Other aims of this study are: (1)to identify and standardize the most appropriate sham acupuncture points for CTS, (2)to develop a manual that standardizes the administration of true and sham acupuncture that can be used at any study site performing a randomized clinical trial (RCT), (3)to demonstrate that patient recruitment for and retention in an RCT of acupuncture for CTS is sufficient to justify a full-scale RCT, (4)to deter-mine, in a small Phase II RCT, whether true acupuncture provides meaningful benefit for pain in CTS compared to sham acupuncture and whether the frequency of administration of acupuncture influences the outcome.

Usual Care vs. Choice of Alternative Therapy for Low Back Pain   (David M. Eisenberg, MD, Beth Israel Deaconess Medical Center)—Patients with uncomplicated acute low-back pain will be randomized in this Phase III trial to either usual care or choice of expanded benefits (chiro-practic,acupuncture, or massage therapy). It is hypothesized that patients offered their choice of expanded benefits will experience a more rapid improvement in symptoms, a faster return to base-line functional status, a decrease in utilization of conventional medical services, and will be more satisfied with their care.

NEUROLOGICAL DISORDERS

Ginkgo biloba **Prevention Trial in Older Individuals**   (Steven DeKosky, MD, University of Pittsburgh)—*Cofunded with the National Heart, Lung, and Blood Institute, the National Institute on Aging, and the National Institute of Neurological Disorders and Stroke*—This is a multicenter, randomized, double-blind, placebo-controlled Phase III trial to determine the effect of 240mg/day of *Ginkgo biloba* in decreasing the incidence of dementia, in general, and Alzheimer's disease, specifically. The subjects will be aged 75 years and older. Secondary outcomes,

including changes in cognitive function, incidence of cardiovascular disease and total mortality, will also be measured.

Melatonin for Sleep Disorders in Parkinson's Disease   (Glenna Dowling, RN, PhD, University of California, San Francisco) *Cofunded with the National Institute of Nursing Research*—The purpose of this Phase III, multisite, double-blind study is to compare the effects of melatonin given at two different doses (5mg and 50mg)and placebo on nocturnal sleep. The clinical design, a placebo-controlled, double crossover trial, will also allow for assessment of any adverse events associated with melatonin related to its safety and tolerance. This research may lead to the development of safer, more physiologic therapies for treating sleep disturbances in patients with Parkinson's Disease.

Neurobiology of Acupuncture Analgesia   (Ji-Sheng Han, MD, Beijing Medical University)—This study is examining the effects of elec-troacupuncture on gene and protein expression in a rat model by exploring the regulation of the endogenous opioid system in the nervous system.

Neuroprotective Agents from Oriental Medicines   (Tae H.Oh, PhD, University of Maryland)—These studies are designed to elucidate and establish the mechanism(s)of neuroprotection demonstrated by isolates of oriental medicines (*Panax ginseng, Cynanchum wilfordii, Scrophularia buergeriana*). Specifically, this project investigate whether Rg3 (a gingenoside fraction prepared from *Panax ginseng*) and MCA (a p-methoxy-trans_cin-namic acid prepared from *Scrophulara buergeriana*) exert neuroprotective activities by inhibiting Ca++ influx by determining their effects on Ca++ influx in vitro; whether Rg3, cynandione A and MCA exert neuroprotective activity by inhibiting neuronal apopotosis by assessing their effects on apoptosis and its markers *in vitro* and *in vivo*; and whether neoline ameliorates deficits in short-term memory by influencing central cholinergic transmission in the brain. In addition, the study addresses issues involved in drug delivery across the blood brain barrier.

UROLOGICAL

Saw Palmetto Extract in Benign Prostatic Hyperplasia (BPH)   (Andrew Avins, MD, Veterans Medical Center, San Francisco) *Cofunded with* *the National Institute of Diabetes and Digestive and Kidney Diseases*—This is a Phase III, double-blind placebo-controlled, randomized clinical trial of the effect of 160 mg (taken twice daily) of saw palmetto extract on symptoms, objective parameters of disease severity, and quality of life in men with moderate-to-severe BPH. The primary outcome measurement is the American Urological Association Symptom Index score; the secondary outcome measures are peak urinary flow rate, post-void residual urine volume, and BPH Impact Index.

WOMEN'S HEALTH

Study of Women's Health Across the Nation (SWAN) (Ellen B. Gold, MD, University of California, Davis) *Cofunded with the National Institute on Aging and the National Institute of Nursing*—A multisite study to describe and contrast menopausal transition in relation to ethnicity, SWAN aims to contribute substantive new knowledge on the menopause transition through its prospective design,multiethnic/racial composition, representativeness of defined populations, and comprehensive measurement and power. A major goal of the project is to collect and analyze data on demographics, health and social characteristics, race/ethnicity, reproductive history, pre-existing illness, physical activity (includes activity limitations), health practices (includes diet, smoking, use of over-the-counter medications, use of CAM treatments) as potential predictor variables and to describe the multiethnic community-based samples of mid-life women.

Acupuncture Treatment of Depression During Pregnancy (Rachel Manber, MD, Stanford University) *Cofunded with the Agency for Healthcare Research and Quality*—The primary study objective of this Phase II trial is to determine if the efficacy of acute (short-term) acupuncture treatment for depression during pregnancy or postpartum is substantial enough to warrant a large-scale clinical trial. Since it is known that the mother's psychological state affects the infant's health, the trial will also assess the effect of treatment on infant well-being.

RESEARCH CENTERS

NCCAM supports a number of centers. CAM Specialized Centers provide focal points for initiating and maintaining state-of-the-art multidisciplinary CAM research, developing core research resources, careers of new CAM investigators, and expanding the research base through collaborative research with scientists and clinicians. Botanical Centers, cofunded with the NIH Office of Dietary Supplements, the Office of Research on Women's Health, and the National Institute of General Medical Sciences, foster multidisciplinary research to identify potential health benefits and develop a systematic evaluation of the safety and effectiveness of botanicals available as dietary supplements.

SPECIALIZED RESEARCH CENTERS

Pediatric Center for Complementary/Alternative Medicine (Fayez Ghishan, MD, University of Arizona)—The goal of this Center is to study integrative approaches in pediatrics. Three Phase II trials investigate the role of alternative approaches to treating very common pediatric problems for which there are no good conventional medical therapies. Included are randomized, controlled trials in children to evaluate:

- Craniosacral osteopathic manipulation and botanical treatment of recurrent otitis;
- Relaxation/guided imagery and chamomile tea as therapeutic modalities to treat functional abdominal pain; and
- The use of self-hypnosis, acupuncture, and osteopathic manipulation on muscle tension in children with spastic cerebral palsy.

Center for Addiction and Alternative Medicine Research (Thomas Kiresuk, PhD, Minneapolis Medical Research Foundation)—This Center will focus on the utilization, applicability, and effectiveness of selected CAM modalities in the treatment of addictive, health and psychological complications of substance abuse. The Center is studying:

- Herbal treatment of hepatitis C in methadone maintained patients (Phase I clinical trial);and
- Electroacupuncture examined for its effects and mechanisms of action.

CAM Center for Cardiovascular Diseases (Steven Bolling, MD, University of Michigan)—This center focuses on the investigation of CAM modalities to treat and prevent cardiovascular disease. Additionally, the Center will stress CAM education and promotion of validated CAM treatments for cardiovascular well-being. Individual research projects being conducted within the Center include Phase II clinical trials to determine the:

- Effectiveness of Hawthorn in the treatment of heart failure;
- Effect of Reiki on noninsulin dependent diabetes mellitus patients with chronic diabetic painful neuropathy or deficits in cardiovascular autonomic function; and
- Effect of Qi gong and spirituality/psychosocial factors on wound closure, pain, medication usage and hospital stay in post-operative cardiac patients.

Oregon Center for CAM in Neurological Disorders (Barry Oken, MD, Oregon Health Sciences University)—The Center is investigating whether:

- Three antioxidant regimens, *Ginkgo biloba*, alpha-lipoic acid/essential fatty acids and vitamin E/selenium are effective in decreasing multiple sclerosis disease activity (Phase I clinical trial);
- A standardized Ginkgo biloba extract can prevent or delay cognitive decline in elderly patients (Phase II clinical trial);
- Hatha yoga has palliative benefits on the cognitive and behavioral changes associated with aging and neurological disorders in multiple sclerosis patients and in the healthy elderly (Phase III clinical trial); and
- Vitamin E and Ginkgo biloba extract will be as effective as sodium azide and no treatment in reducing oxidative end-products in transgenic and wild-type mice.

Craniofacial CAM Center (Alexander B. White, DDS, DrPH, Kaiser Center for Health Research)—The Center will investigate via Phase II clinical trials to determine whether:

- Acupuncture, chiropractic therapy, and body-work therapy are as effective as standard treatment for tenderness and pain caused by temporomandibular disorders (TMDs);
- Naturopathic medicine and traditional Chinese medicine are as effective as standard treatment for tenderness and pain caused by TMD;and
- Three naturopathic medicines (glutamine, Connective Tissue Nutrient Formula, and adaptogenic herbs) are as effective as a placebo in alleviating clinical signs and symptoms of adult periodontitis.

Center for CAM, Minority Aging and Cardiovascular Disease (Robert Schneider MD, Maharishi University of Management)—This Center focuses on Vedic Medicine, a form of traditional Ayurvedic Indian medicine that incorporates herbal formulations and meditation, in the older African American population. The emphasis of the Center's research is on testing the efficacy and effectiveness of Vedic medicine for reducing mortality and morbidity associated with cardiovascular disease (CVD).The Center is conducting three single-blind, randomized, controlled Phase II clinical trials to determine the:

- Basic mechanisms of meditation and CVD in older blacks;
- Effect of transcendental meditation on carotid artery intima-media thickness toward reducing hypertension; and
- Effects of herbal antioxidants on CVD in older blacks.

Center for Alternative Medicine Research of Arthritis (Brian Berman, MD, University of Maryland)—The center will investigate the:

- Cost effectiveness of and long-term outcomes following acupuncture treatment for osteoarthritis of the knee (Phase III clinical trial);
- Effectiveness of mind/body therapies for fibromyalgia (Phase II clinical trial);
- Mechanism of action and effects of electroacupuncture on persistent pain and inflammation; and

- Mechanism of action of an herbal combination with immunomodulatory properties.

Center for CAM Research in Aging (Fredi Kronenberg, PhD, Columbia University)—The Center will investigate:

- The influence of a macrobiotic diet, as compared with the American Heart Association (AHA)Step 1 Diet, and an AHA diet plus flaxseed, on various endocrine, biochemical and cardiovascular parameters that might bc influenced by estrogens and phytoestrogens (Phase II randomized clinical trial);
- Whether phytoestrogens provided in a macrobiotic diet influence bone metabolism in postmenopausal women (Phase II randomized trial);
- Whether treatment with black cohosh (*Cimicifuga racemosa*)reduces the frequency and intensity of menopausal hot flashes and other menopausal symptoms (Phase II, double-blind, randomized, clinical trial); and the biological activities and mechanism of action of a Chinese herbal formula (whole formula and individual component herbs)on breast cancer cells in vitro and in vivo, as well as possible risks and/or benefits for women with breast cancer.

Consortial Center for Chiropractic Research (William Meeker, DC, MPH, Palmer College of Chiropractic)—The faculty and administrators of the Palmer Center for Chiropractic Research,Palmer College of Chiropractic; University of Iowa, Los Angeles College of Chiropractic, National College of Chiropractic, Kansas State University, and Wolfe-Harris Center for Clinical Studies, Northwestern College of Chiropractic have formed the Center to provide an infrastructure to examine the potential effectiveness and validity of chiropractic healthcare and to provide the appropriate clinical, scientific, and technical assistance to chiropractic researchers in developing high-quality research projects The Center is investigating the:

- Load distribution during bilateral thoracic manipulation;
- Effectiveness of chiropractic for chronic pelvic pain (Phase I clinical trial);

- Effectiveness of chiropractic relative to conservative medical care for sciatica and neck pain;
- Effects of spinal manipulation on immune function;
- Utility of joint end-play assessment (palpation);
- Effect of spinal manipulation on muscle excitability;
- Effect of vertebral loads on sympathetic nerve regulation; and
- Facet capsule biomechanics.

BOTANICAL CENTERS

Botanical Dietary Supplements for Women's Health (Norman Farnsworth, PhD, University of Illinois at Chicago)—This Center is studying the clinical safety and efficacy of botanicals used to treat women's health with particular emphasis on therapies for menopause. Additional studies are addressing mechanisms of action, identification of active compounds, and characterization of metabolism, bioavailability and pharmacokinetics of active species contained in these botanicals. The Center also provides information about botanicals to the public and health professionals. Four research projects are underway to:

- Standardize botanical dietary supplements and elucidate the structure of active compounds using bioassay-guided fractionation;
- Isolate active compounds for structure elucidation by bioassay-guided fractionation and carry out biochemical studies to determine the mechanism(s)of botanicals used for women's health;
- Develop and apply novel in vitro methods for the study of metabolism, absorption and toxicity of active compounds in botanicals, and to evaluate immunotoxicity of botanical preparations; and
- Carry out Phase I and Phase II clinical trials ot black cohosh (*Cimicifugae racemosa*) and red clover (*Trifolium pratense*).

UCLA Center for Dietary Supplements Research on Botanicals (CDSRB) (David Heber, MD, PhD, University of California, Los

Angeles)—The UCLA Center fosters interdisciplinary research to develop systematic evaluation of the safety and efficacy of botanical dietary supplements. The CDSRB is:

- Determining the effects of putative active ingredients (lovastatin in Chinese Red Yeast Rice, EGCG in Green Tea, Hypericin in St. John's wort)compared to the combination of compounds (*Monacolin, Catechins, Hyperforin/Hypericin*) that naturally occur in these botanicals;

- Examining the specific immune-enhancing actions of Echinacea;

- Establishing a screening assay for plant estrogens;

- Developing information on the bioavailability of flavonoids; and

- Assessing the inhibitory effects of soy isoflavones compared to genistein on prostate cancer growth.

RESEARCH TRAINING

POSTDOCTORAL FELLOWSHIPS

NCCAM provides individual National Research Service Awards (NRSAs)to postdoctoral fellows with aim of developing a cadre of investigators capable of conducting rigorous CAM research.

Yihui He, PhD, Beth Israel Deaconess Medical Center
Antihyperglycemic Activities of Bamboo Shoot Phytosterol—Dr. He will examine a potential antihyperglycemic effect of bamboo shoot and its ethanol and methanol extracts using diabetic rodent models 3T3-L1 (preadipocyte)and L6 (myoblast)cell lines. The proposed study aims at (1)identifying active antihyperglycemic phytosterols present in the solvent extracts using a genetic diabetic mouse model; (2) the active phytosterols for their effects on oral glucose tolerance and insulin sensitivity in streptozotocin diabetic rats fed a high-fructose diet; and (3) examining the effects of the phytosterols on glucose uptake GLUT4 mRNA levels in both the adipocyte and muscle cell lines.

Shujia Pan, PhD, University of Texas at Austin
Ginseng's Effects on mRNA Profiles in a Diabetes-2 Model—The objectives of this postdoctoral fellowship training are to study (1) the effects of herbal medicine on diabetes and metabolism; (2) the effects complementary intervention (including diet and exercise); and (3) molecular biology techniques on the control of gene expression.

CAREER DEVELOPMENT AWARDS

Mentored Research Scientist Development Award—(provides support of a scientist, committed to research, in need of both advanced research training and additional experience)

Raymond G. Devries, PhD, St. Olaf College
An Ethnographic Study of Institutional Review Boards—This Mentored Research Scientist Development Award in Research Ethics focuses on describing the social influences on Institutional Review Boards (IRBs) and the decisions they generate.The research has two aims:(1) to promote the development of the applicant as a scholar in the ethics of research on human subjects and (2) to address the behavior and effectiveness of IRBs.

Mentored Patient-Oriented Research Career Development Award—(provides support for the career development of an investigator who has made a commitment to focus his/her research endeavors on patient-oriented research, for three to five years of supervised study and research for clinically trained professionals who have the potential to develop into productive, clinical investigators)

Bruce Barrett, MD, PhD, University of Wisconsin Medical School
Mentored Patient-Oriented Research Career Development—Dr. Barrett will design and implement randomized trials of Echinacea for upper respiratory infection (URI)to test the efficacy of early Echinacea as treatment for URI.

INSTITUTIONAL TRAINING GRANTS

NCCAM awards grants to institutions to establish programs for individuals to train for careers in

CAM-related research. Where opportunity exists, NCCAM also supplements grants awarded by other Institutes and Centers to support trainees whose specific focus is CAM-related research.

Fellowship Training Program in Alternative Medicine   (Russell Phillips, MD, Beth Israel Deaconess Medical Center)—The overall goal of this program is to prepare general internists for careers as academic research faculty and educators in general and complementary-alternative internal medicine.

Cardiovascular Disease Prevention Training Program—(William L. Haskell, PhD, Stanford University School of Medicine, *Cofunded with the National Heart, Lung, and Blood Institute*)—NCCAM provides support for two postdoctoral fellows to receive research training in cardiovascular disease prevention with an emphasis on complementary and alternative therapies.

Multidisciplinary Respiratory Diseases Research Training—(Marvin I. Schwarz, MD, University of Colorado Health Sciences Center (UCHSC), *Cofunded with the National Heart, Lung, and Blood Institute*)—NCCAM provides funds for a nurse anaesthetist to fulfill the requirements of the UCHSC School of Nursing's doctoral program, with a focus on the use of complementary and alternative medicine as it relates to operative and perioperative anaesthesiology.

UCLA/RAND Health Services Research Training Program—(Ronald M. Anderson, PhD., *Cofunded by the Agency for Healthcare Research and Quality [AHRQ]*)—NCCAM provides funds for one postdoctoral trainee, working in the area of chiropractic research, to complete the two-year master's degree program in the Department of Epidemiology in the UCLA School of Public Health.

APPENDIX V

NCCAM OUTREACH ACTIVITIES

NCCAM Clearinghouse P.O. Box 7923,Gaithersburg, MD 20898, Phone: 888-644-6226, Fax:866-464-3616—The NCCAM Clearinghouse disseminates information to the public and healthcare providers about the NCCAM's programs and research findings through CAM fact sheets, information packages, publications, and a quarterly newsletter distributed to 6,000 public subscribers. During the first 10 months of FY 1999, the Clearinghouse received more than 18,000 requests for information, distributed more than 37,000 copies of publications, and made nearly 13,000 referrals to other NIH organizations, NCCAM's research centers, other governing agencies, or CAM organizations.

Web Site—(*http://nccam.nih.gov*) Established in 1996,the NCCAM's Web site, which receives nearly 500,000 hits per month, offers comprehensive information of interest to healthcare consumers and practitioners, and to researchers.

Combined Health Information Database (CHID) (*http://chid.nih.gov*)—In February 1999, NCCAM joined CHID, a cooperative effort of several Federal agencies organized to consolidate information related to health and disease contained in individual government databases within a single database. CHID also contains some health information materials not available in other government databases. Currently, CHID contains approximately 1,000 records covering the spectrum of CAM assembled by the NCCAM Clearinghouse or that are publicly available elsewhere.

Town Meetings—NCCAM holds town meetings for CAM consumers and practitioners. The first such meeting was held on March 15,2000 in Boston in collaboration with the Center for Alternative Medicine Research and Education, Beth Israel Deaconess Medical Center, Harvard University.

Conferences—The Center sponsors conferences in areas of CAM practice and research, for example:

- *Placebo and Nocebo Effects:Developing a Research Agenda*, December 1996

- *Complementary and Alternative Medicine in Chronic Liver Disease*, August 22–24, 1999, with the National Institute of Diabetes and Digestive and Kidney Diseases (NIDDK)and the Office of Dietary Supplements (ODS), NIH, and the American Association of Naturopathic Physicians.

- *The Science of the Placebo: Toward an Interdisciplinary Research Agenda*, November 19–21, 2000, a trans-NIH/DHHS conference.

APPENDIX VI

EVIDENCE-BASED REVIEWS

To help identify fertile areas for clinical investigation and the appropriate level of investment in each, NCCAM examines the scientific evidence regarding the effectiveness of CAM treatments. This hierarchy of evidence ranges from those considered to provide the weakest evidence, for example, anecdotes and case studies, through observational studies, uncontrolled trials, small randomized controlled trials to large randomized clinical trials, considered the gold standard in terms of level of evidence. Systematic reviews may be conducted at and across all levels. NCCAM taps a number of resources to obtain evidence-based reviews.

Centers for Disease Control and Prevention (CDC)—NCCAM has engaged the CDC to develop effective methods of identifying and enlisting the cooperation of practitioners who claim to have observed effective new therapies and subsequently will work with CDC representatives to review their case files in a systematic fashion. The goal of this activity is to identify practices worthy of scientific study by NCCAM.

Cancer Advisory Panel for Complementary and Alternative Medicine (CAPCAM)— NCCAM, in collaboration with the National Cancer Institute (NCI), established the federally chartered CAPCAM to enable discovery of new, promising CAM cancer treatments. Members of the 15-person panel (listed in Appendix VII) represent a cross section of expertise from the CAM and mainstream oncology communities. CAPCAM's members review and assess clinical data submitted by CAM scientists and clinicians, including evaluation of best-case series (retrospective analyses of data from patients treated with a specific modality in order to assess specific therapeutic benefit). Based on these evaluations, CAPCAM will identify therapies worthy of more rigorous scientific study by NCCAM.

Agency for Healthcare Research and Quality (AHRQ), formerly the Agency for Health Care Policy and Research (AHCPR)—NCCAM contracts with AHRQ to carry out systematic reviews though the Agency's Evidence-based Practice Program, which supports 12 Evidence-based Practice Centers (EPCs) in the United States and Canada. Under this program, the EPC at the University of Texas, San Antonio evaluated the use of garlic for cardiovascular disease and the use of Silybum marianum (milk thistle) for treatment of liver disease and cancer. Currently, the Southern California Evidence-based Practice Center-RAND, Santa Monica, CA is surveying the state of CAM science to identify promising "frontiers of CAM investigation" for which they will subsequently conduct full systematic reviews.

The Cochrane Collaboration (CC)—The Cochrane Collaboration (*http://www.cochrane.dk*) is an international nonprofit organization that emphasizes the need to rely on systematic reviews of scientific evidence, rather than on beliefs, traditions, common practices or case histories. The CC's mission is to prepare, maintain, and disseminate systematic, up-to-date reviews of randomized controlled clinical trials across all areas of health care. A group of Fields/Networks represents the interests of specific groups of patients or specific types of treatment (such as child health, vaccines, and rehabilitation and related therapies). The Complementary Medicine (CM) Field, supported by NCCAM and coordinated by Brian Berman, MD, was added in 1996 (*http://www.compmed.ummc.umaryland.edu*).

The Cochrane Field Groups work in collaboration with approximately 50 Cochrane Research Groups (CRGs),arranged by disease specialty, to carry out systematic reviews related to their disease specialty. The CRG with which the Field works is determined by the research question. For example, examining whether massage is effective in increasing the weight of low birth weight infants is being done in collaboration with the Neonatal CRG, whereas exploring whether homeopathy is effective for asthma is being done in collaboration with the Airways CRG. Since formation of the CM Field, staff have produced the Cochrane Registry of Randomized Controlled Trials in Complementary Medicine. As of March 2000 the registry holdings include approximately 4,700 RCTs, 5,400 possible RCTs, 204 systematic reviews, and 1,812 hard copy reports in the archive. The registry is available in the Cochrane Library Controlled Clinical Trials Registry (CCTR).

NIH Consensus Development and Technology Assessment Conferences—NCCAM supports NIH consensus conferences on CAM-related areas through the Office of Medical Applications of Research at the NIH. *Integration of Behavioral and Relaxation Approaches Into the Treatment of Chronic Pain and Insomnia,* a technology assessment conference held in October 1995, was cosponsored with nine NIH components.[4] Acupuncture: An NIH Consensus Development Conference was held in 1997 to review the efficacy of acupuncture in therapeutic and preventive medicine, jointly sponsored with eight components of the NIH.[5]

APPENDIX VII

NCCAM Cancer Advisory Panel for Complementary and Alternative Medicine 1999

CHAIR
HAWKINS, Michael, MD
Washington Cancer Institute
Washington Hospital Center
Washington, D.C. 20010

MEMBERS
CHOYKE, Peter L., MD
Chief, Magnetic Resonance Imaging
Diagnostic Radiology Department
Warren G. Magnuson Clinical Center
National Institutes of Health
Bethesda, Maryland 20892

COULTER, Ian D., PhD
Research Professor and Health Consultant
RAND Corporation
Santa Monica, California 90407

ELLENBERG, Susan S., PhD
Director
Division of Biostatistics and Epidemiology
Center for Biology Evaluation
and Research
Food and Drug Administration
Rockville, Maryland 20852

FAIR, William R., MD
Attending Surgeon,
Urology (Emeritus)
Memorial Sloan-Kettering
Cancer Center
Chairman, Clinical
Advisory Board
Health, L.L.C.
New York, New York 10021

GORDON, James S., MD
Director
Center for Mind-Body Medicine
Georgetown University
School of Medicine
Washington, D.C. 20015

HUFFORD, David J., PhD
Professor
Medical Humanities,
Behavioral Science,
and Family Medicine
The Pennsylvania State University
College of Medicine
Hershey, Pennsylvania 17033

JACOBS, Frances A., RN
Clinical Nurse Coordinator
Adult Oncology Unit
Rush-Presbyterian-St. Luke's
Medical Center
Chicago, Illinois 60612

MOSS, Ralph W., PhD
Director
The Moss Reports
Brooklyn, New York 11217

WEED, Douglas L., MD, PhD
Chief, Preventive Oncology Branch
Division of Cancer Prevention
National Cancer Institute, NIH
Bethesda, Maryland 20892

WOOD, Lauren V., MD
Senior Clinical Investigator
HIV and AIDS Malignancy Branch
National Cancer Institute, NIH
Bethesda, Maryland 20892

EX OFFICIO

STRAUS, Stephen E., MD
Director
National Center for
Complementary and
Alternative Medicine, NIH
Bethesda, Maryland 20892

WHITE, Jeffrey D., MD
Director
Office of Cancer Complementary
and Alternative Medicine
Office of the Deputy Director
for Extramural Science
National Cancer Institute, NIH
Bethesda, Maryland 20892

EXECUTIVE SECRETARY

NAHIN, Richard, PhD
Director,Division of Extramural
Research and Training
National Center for Complementary
and Alternative Medicine, NIH
Bethesda, Maryland 20892

APPENDIX VIII

STRATEGIC PLANNING PROCESS

The NCCAM Strategic Plan builds upon the Strategic Plan originally drafted by OAM. The OAM strategic planning process benefited from significant input from a broad base of stakeholders garnered through a series of meetings. These include the 1993 "Chantilly Meeting," which resulted in a report to the NIH, *Alternative Medicine, Expanding Medical Horizons;* meetings in 1994 of the Alternative Medicine Program Advisory Council (AMPAC); and several strategic planning workshops in 1995–1996 to outline the challenges for CAM research and how they might be addressed by the OAM. The draft report was reviewed in 1997 and 1998 by a Strategic Planning Advisory Group and AMPAC. Members of these groups included representatives of the CAM and conventional scientific communities, both from within and outside NIH. A subsequent draft Report and Plan were distributed to a wide variety of organizations for review. The final revision served as a departure point for this document.

NCCAM's Strategic Plan has also been shaped at each stage of the process by input from the Center's broad range of stakeholders. Evolving drafts have been reviewed by NCCAM staff, members of the National Advisory Council on Complementary and Alternative Medicine, senior officials at NIH, and opinion leaders within the conventional and CAM communities. The public-at-large and the broad research community also were afforded the opportunity to help shape the final report. Indeed, this document was modified to reflect the thoughtful comments contributed by over 200 individuals and organizations who, representing the diversity of our stakeholders, reviewed the penultimate draft during the six-week period it was posted on NCCAM's Web site.[6]

With completion of this first five-year plan, NCCAM will initiate an ongoing planning process that will be employed periodically to refine priorities in the coming years to assure that its priorities match developments as the field matures, and that they reflect an appropriate balance between pursuing scientific opportunity and addressing public health needs. Throughout the process, NCCAM will continue to rely significantly on input from the public and our many other diverse stakeholders.

APPENDIX IX

National Advisory Council for Complementary and Alternative Medicine 1999

CHAIR

STRAUS, Stephen E., MD
Director
National Center for
Complementary and
Alternative Medicine
National Institutes of Health
Bethesda, Maryland 20892

MEMBERS

CANTWELL, Michael F., MD,
MPH
Complementary Medicine Physician

Complementary Medicine
Research Institute
San Francisco, California 94115

CHUNG, Mary K.
President and CEO
National Asian Women's
Health Organization
San Francisco, California 94104

GRIMM, Richard H., Jr., MD, PhD
Director
Department of Internal Medicine
Berman Center for Outcomes and
Clinical Research
Hennepin County Medical Center
Minneapolis Medical Research
Foundation
Minneapolis, Minnesota 55415

HOLLORAN, Susan
Researcher and Writer
Bluemont, Virginia 20135

KAHN, Janet R., PhD, LMT
Senior Research Scientist
Wellesley College Center for
Research on Women
Silver Spring, Maryland 20910

KAIL, Konrad, ND
Naturopathic Physician
Naturopathic Family Care, Inc.
Phoenix, Arizona 85032

KAPTCHUK, Ted J., OMD
Assistant Professor of Medicine
Harvard Medical School
Beth Israel Deaconess Medical Center
Boston, Massachusetts 02215

LAWRENCE, Dana J., DC
Director
Department of Publications and
Editorial Review
National College of Chiropractic
Lombard, Illinois 60148

MANLEY, Diane C.
Massage Therapist
New Bern, North Carolina 28560

MEEKER, William C., DC, M.P.H.
Director of Research
Palmer Center for Chiropractic Research
Palmer Chiropractic University Foundation
Davenport, Iowa 52803

OLNESS, Karen N., MD
Professor
Department of Pediatrics
School of Medicine
Case Western Reserve University
Rainbow Babies and Children's Hospital
Cleveland, Ohio 44106-6038

PARDES, Herbert, MD
President and CEO
New York Presbyterian Hospital
New York, New York 10032

RAMIREZ, Gilbert, PhD
Associate Director, San Antonio
Evidence-based Practice Center and
San Antonio Cochrane Center
University of Texas Health Science
Center–San Antonio
San Antonio, Texas 78229

RHOADES, Everett R., MD
Associate Dean for
Community Affairs
University of Oklahoma
School of Medicine
Oklahoma City, Oklahoma 73104

SCHLITZ, Marilyn J., PhD
Director of Research
Department of Research
Institute of Noetic Sciences
Sausalito, California 94965

STANDISH, Leanna, ND, PhD, LAc
Director of Research
Bastyr University
Kenmore, Washington 98028

WILLIAMS, James E., Jr.
Jim Williams and Associates
Camp Hill, Pennsylvania 17011-1049

EXECUTIVE SECRETARY
NAHIN, Richard, PhD
Director, Division of Extramural
Research and Training
National Center for Complementary
and Alternative Medicine
Bethesda, Maryland 20892

ENDNOTES

1 The term *conventional medicine* refers to medicine as practiced by holders of M.D. (medical doctor) or D.O. (doctor of osteopathy) degrees and their allied health professionals, who may also practice complementary and alternative medicine.

2 Readers interested in obtaining additional information are referred to the NCCAM Clearinghouse *(http://nccam.nih.gov/nccam/fcp/clearinghouse)*, P.O.Box 7923,Gaithersburg,MD 20898, Phone:888-644-6226, Fax:866-495-4957).

3 As of October 1,1999.

4 Office of Medical Applications of Research; National Cancer Institute; National Heart, Lung, and Blood Institute; National Institute on Aging; National Institute of Arthritis and Musculoskeletal and Skin Diseases; National Institute of Dental and Craniofacial Disorders; National Institute of Mental Health; National Institute of Neurological Disorders and Stroke; and National Institute of Nursing Research.

5 Office of Medical Applications of Research; Office of Research on Women's Health; National Cancer Institute; National Heart, Lung, and Blood Institute; National Institute of Allergy and Infectious Diseases; National Institute of Arthritis and Musculoskeletal and Skin Diseases; National Institute of Dental and Craniofacial Disorders; and National Institute on Drug Abuse.

6 Many respondents contributed comments related to policy issues, such as licensing, insurance, and regulation. Such issues are not within the purview of NCCAM's mission. These comments have been transmitted to the White House Commission on Complementary and Alternative Medicine Policy, which has been constituted specifically to make recommendations on these matters.

APPENDIX VI
HISTORIC TIMELINE OF ALTERNATIVE AND COMPLEMENTARY THERAPIES

Prehistoric healing methods which may have been used in Paleolithic, Mesolithic, and Neolithic times, have been thought of as part of the compelling forces that helped people find food and other substances they needed to survive. Evidence of disease and injury has been discovered in bodies and organs from as early as 4000 B.C. By the Neolithic period, people began to produce food and were possibly aware that certain foods had medicinal properties. Trephined skulls of the Neolithic period may indicate either a medical or a mystical operation, which some believe was done to let havoc-causing demons escape.

Primitive medicine among peoples including Native Americans, Inuit (Eskimo), and Siberian tribes emerged through the appointment of shamans, witch doctors, and medicine men and women, some of whom were chosen because they seemed to possess psychic ability. Illness of any kind was treated with a variety of therapies—herbal remedies, religious rites, chants, prayers, elaborate ceremonies, and techniques of cupping, sucking, bleeding, fumigating, steam baths, cautery, tourniquet, reduction of dislocations, wound care, and others.

Ancient Greeks, Romans, Chinese, Egyptians, Indians, Mesopotamians, and other peoples practiced herbalism and holistic medicine. Using natural methods including massage, nutrition, meditation, exercise, and herbal and other therapies, healers focused on balancing a main life force, or vital energy, present in the human body to restore or maintain health.

2000–1501 B.C.
Four basic elements are acknowledged in India: earth, air, fire, and water.

Fourth century B.C.
The Greek physician Hippocrates advocates natural remedies and a holistic approach to medical treatment. He is known as the "Father of Medicine."

Second century A.D.
Galen uses holistic methods in his medical practice. During the years 151–200 he extracts plant juices for medicinal purposes.

The Greek physician Asclepiades practices nature healing in Rome.

11th century
Trotula, of Salerno, Italy (d. 1097), a woman surgeon, practices medicine using nutrition, herbal baths, and herbalism as therapy.

The German abbess Mechthild of Magdeburg (1212–1283) practices preventive medicine, employing sunlight, music, the natural world, and hygiene.

12th century
The abbess, musician, artist, and healer Hildegard von Bingen, Germany, writes *Physica* (The Book of Simples), which describes more than 300 medicinal plants. Hildegard believes disease stems from

imbalances in the body and called health *viriditas*, meaning the "green life force of the flesh." Her medical observations are still recognized; her healing techniques included physical ministration, herbalism, laying on of hands, prayer, blessed waters, amulets, and exorcism.

1322
The itinerant healer Jacoba Felice de Almania is convicted in Paris of practicing medicine, including laying on of hands and examining urine, without a license.

Pre-Columbian cultures in Mesoamerica combine magic, religion, and science in a medical system. The pre-Columbian native believes the cause of disease is imbalance of favorable and unfavorable forces. Shamans are relied upon as healers. In the Mayan culture, for example, *hemenes*, or priests, are members of a respected organized medical society, and *hechiceros* are individuals designated to perform bleeding, treating wounds, lancing abscesses, and reducing fractures.

11th, 12th, and 13th centuries
During the Crusades medical care orders and hospitals are established, and soldiers recognize and trade in the Islamic East's array of pharmacological treasures, new to the West. The practice of medicine during the Middle Ages draws upon both science and mysticism, concepts that survived into the 1800s.

15th century
During the 1600s in Scotland women healers and herbalists such as Bessie Paine and Margaret Provost are persecuted for witchcraft.

16th century
The German-Swiss physician and alchemist Paracelsus (1493-1541) favors holistic treatment of patients. In 1536 he writes *Der grossen Wundartzney* (Great Surgery Book), which includes what was to become known later as homeopathy.

The Swiss physician Barbara von Roll (1502–71) pioneers treatment of mental illness now known as psychosomatic medicine.

17th century
The period known as "the age of the Scientific Revolution," in which Aristotle, Galen, and Paracelsus are still influential, but under the attack that marks the beginning of the idea of separation of mind and body, and that disease exists only on a physical level. The iatromechanist Giorgio Baglivi (1669–1707) describes each bodily organ as though it were a specific type of machine. And Antony van Leeuwenhoek (1632–1723) uses a microscope to discover male spermatozoa and establish embryology. With each stride in anatomical and physiological science, holistic approaches to medical practice seem to fade or to be scorned as quackery.

1737
The New York physician and obstetrician Elizabeth Blackwell writes the *Curious Herbal*.

1810
The German physician and chemist Samuel Hahnemann founds homeopathy, a system of medical practice based on holistic and scientific principles including the approach favoring the "like cures like" theory, used in immunization and vaccination therapies.

mid-1800s
Naturopathic medicine develops from the European practice of using natural springs and spas as therapy. Early naturopaths include Dr. John Kellogg, who establishes the Battle Creek Sanitarium in Michigan, and his brother, Will Kellogg, who operates a health-food factory along with C. W. Post.

Chinese immigrants introduce the practice of acupuncture to the United States.

Vincenz Priessnitz (1799–1851) becomes known as a major proponent of all types of hydrotherapy.

The German-born clinician Franz Joseph Gall (1758–1828) develops phrenology, soon considered a pseudoscience.

Franz Anton Mesmer (1733–1815), a graduate physician of Vienna, demonstrates his theory of animal magnetism and unwittingly introduces the use of hypnotic suggestion. He operated the Magnetic Institute in Paris but lost favor in France. His theories led to hypnosis as a therapy.

The mesmerist Phineas P. Quimby (1802–1866) allegedly cures Mary Baker Eddy, who later founds the Christian Science Church, of long-standing illness.

James Braid introduces the term *hypnotism* in 1843.

1858

Bernadette Soubirous is reported to have had a vision of the Blessed Virgin Mary at Lourdes, France, since a pilgrimage destination for the faithful who believe the waters there have curative properties.

1859

Florence Nightingale, the founder of modern nursing and a major proponent of holistic practice, writes *Notes on Nursing*, published in London and later by Lippincott in the United States.

1861

The French chemist and microbiologist Louis Pasteur develops the germ theory of disease, heralding the birth of modern medicine based on the concept of infectious disease. Although his contributions had significant influence in allopathic medicine, the concept of vaccination and immunization using like substances added to the body of knowledge that evolved into homeopathy.

1865

Ivan M. Sechenov, known as the founder of Russian physiology, writes *Reflexes of the Brain*, on the physiological basis of psychic processes.

1873

The German psychologist Wilhelm Wundt, often called the founder of modern psychology, writes *Physiological Psychology*.

1874

A. T. Still, of Kansas, founds osteopathy, a system of medical practice based on the theory that disease is mainly attributable to dysfunction or loss of the body's structural integrity and the dysfunctional parts may be treated by manipulation, medicine, and surgery.

1881

Mary Baker Eddy (1821–1910) founds the Massachusetts Metaphysical College. Eddy, who was cured of illness by a charismatic healer from Maine, is also founder of the Christian Science Church, which espouses the spiritual basis of disease.

1882

The Viennese physician Joseph Breuer uses hypnosis to treat hysteria.

1892

The German physician Benedict Lust founds the prototype of the modern health food store.

Sir William Osler, an influential Canadian physician who also practices in the United States and Great Britain, writes *The Principles and Practice of Medicine*, which includes the recommendation that physicians embrace social concern, compassion, optimism, generosity, and other desirable qualities in their practices.

1895

Dr. Daniel David Palmer founds chiropractic, a system of treatment based on Hippocrates' idea that disease emanates from dysfunction or subluxations of the spine, which can be adjusted by hands-on manipulation of the neuroskeleton, and the concept of the body's "innate intelligence" to heal itself.

1912
The Swiss psychiatrist and philosopher Carl Jung writes *The Theory of Psychoanalysis*.

1921
The National Institute for Industrial Psychology is founded in London.

The German psychiatrist Ernst Kretschmer writes *Physique and Character*.

1926
The South African statesman, biologist, and philosopher Jan Christian Smuts coins the term *holism*, in the belief that whole organisms, rather than their separate components, establish the determining factors in nature and evolution.

1930s
The English physician Edward Bach develops Bach's Flower Essences for treating emotional problems that may lead to disease.

1940s
The American psychiatrist Helen Flanders Dunbar researches psychosomatic medicine and establishes the "personality profile (or personality constellation)."

1950s
The Canadian physiologist Hans Selye develops his theory of stress, known as the "general adaptation syndrome," which involves the stimulation of the hypothalamic-pituitary-adrenal axis when exposed to stress (the fight-or-flight response).

1952
Dr. Norman Vincent Peale writes *The Power of Positive Thinking*.

1960s
The researchers Thomas Holmes and Richard Rahe develop an assessment tool called the Social Readjustment Rating Scale, based on the concept that illness may be caused by a person's positive and negative experiences and changes in lifestyle.

1961
Halbert Dunn writes *High-Level Wellness*, which addresses the idea of fighting for wellness rather than fighting against disease.

1970s
The hippie movement encourages recreational use of drugs, but also of vegetarianism and organically grown foods, transcendental meditation, Eastern philosophies geared toward peace and inner balance, and "back-to-basics" treatment modalities such as massage and aromatherapy.

1973
Dolores Krieger and Dora Kunz develop Therapeutic Touch as an alternative healing technique.

1974
The Canadian Ministry of Health and Welfare reports evidence indicating a link between lifestyle and environment and the presence of health or disease.

1975
The Nobel Prize–winning scientist Linus Pauling receives the U.S. National Medal of Honor.

1976
The sociobiologist and philosopher D. C. Phillips identifies principles of holism, including that the whole is more than the sum of its parts, the whole determines the nature of its parts, and the parts are dynamically interrelated or interdependent.

The United States Select Senate Committee issues a report acknowledging the relationship between nutrition and disease, which leads to widespread reduction of red-meat and fat intake.

1977
Dr. C. Norman Shealy founds the American Holistic Medical Association.

1980

The Texas nurse Charlotte McGuire founds the American Holistic Nurses' Association.

1980s to the present

The American public begins to show signs of disillusionment with conventional health care and turns to newly flourishing alternatives including chiropractic, homeopathy, herbalism, massage, Reiki, aromatherapy, bodywork, bioenergetic modalities, and other disciplines embracing the idea of mind-body connection.

BIBLIOGRAPHY

"About the Feldenkrais Method of Somatic Education." Feldenkrais Guild of North America. Available on-line. URL: www.feldenkrais.com/aboutfm.html. Downloaded December 2000.

"Alternative Medicine," *Audio-Digest Internal Medicine* 49, no. 14 (July 21, 2002). Downloaded November 2002.

American Medical Association. "Alternative Medicine: Report 12 of the Council on Scientific Affairs (A-97)." Available on-line. URL: http://www.ama-assn, org/ama/pub/article/2036-2432.html. Last updated January 23, 2003.

Ask NOAH About Complementary and Alternative Medicine. Available on-line. URL: http://www.umdnj.edu /csacmweb/index.shtml#top. Downloaded 2002.

Ballentine, Rudolph, M.D. *Radical Healing: Integrating the World's Great Therapeutic Traditions to Create a New Transformative Medicine.* New York: Harmony Books, 1999.

Beinfield, Harriet, L.Ac., and Korngold, Efrem, L.Ac., O.M.D. *Between Heaven and Earth: A Guide to Chinese Medicine.* New York: Ballantine Books, 1991.

Benson, Herbert, M.D. *Timeless Healing: The Power and Biology of Belief.* New York: Scribner, 1996.

———. *The Mind/Body Effect: How Behavioral Medicine Can Show You the Way to Better Health.* New York: Simon & Schuster, 1979.

Bradford, Nikki, ed. *The One Spirit Encyclopedia of Complementary Health.* London: Hamlyn, 1996.

Brooke, Elisabeth. *Medicine Women: A Pictorial History of Women Healers.* Wheaton, Ill.: Quest Books, Theosophical Publishing House, 1997.

"Cell-Molecular Nutrition." Available on-line. URL:http://nutrition.tufts.edu/programs/emn/.

Chopra, Deepak, M.D. *Quantum Healing: Exploring the Frontiers of Mind/Body Medicine,* New York: Bantam Books, 1989

Clayman, Charles, B., M.D., ed. *The American Medical Association Encyclopedia of Medicine.* New York: Random House, 1989.

Cohen, Kenneth. *Honoring the Medicine: The Essential Guide to Native American Healing,* New York: Ballantine Books, 2003.

Coles, Robert, M.D. *The Spiritual Life of Children,* Boston: Houghton Mifflin Company, 1990.

Complementary Medicine: What Patients Are Doing, What You Should Be Asking, Network for Continuing Medical Education (NCME), Secaucus, New Jersey, 1999, Program Number 751, 60-minute videotape.

Curtis, Edward. "The Curtis Collection: Cheyenne Sweat Lodge," From *North American Indian.* Vol. 6. Available on-line. URL: http://curtis-collection.com/cheyanne sweatlodge.html. Downloaded 2001.

De Schepper, Luc, M.D., Ph.D. *The People's Pharmacy: Your Guide to Safe, Effective Homeopathic Remedies.* Santa Fe, N. Mex.: Full of Life Publishing, 1998.

Dossey, Larry, M.D. *Reinventing Medicine: Beyond Mind-Body to a New Era of Healing.* San Francisco: Harper-SanFrancisco, 1999.

———. *Healing Words: The Power of Prayer and the Practice of Medicine.* San Francisco: HarperSanFrancisco, 1993.

Fischer-Rizzi, Susanne. *Complete Aromatherapy Handbook: Essential Oils for Radiant Health,* New York: Sterling Publishing, 1989.

Fleming, Yolanda. *The Encyclopedia of Yoga.* New York: Sterling Publishing, forthcoming 2004.

"Food as a Cure." Available on-line. URL: http// www.itppeople.com/macrobio.htm. Downloaded 2002.

Frawley, Dr. David, and Lad, Dr. Vasant, *The Yoga of Herbs: An Ayurvedic Guide to Herbal Medicine.* Twin Lakes, Wisc.: Lotus Press, 1988.

Georgi, Kristen. "The Healing Power of Qigong: Qigong and Cancer," *Traditional Chinese Medicine,* 5, no. 1, (Spring 2003).

Gerber, Richard, M.D. *A Practical Guide to Vibrational Medicine: Energy Healing and Spiritual Transformation.* New York: Quill/HarperCollins Publishers, 2000.

Hale, Gill. *The Practical Encyclopedia of Feng Shui.* London and New York: Lorenz Books/Anness Publishing Limited, 1999.

Hammerschlag, Carl A., M.D. *The Dancing Healers: A Doctor's Journey of Healing with Native Americans.* San Francisco: HarperSanFrancisco, 1988.

HealthFinder: Alternative Medicine. Available on-line. URL: http://www.healthfinder.gov/scripts/Topics.asp? context=5&keyword=114&Branch=5. Downloaded 2002.

HealthyNJ: Alternative and Complementary Medicine. Available on-line. URL: http//www.healthynj.org/health-wellness/altmed/main.htm. Downloaded 2002.

Healthy People 2010. Washington, D.C.: U.S. Department of Health and Human Services, November 2000, Vol. 1.

Holistic-Online Philosophy of the Synergy of Alternative and Traditional Medicine. Available on-line. URL: http://www.holisticonline.com/Alt_Medicine/altmed_philosophy.htm.

Hulse, Janet R., MSN, RN, CS. "Drugstore Dangers," *Advance for Nurses, Greater New York/New Jersey 3*, no. 8 (March 31, 2003) 22–24.

Huth, Edward J., M.D., and Murray, T. Jock, O.C., M.D. *Medicine in Quotations: Views of Health and Disease Through the Ages*. Philadelphia: American College of Physicians, 2000.

Hyman, Jane Wegscheider. *The Light Book: How Natural and Artificial Light Affect Our Health, Mood, and Behavior*. New York: Ballantine Books, 1990.

The International Center for Reiki Training "What Is Reiki?" International Center for Reiki Training. Available on-line. URL: www.reiki.org. Posted 2000.

The Institute of Noetic Sciences. *The Heart of Healing*. Atlanta: Turner Publishing, 1993.

Johnson, Michael, L., M.D. "How acupuncture Works: MCI Offers Unique Insight," *Traditional Chinese Medicine* 4, no.4, (Winter) 2002.

Kaufman, Barry Neil, *Happiness Is a Choice*. New York: Fawcett Columbine/Ballantine Books, 1991.

Krieger, Dolores, Ph.D., R.N. *Accepting Your Power to Heal: The Personal Practice of Therapeutic Touch*. Santa Fe, N. Mex.: Bear & Company Publishing, 1993.

Kübler-Ross, Elisabeth. *On Children and Death*. New York: Macmillan, 1983.

Lad, Dr.Vasant. *Ayurveda: The Science of Self-Healing*. Twin Lakes, Wisc.: Lotus Press, 1985.

Linn, Denise. *Sacred Space: Clearing and Enhancing the Energy of Your Home*. New York: Ballantine, 1995.

Lock, Dr. Margaret M. *East Asian Medicine in Urban Japan: Varieties of Medical Experience*. Berkeley: University of California Press, 1980.

Lyons, Albert S., M.D., and Petrucelli, R. Joseph, II, M.D. *Medicine: An Illustrated History*. New York: Harry N. Abrams, 1987.

Marcolina, Susan T., M.D. "Apitherapy: What's the Buzz? Bee Venom Therapy for Arthritis and Multiple Sclerosis," *Alternative Medicine Alert* 6, no. 2 (February 2003).

Martin, Harvey J., III. "Unraveling the Enigma of Psychic Surgery," Available on-line. URL: www.metamind.net/enigmaipsysur.html. Posted 1999.

"Massage Therapy" Available on-line. URL: www.health.yahoo.com/health/Alternative_Medicine/Alternative_Therapies/Massage_Therapy/. Downloaded 2002.

McCarty, Meredith. *American Macrobiotic Cuisine*. Eureka, Calif.: Turning Point Publications, Eureka, 1986.

McGraw, Phillip C., Ph.D., *Self Matters: Creating Your Life from the Inside Out*. New York: Simon & Schuster, 2001.

McKenzie, Eleanor, *Healing Reiki: Reunite Mind, Body and Spirit with Healing Energy*. Berkeley, Calif.: Ulysses Press, 1999.

MEDLINEPlus: Alternative Medicine. Available on-line. URL: http//www.nlm.hih.gov/medlineplus/alternativemedicine.html.

Moskovitz, Reed C., M.D. *Your Healing Mind*. New York: William Morrow, 1992.

"The National Council Against Health Fraud: Enhancing Freedom of Choice through Reliable Health Information" Available on-line. URL: http://www.ncahf.org/index.html.

Navarra, Tova, B.A., R.N., and Lipkowitz, Myron A., M.D., *Encyclopedia of Vitamins, Minerals and Supplements*. New York: Facts On File, 1996.

"NCAHF Consumer Information Statements on Faith Healing and Psychic Surgery" Available on-line. URL: http://www.ncahf.org/pp/faith.html.

New Zealand Health Information Network. "The History of Massage" New Zealand Health Information Network. Available on-line. URL: www.nzhealth.net.nz/healing/massage-def.html.

Nurse's Handbook of Alternative & Complementary Therapies. 2d ed. Philadelphia: Lippincott Williams & Wilkins, 2003.

Ornish, Dean, M.D. *Dr. Dean Ornish's Program for Reversing Heart Disease,* New York: Ballantine, 1990.

"Patient/Public Info-Unconventional Therapies" Available on-line. URL: http.//www.bccancer.bc.cs/a/PPI/Unconventional Therapie.

Peale, Dr. Norman Vincent. *Positive Imaging: The Powerful Way to Change Your Life*. New York: Fawcett Crest/Ballantine, 1982.

Perlman, Adam, M.D., M.P.H., ed. *The Medical Clinics of North America: Complementary and Alternative Medicine*. Philadelphia: W.B. Saunders Company, January 2002.

Rakel, David. "Center combines traditional, complementary techniques" Available on-line. URL: http://www.wisc.edu/grad/catalog/cals/nutritio.html.

Rector-Page, Linda G., N.D., Ph.D. *Healthy Healing: An Alternative Healing Reference*. Carmel Valley, Calif.: Healthy Healing Publications, 1994.

Restak, Richard, M.D. *The Brain Has a Mind of Its Own: Insights from a Practicing Neurologist*. New York: Harmony Books, 1991.

Ritacco. Barbara. "Be care free in a flotation tank," *Options for a Healthy Mind, Body and Spirit,* October 2002, p. 21.

"Rudolf Steiner" Available on-line. URL: www.elib.com/Steiner/RSBio.php3.

Shealy, C. Norman, M.D., Ph.D. *The Illustrated Encyclopedia of Natural Remedies,* Boston: Element Books, 1998.

Siegel, Bernie S., M.D., *Love, Medicine & Miracles: Lessons Learned About Self-Healing from a Surgeon's Experience with Exceptional Patients.* New York: Harper & Row Publishers, 1986.

———. "Conscious Healing," Available on-line. URL: www.ethoschannel.com/ersonalgrowth/voices/bs_voices.html.

Sifton, David W., ed. *The PDR Family Guide to Natural Medicines and Healing Therapies,* New York: Ballantine, 1999.

Smolan, Rick, Moffitt, Phillip, and Naythons, Matthew, M.D. *The Power to Heal: Ancient Arts & Modern Medicine.* New York: Prentice Hall Press, 1990.

"Special Theme: Complementary, Alternative, and Integrative Medicine," *Academic Medicine* (The Journal of the Association of American Medical Colleges), Washington, D.C., 77, no. 9 (September 2002).

Stewart, Isabel M., and Anne L. Austin, *A History of Nursing: From Ancient to Modern Times, A World View.* 5th ed. New York: G.P. Putnam's Sons, 1962.

Taber's Cyclopedic Medical Dictionary, 17th ed. Philadelphia: F.A. Davis, 1993.

"Thai Massage Nuad Bo'Rarn, The History of Thai Traditional Massage," Available on-line. URL: www.thai-traditional-massage.org/history.html.

"Therapeutic Touch: Healing Therapy or Hoax?" Available on-line. www.religioustolerance.org/ther_tou.htm.

Tierra, Michael, C.A., N.D. *The Way of Herbs.* New York: Pocket Books, 1990.

Trivieri, Larry, Jr., and Anderson, John W., eds. *Alternative Medicine: The Definitive Guide.* Berkeley, Calif.: Celestial Arts, 2002.

Weil, Andrew, M.D. *Health and Healing.* Boston: Houghton Mifflin Company, 1988.

Weiss, Brian L., M.D. *Through Time into Healing.* New York: Simon & Schuster, 1992.

"What Is Sound Therapy?" Available on-line. URL: www.biowaves.com/Info/WhatIsSound.cfm.

Wilde, Stuart, *Affirmations.* New South Wales, Australia: Nacson & Sons PTY LTD, 1987.

Wynn, Susan G., Marsden, Steve. *Manual of Natural Veterinary Medicine: Science and Tradition,* St. Louis: Mosby 2003.

Zak, Victor, "Sleeping prophet's legacy lives on in Virginia Beach," *Asbury Park Press,* February 23, 1997, page F2.

Zukav, Gary, *The Seat of the Soul.* New York: Simon & Schuster, 1989.

Selected Reading

Barnes, Joanne, et al. Herbal Medicines: *A Guide for Health Care Professionals,* 2d ed. London: Pharmeceutical Press, 2002.

Beckner, William Mac, and Berman, Brian M. *Complementary Therapies on the Internet.* St. Louis: Churchill Livingstone, 2003.

Borysenko, Joan, *Minding the Body/Mending the Mind.* New York: Bantam Books, 1988.

Buckle, Jane, *Clinical Aromatherapy.* Edinburgh, N.Y.: Churchill Livingstone, 2003.

Carlson, Michael, *Classical Homeopathy.* Edinburgh, N.Y.: Churchill Livingstone, 2003.

Cousins, Norman, *Head First: The Biology of Hope and the Healing Power of the Human Spirit.* New York: Penguin Books, 1989.

Hahnemann, Samuel. *Organon of Medicine.* Translated by W. Boericke, M.D. New Delhi, India: B. Jain Publishers, 1992.

Huard, P., and Wong, M., *Chinese Medicine.* New York: World University Library, 1968.

McKenna, Dennis J., PhD; Jones, Kenneth; and Hughes, Kerry, MSc. *Botanical Medicines: The Desk Reference for Major Herbal Supplements.* 2d ed. New York: The Haworth Press, 2002.

Moyers, Bill, *Healing and the Mind.* New York: Doubleday, 1993.

Oschmen, James L., *Energy Medicine in Therapeutics and Human Performance.* Edinburgh, N.Y.: Butterworth-Heinemann, 2003.

Rakel, David, M.D., *Integrative Medicine.* New York: Saunders, 2003.

Rich, Grant Jewell, ed. *Massage Therapy: The Evidence for Practice.* Philadelphia: Mosby, 2002.

Spencer, John W., and Jacobs, Joseph J. *Complementary and Alternative Medicine.* St. Louis: Mosby, 2003.

Visalli, Gayla, et al. *Health and Healing the Natural Way: Hands on Health.* Pleasantville, N.Y.: Reader's Digest, 1999.

Wainapel, Stanley F., and Fast, Avital, eds. *Alternative Medicine and Rehabilitation.* New York: Demos, 2003.

Weil, Andrew, M.D. "A New Look at Botanical Medicine," *Whole Earth Review* 64 (1989: 3–8).

Yuan Chung-Su, and Bieber, Eric J., eds. *Textbook of Complementary and Alternative Medicine.* Boca Raton, Fla: Parthenon, 2003.

INDEX

Note: Page numbers in **boldface** indicate the main discussion of a subject.

A

AABD. *See* American Academy of Biological Dentistry
aama **1,** 161
aamdosh 1
AAS. *See* American Apitherapy Society
abortifacient **1**
Abrams, Albert 135, 136
An Abridged Therapy Manual for the Biochemical Treatment of Disease (Schuessler) 24
Academy for Guided Imagery 177
Accepting Your Power to Heal (Krieger) 72
accident-prone personality 35
Accreditation Commission for Acupuncture and Oriental Medicine 177
acupoints (trigger points) **1**
  in acupuncture 2–3, 4
  in Bonnie Prudden Myotherapy 21
  definition of 1
  in ear 4
acupressure **1–2,** 82
  meridians in 1, 2
  in reflexology 137
  vs. shiatsu 2
Acupressure Institute 177

acupuncture **2–5**
  AMA on 195–196
  auricular therapy 4, **12**
  body units in **20**
  cupping 3–4, 67
  for dental pain 232
  for depression 233, 235
  electroacupuncture **38**
  in Islamic Sufi healing practices 67
  meridians in 2
  moxibustion 4, **87**
  NCCAM on 95, 216, 217, 231, 232, 233–234, 235
  oral 19
  practitioners of 4
  scientific studies on 3, 4, 95
  types of 3–4
  uses for 3, 4
Acupuncture Foundation of Canada 177
acupuncture points 1
adaptation syndrome, general (GAS) 141–142
adrenal glandular 50
Advaita Vedanta 165
Advanced Health Research Institute 177
affirmations **5**
Affirmations (Wilde) 5
A4M. *See* American Academy of Anti-Aging Medicine
Africa
  bush medicine of 107
  sangomas of **141**
Agency for Healthcare Research and Quality (AHRQ) 240

agni **5**
Agpaoa, Tony 129
agrimony 16
ahara rasa **5**
AHMA. *See* American Holistic Medical Association
AHRQ. *See* Agency for Healthcare Research and Quality
Aidan Incorporated 177
AIDS Alternative Health Project 177
air, in Five Elements 46
ajowan oil 107
AK (applied kinesiology). *See* kinesiology
Alexander, Franz 35–36
Alexander, Frederick Matthias 5–6
Alexander Technique **5–6**
alfalfa 50
algae 50
allopathy **6**
allspice berry oil 107
almond oil 107
aloe vera 50
alpine mint bush 12
alteratives **6**
Alternative Health Benefit Service xix
alternative medicine **6**.
  See also complementary and alternative medicine
  AMA on 189–203
  definitions of xvii, 6, 89, 189
  historic timeline of 245–248

Alternative Medicine (journal) xxii

Alternative Medicine: A Definitive Guide (Goldberg) xviii
  on acupuncture 3
  on cell therapy 24
  on homeopathy 57

Alternative Therapies in Health and Medicine (journal) xxii

AMA. *See* American Medical Association

ama **6**

amaroli. See urine therapy

ambrete seed oil 107

American Academy of Anti-Aging Medicine (A4M) 76, 177

American Academy of Biological Dentistry (AABD) 177

American Academy of Environmental Medicine 177

American Academy of Medical Acupuncture 177, 195

American Academy of Neural Therapy 102, 178

American Academy of Osteopathy 178

American Alliance of Aromatherapy 178

American Alternative Medicine Association 178

American and International Boards of Environmental Medicine 178

American Apitherapy Society (AAS) 8, 178

American Aromatherapy Association 178

American Art Therapy Association 178

American Association for Therapeutic Humor 178

American Association of Acupuncture and Bioenergetic Medicine 178

American Association of Acupuncture and Oriental Medicine 178

American Association of Ayurvedic Medicine 29

American Association of Drugless Practitioners 178

American Association of Naturopathic Physicians 44, 178

American Association of Oriental Medicine 178

American Association of Orthopedic Medicine 178

American Association of Professional Hypnotherapists 178

American Board of Chelation Therapy 178

American Board of Hypnotherapy 179

American Bodywork and Massage Professionals 179

American Botanical Council 179

American Cancer Society xvii–xviii

American Center for the Alexander Technique 179

American Chiropractic Association 28–29, 179

American Chronic Pain Association 179

American College of Addictionology and Compulsive Disorders 179

American College of Advancement in Medicine 179

American College of Hyperbaric Medicine 179

American College of Nutrition 179

American College of Osteopathic Pain Management and Sclerotherapy 179

American College of Traditional Chinese Medicine 179

American Colon Therapy Association 179

American Council of Hypnotist Examiners 179

American Council on Science and Health 179

American CranioSacral Therapy Association 179

American Dietetic Association 40, 180

American Foundation for Homeopathy 180

American Health Institute 180

American Herbalists Guild 180

American Herbal Pharmacopoeia 180

American Herbal Products Association 180

American Herb Association 180

American Holistic Health Association 180

American Holistic Medical Association (AHMA)
  address of 180
  establishment of xxi, 142
  mission of xxi
  principles of xxi

American Holistic Nurses Association 180

American Holistic Veterinary Medical Association 180

American Imagery Association 180

American Imagery Institute 180

American Institute of Hypnotherapy 179, 180

American Massage Therapy Association (AMTA) 83, 180

American Medical Association (AMA) xviii, xx
  contact information for 180
  Council on Scientific Affairs, text of report by 189–203
  on Hoxsey therapy 57–58
  on hypnosis 63

American Music Therapy Association 180

American Oriental Bodywork Therapy Association 180–181
American Osteopathic Association 181
American Physical Therapy Association 181
American Polarity Therapy Association 181
American Psychiatric Association (APA) 120
American Psychiatric Association Journal 120
American Psychosomatic Society 36
American Psychotherapy and Medical Hypnosis Association 181
American Qigong Association 181
American Reflexology Certification Board 181
American Shiatsu Association 181
American Society for Clinical Nutrition 181
American Society of Bariatric Physicians 181
American Society of Clinical Hypnosis 181
American Society of the Alexander Technique 181
American Speech-Language-Hearing Association 181
American Vegan Society 181
American Yoga Association 181
amethyst 32
amma therapy **7**. *See also* shiatsu
AMTA. *See* American Massage Therapy Association
amyris oil 107
analgesia 232
Anandashram 167
Ananda yoga 168
Anatomy of the Spirit (Myss) 87
Anchor Point Institute 181

Ancient Secrets of the Fountain of Youth (Kelder) 171
Andrus, Veda xix
angelica root oil 108
animal(s). *See also* pet(s)
  cells from, therapy with **24–25**
  glandulars from **50**
animal-assisted therapy **7**. *See also* pet(s)
aniseed oil 108
anise oil 108
ankylosing spondylitis xxi
Anthroposophical Medicine (Bott) 21, 146
anthroposophy 21, 146
antibiotics, herbal **7**
Anusara yoga 168
anxiety **7–8**
  symptoms of 7
  transcendental meditation for 154
  treatment of 7–8, 154
APA. *See* American Psychiatric Association
aphasia 103
apitherapy **8**
applications, healing **8**
applied kinesiology (AK). *See* kinesiology
apricot kernel oil 108
apricots 47
aquamarine 32
aquasonics **8,** 32
Arcier, Micheline 9
A.R.E. *See* Association for Research and Enlightenment
arjowan oil 108
arm bath 60
arm douche 59
armoise oil 108, 115
Armstrong, John W. 155
Arnica montana 154
Arnold, Joan 6
aromatherapy **9–10**
  for anxiety 8
  coining of term 9, 49

in Islamic Sufi healing practices 67
  with massage 83
Aromatherapy Institute and Research 182
Aromatherapy Seminars 182
aromatic substance **10**
artav (reproductive tissue) **10**
Artharva-Veda 165
arthritis, NCCAM on 230–231
Arthritis Trust of America 182
The Art Spirit (Henri) 10
art therapy **10**
asanas **10,** 164, 165, 166
Asbury Park Press (newspaper) 142
ascorbic acid flush **10–11**
ashtanga yoga **11,** 168, 170
aspen 16
Association for Applied Psychophysiology and Biofeedback 182
Association for Research and Enlightenment (A.R.E.) 23, 24
Association of Vegetarian Dietitians & Nutrition Educators 182
asthi (bone) **11,** 34
asthma
  Buteyko breathing technique for 22
  Chinese herbs for 27
  magnesium therapy for 97
Aston, Judith 11
Aston-Patterning **11**
Aston Training Center 11, 182
astringent **11**
atherosclerosis, carotid, vitamin E for 231
athma **11**
attars 67
attunement **11**
aura **11–12**
auricular therapy 4, **12**
Aurobindo Ashram 167
Aurobindo Ghose, Sri 167

Australian Bush Flower
    Essences **12**
autism, Options Institute on
    118–119
Autism Research Institute 182
Autism Services Center 182
Autism Society of America 182
Autobiography of a Yogi
    (Yogananda) 167
autogenic training **12–13**
autonomic nervous system
    autogenic training of 12–13
    Bowen Method for 21–22
    neural therapy for 19, 102
avocado oil 108
Awareness Through Movement
    45
Ayurveda **13**
    aama in 1, 161
    agni in 5
    ahara rasa in 5
    ama in 6
    AMA on 197
    astringents in 11
    athma in 11
    chakras in 25–26
    color in 30
    definition of 13
    development of 13
    dina chariya in 34
    doshas in 34, 154
    energy in 38
    exercise in 40
    face analysis in 43
    fasting in 44
    Five Elements in 46
    fomentations in 47
    gunas in 50–51
    Law of Contraries in 75
    Law of Similars in 56, 75
    malas in 81
    mantra in 81
    marma in 81
    marma puncture in 82
    nasya in 89
    NCCAM on 227
    oja in 118
    panchakarma in 124

prakruti in 127
pulse analysis in 131
purvakarma in 131
rajasic in 136
rakta moksha in 136
rasayana in 136
refrigerants in 137
samagni in 141
scientific studies on 13
shad rasa in 142
stomach wash in 146
tongue analysis in 151
urine therapy in 155–156
xenobiotics in 161
Ayurveda Institute 182
Ayurvedic Institute 182
Ayurvedic & Naturopathic
    Medical Clinic 182

B

babassu oil 108
Bach, Edward **15**
    Heal Thyself 15
    *The Twelve Healers and Other
        Remedies* 15
Bacha, Jibaka Kumaru 82
Bach Centre 15, 183
Bach Flower Remedies **15–17**
Bach Healing Society 183
back douche 60
back pain 234
Bagua map 45
Baily, Philip M. **17**
Balancing Your Body (Bond) 21
Balch, James **17**
Balch, Phyllis **17**
Ballentine, Rudolph M. **17–18**
    Radical Healing xviii, 135
        on allopathy 6
        on flower remedies
            15–16
        on Hering's Law of Cure
            55
        on sweat lodges
            147–148
balsam peru oil 108

Banerjee, P. N. **18**
Banksi Robur 12
barley grass 50
Barondess, Jeremiah 201
Barral, Jean Pierre 18
Barral visceral manipulation
    18
Barrett, Stephen 146
Barzini, Luigi xx
basil oil 108
Bates, William H. 18
Bates Method for Improving
    Eyesight **18**
baths
    as healing application 8
    hydrotherapy with 59–61
    pranic 161
    purvakarma 131
bay leaf oil 108
Becker, Robert O. 3
Beebe, Kenneth 125
beech, in Bach Flower
    Remedies 15, 16
Beecher, Henry 130
beechnut oil 108
bee products 8, 47, 141
behavioral medicine **18**
Beinfield, Harriet **18**
    Between Heaven and Earth
        4–5, 18, 133
Bellavite, Paolo **18–19**
    *Homeopathy, a Frontier in
        Medical Science* 18–19
benign prostatic hyperplasia
    (BPH) 234–235
ben oil 108
Benson, Herbert **19**
    The Mind/Body Effect 18
    on relaxation response
        138
    Timeless Healing xx
        on acupuncture 4
        on faith healing 43
benzoin tincture 108
Berard, Guy 145
Berard Method 145
Berch, Rama 170–171
bergamot oil 108

Between Heaven and Earth: A Guide to Chinese Medicine (Beinfield and Korngold) 4–5, 18, 133
Bhagavad-Gita 166
Bhajan, Yogi 169–170
Bikram yoga **19,** 168
bile, as humor 58
biodynamics 38
Bio-Electro-Magnetics Institute 182
bioenergetics **19**
    definition of 19, 38
    effects of depression in 33–34
    of plants 126
bioenergies, types of 38
bioentrainment **19**
biofeedback **19**
biological dentistry **19–20**
Bio-Medical Center 58
Bio-Resonance Therapy 145
bipolar disorder 233
birch
    sweet 108
    white 109
Birch, Beryl Bender 170
Bircher-Benner, Max 69
bitter **20**
blackberry flower essence 15–16
black bile 58
black currant seed and bud 109
black pepper 109
Bleuler, Eugen 70
blood, as humor 58
blood cleansing **20**
    with depurgative 34
blood flow, cerebral, melatonin and 232
bloodletting, in Ayurveda 136
blood pressure, high
    acupuncture for 231
    transcendental meditation for 153
A Blue Fire (Hillman) 86
body fluids
    four humors of 58
    as *jing ye* 69

body maps **20**
body types, in Ayurveda *(doshas)* **34**
body unit **20**
Bodywise (Heller and Henkin) 54
bodywork **20**
    for anxiety 8
    Aston-Patterning **11**
    Barral visceral manipulation **18**
    hakomi **53–54**
    Hellerwork **54**
    polarity therapy **126–127**
Boericke, William **20–21**
    The Twelve Tissue Remedies of Schuessler 21
Bogart, Greg **21**
    Therapeutic Astrology 21
Bohm, David **21**
    Wholeness and the Implicate Order 21
Bond, Mary **21**
    Balancing Your Body 21
Bonnie Prudden Myotherapy **21**
Bonnie Prudden Pain Erasure 182
borage oil 109
botanicals, NCCAM on 96–97, 237–238
botanic physicians **21**
Bott, Victor **21**
    Anthroposophical Medicine 21, 146
Bowen, Thomas 21
Bowen Method **21–22**
Bowen Research and Training Institute 182
Bower, Peter **22**
BPH. *See* benign prostatic hyperplasia
brahman 165
Braid, James 63
brain oxygenators, for anxiety 8
bran 47
Brazil, Museum of Images from the Unconscious in 10
brazil nuts 47, 109

breast cancer
    NCCAM on 231
    soy supplements for 96–97
breast milk secretion 49
breathing techniques **22**
    Buteyko **22**
    kappalbhati 161
    PowerBreathing 170
    pranayama **127**
breathwork **22**
Breiling, Brian Joseph **22**
    Light Years Ahead 22
Brennan, Barbara Ann **22**
broccoli 47
broth, cleansing **22**
Buegel, Dale **22**
    Homeopathic Remedies for Health Professionals and Laypeople 22
Buhner, Stephen Harrod **22**
    Sacred Plant Medicine 22
Bush Fuschia 12
Buteyko technique **22**
Byers, Dwight 137

C

cabbage, savoy 47
cabreuva oil 109
cade oil 109
cajaput oil 109
calamit 109
calamus 109
Calbom, Cherie, *Juicing for Life* 69
calcium fluoride 24
calcium phosphate 24
calcium sulfate 24
calendula oil 109
calmative **23**
calophyllum 109
CAM. *See* complementary and alternative medicine
camphor white 109
Canadian Association of Ayurvedic Medicine 182

Canadian Holistic Medical
   Association 182
Canadian Institute of Stress
   (CIS) 141, 182
cananga oil 109
cancer
      AMA on 199
      Ayurvedic treatment of 13
      chelation therapy for
         26–27
      Hoxsey therapy for **57–58**
      insulin potentiation therapy
         for **65**
      Issels's fever therapy for
         67–68
      Native American treatment
         of 100
      NCCAM on 93–95, 231
Cancer Advisory Panel for
   Complementary and
   Alternative Medicine
   (CAPCAM) 240, 241–242
canola oil 109
CAPCAM. *See* Cancer Advisory
   Panel for Complementary and
   Alternative Medicine
caraway oil 109–110
cardamom seed oil 110
cardiovascular disease, NCCAM
   on 231–232
Care of the Soul (Moore) 46
carminative **23**
carnation oil 110
carpal tunnel syndrome,
   acupuncture for 233–234
Carroll, Robert Todd, *The
   Skeptic's Dictionary* 81
carrot seed and root 110
cascarilla bark 110
Casey, the Reverend Solanus
   23
cashew nut oil 110
cassia 110
cassie 110
castor oil 110
cathartic **23**
catnip 109, 110

caustic **23**
Cayce, Edgar **23–24**
Cayola, Renato 9
CC. *See* Cochrane Collaboration
CDC. *See* Centers for Disease
   Control and Prevention
cedar leaf oil 110
cedarwood oil 110
celery seed oil 110
celiac plexus. *See* solar plexus
cell salts **24**
cell therapy **24–25**
cellulase 39–40
centaury 16
Center for Applied
   Psychophysiology 183
Center for Mind/Body Medicine
   183
Center for the Study of
   Alternative and
   Complementary Medicine
   (CSACM) xi
centering, in Therapeutic Touch
   150
Centers for Disease Control and
   Prevention (CDC) 240
centesimal scale, homeopathic
   25
cerato 16
cerebral blood flow, melatonin
   and 232
chair massage 82
chakras **25–26**
   color of 30
   definition of 25
   origin of term 25
   root (sexual) 25, **139, 142**
chamomile
   German 110
   Roman 110–111
chamomile Moroc 111
Champaca flower and leaf 111
Chang San-feng 149
channels **26**. *See also* meridians
Charak (physician) 51
chelation therapy **26–27**
   NCCAM on 95

Chernin, Dennis **22**
   *Homeopathic Remedies for
   Health Professionals and
   Laypeople* 22
cherry plum 16
chest douche 59
chestnut
   red 17
   sweet 17
   white 17
chestnut bud 16
ch'i. See qi
chicory 16
Chinese herbalism **27**
Chinese medicine
   acupuncture in 2
   eight principal patterns in
      37, 163
   Empty Heat in **38**
   externals in 41
   Five Elements in 46
   herbalism in **27**
   meridians in 83–84
   six stage patterns in **144**
   yin-yang in 163
chiropractic **27–29**
   AMA on 193–194
   development of 27, 28,
      123–124
   mixed 28
   public acceptance of xvii, 28
   straight 28
   X rays in **161**
Chishti, Hakim 66
chlorella 50
chlorophyll 50
cholera 57
chologogue **29**
Chopra, Deepak **29,** 170
Chowka, Peter Berry 101
Christi Order 66
Christy, Martha M. 155
Chronic Disease: Its Cause and Cure
   (Banerjee) 18
cicatrizant **29**
cinchona 56
cinnamon oil 111

circadian rhythm 75, 76
CIS. *See* Canadian Institute of
    Stress
citronella oil 111
clary sage oil 111
cleansing diet 44
clematis 16
clove oil 111
clysis. *See* colonic irrigation
coagulant **29**
Cobb, Leonard 130
Cochrane, Amanda, *The*
    Encyclopedia of Flower Remedies
    46–47
Cochrane Collaboration (CC)
    240
coenzyme A 40
coenzyme Q10 40
coffee oil 111
cold laser therapy 19
Coles, Robert **29**
colonic irrigation **29–30**
color
    in feng shui 30, 45
    in light therapy 30, 75
Colorpuncture 30
color therapy **30,** 75
combination remedies **30**
Commodus 49
Community Nutrition Institute
    183
complementary and alternative
    medicine (CAM)
    definition of 89–90, 215
    effectiveness of 91
    frequently asked questions
        on 89–92
    historic timeline of 245–248
    practitioners of, selection of
        92
    risks with 91–92
    safety of 90–91
    scientific studies on 90, 92,
        93
    testing of 90–91, 92
complementary medicine **30**
    definitions of xvii, 30, 89

Complementary Wellness
    Professional Association 2
Complete Aromatherapy Handbook
    (Fischer-Rizzi) 9
compresses 8, **30**
connective tissue massage 82
constitutional remedies **30**
consultation-liaison psychiatry
    35, 36
Contraries, Law of **75**
cooling foods and herbs 137
copaiba oil 111
Copeland, Royal 196
cordyceps **31**
Cordyceps sinensis 31
core energetics 19
coriander oil 111
cornmint oil 111
coronary heart disease,
    meditation and 231–232
Cosechi, Paolo 120–121
costus oil 111
counterirritant **31**
Cousins, Norman xiii, xxi
crab apple 16
cranberry 47, 97
Cranial Academy 183
craniosacral massage 82
craniosacral therapy (CST) **31**
Creighton, James 144
Crichton, Michael xxii
Crowea 12
crystal therapy **31–32**
CSACM. *See* Center for the
    Study of Alternative and
    Complementary Medicine
CST. *See* craniosacral therapy
cubeb oil 111
Culpeper, Nicholas 32
Culpeper's Herbal **32**
cumin oil 111–112
cupping 3–4, 67
curandera 142
curanderismo **32**
The Cure of Imperfect Eyesight by
    Treatment Without Glasses
    (Bates) 18

Curtis, Edward S. 148
cymatics **32**
    aquasonics in 8, 32
cyperus oil 112
cypress oil 112
cysteine 26

D

DAMS. *See* Dental Amalgam
    Mercury Syndrome
dance therapy **33**
The Dancing Wu Li Masters
    (Zukav) 173
dan tien **33**
Dasgupta, S. 165
Davis, Adelle **33**
decimal scale, homeopathic
    33
decoction **33**
    infusion followed by 65
Deep Tissue massage 82
DeJarnette, B. 31
De La Warr, George 136
Delta Society 7
demulcent **33**
Dental Amalgam Mercury
    Syndrome (DAMS) 183
dentistry
    biological **19–20**
    NCCAM on 232
depression
    acupuncture for 233, 235
    effects of **33–34**
depurgative **34**
Desai, Amrit 169
De Schepper, Luc, *The People's*
    Repertory 56
desensitization 39
Desikachar, T. K. V. 166, 168,
    171
desktop yoga 170
detoxification **34**
developmental disorders,
    Options Institute on 118–119
Devi, Indra 167

Dewey, W. A. **20–21**
  *The Twelve Tissue Remedies of
    Schuessler* 21
dharana 164
dhatus **34**
  artav and *shukra*
    (reproductive tissue) **10,** 34
  asthi (bone) **11,** 34
  majja (nerve) 34
  mamsa (muscle) 34
  meda (adipose tissue) 34
  rakta (blood) 34
  rasa (plasma) 34, **136**
D'Hervilly, Melanie 53
dhyana 164
diabetes, Reiki and 138
diarrhea 232
diathermy 62
diet(s). *See also* nutrition; *specific
  diets*
  AMA on 191
  blood cleansing **20**
  cleansing 44
  macrobiotic **79–80,** 163
  vegetarian **157**
Dietary Supplement Health and
  Education Act (DSHEA)
  (1994) 54, 192
digestive **34**
digestive disorders, NCCAM on
  232
Digitalis purpurea 54
digoxin 54
dill oil 112
dina chariya **34**
distant healing **34**
dogs, used in therapy 7
dolls, *sangoma* use of 141
doshas **34, 154**
  and fasting 44
  kapha 34, **71,** 146, 154, 156
  pitta 34, **126,** 137, 154,
    155–156
  vata 34, 154, 155, **157**
Dossey, Larry **34**
  on Eternity Medicine 40
  on faith healing 43–44

Healing Words 43–44
  journal edited by xxii
  on nonlocal mind 104
  Reinventing Medicine 40, 104,
    133–134
douche(s)
  herbal **34–35**
  in hydrotherapy 59–60
dowser, medical **35**
drama therapy **35**
dreams
  diagnostic **35**
  healing **35**
Drown, Ruth 136
DSHEA. *See* Dietary Supplement
  Health and Education Act
Duke, James 58
Dunbar, Helen Flanders **35–36**
  Emotions and Bodily Changes
    36
Durga (Hindu goddess) 165
Dyer, Wayne W. **36**

E

ear, in auricular therapy 4, **12**
ear-candling **37**
earth, in Five Elements 46
Eastern medicine **37**
EcAP 142
echinacea 7, 54
Eclectic Medical Institute 21,
  150–151
EDTA. *See*
  ethylenediaminetetraacetic
  acid
effleurage **37**
EFT. *See* emotional freedom
  technique
eight principal patterns **37,**
  163
Einstein, Albert xviii, xxii
elecampane oil 112
electroacupuncture **38**
electromagnetic force **38**
elemi oil 112

Elkadi, Ahmed 68
Ellon, Inc. 183
elm 16
EMDR Institute 183
emesis therapy 146
emotional freedom technique
  (EFT) **38**
emotions, negative, Bach's
  seven major 15
Emotions and Bodily Changes
  (Dunbar) 36
Empty Heat **38**
*The Encyclopedia of Flower
  Remedies* (Harvey and
  Cochrane) 46–47
Encyclopedia of Health
  (McFadden) xxii
endorphins **38**
  released by acupuncture 2
  released by laughter 58
enema. *See* colonic irrigation
energetics 38
energy **38–39**
  breathwork and 22
  definition of 38
  Einstein on xviii
  Kirlian photographs of 72
  negative **101–102**
energy medicine **39**
  AMA on 194
  bioenergetics in **19**
  NCCAM on 228
energy psychology, emotional
  freedom technique in 38
enkephalins 2, 38
Environmental Dental
  Association 183
Environmental Health & Light
  Research Institute 183
environmental medicine **39**
enzyme therapy **39–40**
ephedrine 192–193
Erickson, Milton 102
Ericksonian hypnosis 102
ERT. *See* estrogen replacement
  therapy
Esalen Institute 183

Escherichia coli 67
essence(s) **40**
   definition of 16, 40
   flower 12, 15–17, 46
essential oils. *See* oils, essential
estrogen replacement therapy
   (ERT) 96–97
Eternity Medicine **40**
ether, in Five Elements 46
ethylenediaminetetraacetic acid
   (EDTA) 26
eucalyptus oil 112
evening primrose oil 112
exercise **40–41**
external **41**
extracts, herbal **41**
exudative **41**
eyes
   Bates Method for Improving
     Eyesight **18**
   in iridology **65–66**

F

face analysis **43**
face maps 20
facial douche 60
FAIM. *See* Foundation for the
   Advancement of Innovative
   Medicine
faith healing **43–44**
   among Native Americans
     99–100
   NCAHF guidelines on
     130–131
fasting **44**
   in Mayr intestinal therapy
     83
fava beans 47
FDA. *See* Food and Drug
   Administration
febrifuge **44**
feet. *See* foot
Feldenkrais, Moshe 44–45
Feldenkrais Guild of North
   America 183

Feldenkrais method **44–45,**
   82–83
feng shui **45**
   color in 30, 45
   Five Elements in 45, 46
   Interior Realignment in **65**
fennel oil 112
Ferenczi, Michael A. 75–76
ferric phosphate 24
fever therapy 44
   Issels's **67–68**
fibromyalgia, acupuncture for
   233
Finger, Alan 169
Finger, Kavi Yogiraj Mani 169
fire
   as *agni* 5
   in Five Elements 46
fir needle oil 112
Fischer-Rizzi, Susanne, *Complete*
   Aromatherapy Handbook 9
fish 47
Fitzgerald, William 136–137,
   173
Five Elements 45, **46**
The Five Tibetans (Kilham) 171
flotation therapy **46**
Flower Essence Repertory
   (Kaminski and Katz) 46
Flower Essence Society 183
Flower Healing 183
flower remedies **46–47**
   Australian Bush Flower
     Essences **12**
   Bach **15–17**
fluidotherapy 62
flush
   ascorbic acid **10–11**
   liver **76**
folk medicine **47**
folk (home) remedies **57**
   AMA on 197
fomentations, herbal **47**
Food and Drug Administration
   (FDA)
   on acupuncture 3
   on chelation therapy 26

   on herbal remedies 54, 192
   on homeopathy 57
   on Hoxsey therapy 57–58
   and testing of supplements
     90–91, 192
food therapy **47**
   for anxiety 7–8
foot, in reflexology 136–137
foot bath 60
foot chart 137
Footwork 50
Foundation for Christian Living
   125
Foundation for the
   Advancement of Innovative
   Medicine (FAIM) xix–xx
foxglove 54
frankincense oil 112
Franklin, Benjamin 63
Freud, Sigmund **47**
   hypnosis used by 63
   Jung and 70
   Reich and 137
Friend, John 168
Fringed Violet 12
frostbite 75
fruitarians 157
fu 163
Functional Integration 45
fu zheng therapy **47**

G

galactagogue **49**
galangal oil 112
galbanum oil 112–113
Galen, Claudius **49**
gan **49**
Gandhi, Mohandas K.
   (Mahatma) **49**
gan mao ling 49
Gannett, Frank 125
Gannon, Sharon 169
gardenia oil 113
garlic 47
garlic oil 113

Garri, Giovanni 9
GAS. *See* general adaptation
    syndrome
Gattefossé, René-Maurice **49**
    on aromatherapy 9
gemstone therapy **31–32**
general **49**
general adaptation syndrome
    (GAS) 141–142
gentian 16
Georgiana Institute 183
geranium oil 113
Gerber, Richard
    on acupuncture 2–3
    *A Practical Guide to Vibrational
        Medicine* xviii, 47, 80, 135
Gerson, Charlotte 49
Gerson, Max 49
Gerson, Scott 13
Gerson Institute 49, 50
Gerson therapy **49–50**
ghee 44
ginger oil 113
Ginkgo biloba, NCCAM on 219,
    220, 221, 234
ginseng 27, 119
glandulars **50**
Gogh, Vincent van 11–12
glucosamine, NCCAM on 231
Goldberg, Burton
    Alternative Medicine xviii
        on acupuncture 3
        on cell therapy 24
        on homeopathy 57
    Magnet Therapy 80–81
goldenrod oil 113
goldenseal, as herbal antibiotic
    7
The Golden Seven Plus One (West)
    77
Gonzalez, Nicholas 94
Gonzalez Regimen 231
Goodheart, George, Jr. 71
Gorakhnath 165
Goraksa-sataka 165
Gordon Research Institute 183
gorse 16

Grad, Bernard 34
grapefruit 47
grapefruit oil 113
green (color) 75
green drinks 20
green superfoods **50**
Gregorio, Reverend 129
Grinberg, Avi 50
Grinberg Method **50**
Grof, Stanislav 128
guaiac wood oil 113
guided imagery **50**
Guideposts (magazine) 125
Guillotin, Josef de 63
gunas **50–51**

H

Hahnemann, Samuel C. F. **53,**
    56
    on homeopathy 53, 196
    on magnets 80
    on miasms 85
Haiti, Voodoo in 142, 158
hakomi **53–54**
Hakomi Institute 53–54, 184
hands, laying on of **75**
    in faith healing 43
hands-on healing
    in polarity therapy
        126–127
    scientific studies of 34
    in zero balancing 173
Happiness Is a Choice (Kaufman)
    119
Hartwell, Jonathan, *Plants Used
    Against Cancer* 58
Harvey, Clare, *The Encyclopedia
    of Flower Remedies* 46–47
Hatha yoga 164, 165, 168
    types of 168–172
Hatha Yoga Pradipika
    (Svatmarama) 166
Hawaii
    kahuna of 71
    Lomi-Lomi massage in 83

Hay, Louise **54**
    on affirmations 5
Hayes, Diana 101
Healing Touch 150
Healing Touch International 184
Healing Words (Dossey) 43–44
health, definitions of xvii
health disparities 97–98
health insurance coverage 198
*Health Through Inner Body
    Cleansing* (Rauch) 83
*Healthy Healing: An Alternative
    Healing Reference* (Rector-Page)
        on anxiety treatments 7–8
        on ascorbic acid flush 10–11
Heal Thyself (Bach) 15
heart chakra 25–26
heart disease, coronary,
    meditation and 231–232
Heat, Empty **38**
heather 16
heat therapy. *See* hyperthermia
helichrysum oil 113
heliotherapy. *See* solar therapy
Heller, Joseph 54
    Bodywise 54
Hellerwork **54**
Hellerwork International 184
hemorrhoids 60
Henkin, William, *Bodywise* 54
henna oil 113
Henri, Robert, *The Art Spirit* 10
herb(s). *See also specific herbs*
    list of 207–211
herbal antibiotics **7**
herbal douches **34–35**
herbal extracts **41**
herbal fomentations **47**
herbalism **54–55**
    AMA on 191–193
    Chinese **27**
    Native American 99
herbal poultice **127**
herbal tea **149**
herbal vaginal douche 35
herbal vaginal pack **157**
herbal wraps 8, **55,** 61

Herb Research Foundation 184

Hering, Constantine 55

Hering's Law of Cure **55**

Hernandez, Lyla M. 205

Hillman, James 86

Himalayan Institute, Combined Therapy Program of 17–18

Hinduism
  rishis in 139
  yoga in 164

hip bath 60

Hippocrates xvii, **55**
  on aromatherapy 9
  on eyes 66
  on four humors 58
  home remedies of 57
  on massage 82
  as naturopath 100

Hippocratic oath 55

HIV, NCCAM on 232

Hoffer, Abram 119–120

Hoffman, Jeff 171–172

Hohenheim, Philippus Aureolus Theophrastus Bombast von. *See* Paracelsus

Holistic Animal Therapy Association of Australia 184

Holistic Dental Association 184

holistic medicine **55–56**

holly 16

Holmes, Ernest **56**
  The Science of Mind 43, 56

Homeopathic Educational Services 184

Homeopathic Pharmacopoeia of the United States (HPUS) 54

Homeopathic Remedies for Health Professionals and Laypeople (Buegel, Lewis, and Chernin) 22

homeopathy **56–57**
  AMA on 196–197
  centesimal scale in **25**
  combination remedies in **30**

constitutional remedies in **30**

decimal scale in **33**

development of 53, 56, 196

fasting in 44

febrifuge in 44

generals in 49

Hering's Law of Cure in 55

mentals in 83

miasm in 85

NCCAM on 227

nosodes in 104

particulars in 124

peculiars in 125

principles of 56

remedy pictures in 138–139

rubefacients in 139

trauma remedies in 154

Homeopathy, a Frontier in Medical Science (Bellavite and Signorini) 18–19

homeostasis 121

home remedies **57**

honey 8, 47, 57

honeysuckle 16

hops oil 113

Horatio Alger Association 125

hornbean 16–17

hot packs, in hyperthermia 61

hot tonics 22, **151**

hot-water bottles, in hyperthermia 61

Hoxsey, Harry 57–58
  You Don't Have to Die 58

Hoxsey therapy **57–58**

HPUS. *See Homeopathic Pharmacopoeia of the United States*

Hudgings, Carole 198

humectant **58**

humor, use of xxi, **58**

humors, four **58**

Huneke, Ferdinand 102

Huneke, Walter 102

hydrotherapy **58–61,** 62
  for balance of humors 58–59

hydrothermal therapy 58, 59

Hypericum perforatum. See St. John's wort

hypertension
  acupuncture for 231
  transcendental meditation for 153

hyperthermia **61–62**

hypnosis. *See* hypnotherapy

hypnotherapy **62–63**
  Ericksonian 102
  mesmerism and 63, 84
  in past-life regression therapy 124

hypoglycemia, in insulin potentiation therapy 65

hyssop oil 113

I

I Ching 149

imagery, guided **50**

Imaginal Therapy 67

immunizations
  as homeopathy 56
  Law of Similars in 75

impatiens 17

IMSS. *See* International Macrobiotic Shiatsu Society

Inayat Khan, Hazrat 67

Indian. *See* Native American

infusion **65**

infusodecoction 65

Ingham, Eunice 137, 173

Inner Peace Music 184

Insight Meditation Society 184

Instep International 22

Institute of Medicine (IOM) 205–206

insulin potentiation therapy (IPT) **65**

insurance coverage 198

Integral yoga 168
integrative medicine
    definition of xi, xviii
    NCCAM on 98
integrative yoga therapy
    168–169
Interior Realignment **65**
International Academy of Oral
    Medicine and Toxicology
    184
International Alliance of
    Healthcare Education 184
International Apiary Society 8
International Association for
    Colon Hydrotherapy 30
International Association for
    Colon Therapy 184
International Association of
    Professional Natural
    Hygienists 184
International Center for Reiki
    Training 184
International Chiropractors
    Association 184
International Clinical
    Hyperthermia Society 184
International College of
    Advanced Longevity Medicine
    76, 185
International College of Applied
    Kinesiology 71, 185
International Institute of
    Reflexology 185
International Integral Qigong
    and Tai Chi Training Institute
    185
International Macrobiotic
    Shiatsu Society (IMSS) 79
International Medical and
    Dental Hypnotherapy
    Association 185
International Primal Association
    (IPA) 127, 128
*International Review of
    Chiropractic* (journal) 28
International Rolf Institute
    185

International Society for
    Molecular Nutrition and
    Therapy (ISMNT) 85–86
International Society for
    Orthomolecular Medicine 185
intestinal therapy, Mayr **83**
intuitive touch **65**
inyanga 141
IOM. *See* Institute of Medicine
IPA. *See* International Primal
    Association
IPT. *See* insulin potentiation
    therapy
iridology **65–66**
irischromotherapy 66
irritants, in reconstructive
    therapy 136
ISHTA yoga 169
Islamic Sufi healing practices
    66–67
    Zikr in **173**
ISMNT. *See* International
    Society for Molecular
    Nutrition and Therapy
Isopogon 12
Issels, Josef 67–68
Issels's fever therapy **67–68**
Iyengar, B. K. S. 168, 169
Iyengar yoga 169

J

Jacobs, Joseph 199–200
James, William xxii, **69**
Janov, Arthur 127
Japan
    shiatsu in 65
    White Light Reiki in 159
jasmine oil 113
jihva 151
jing 40, **69**
jingluo **69,** 83
jing ye **69**
Jivamukti yoga 169
Johns Hopkins University,
    cancer research at 93–94

Jois, Sir K. Patabhi 168
*Journal of Orthomolecular
    Psychiatry* 120
Journal of Psychosomatic Medicine
    36
Journal of Schizophrenia 119
journals xxii. *See also specific
    journals*
juices and juice therapy **69–70**
    dosha and 44
Juicing for Life (Calbom and
    Keane) 69
Jung, Carl **70**
    *The Psychology of the
    Unconscious* 70
juniper oil 113–114

K

kahuna **71**
Kali Ray TriYoga 169
Kalita, Dwight K., *Magnet
    Therapy* 80–81
Kaminski, Patricia, *Flower
    Essence Repertory* 46
kapha 34, **71,** 146, 154, 156
kappalbhati 161
Karlekar, R. V. 155
Katz, Richard, *Flower Essence
    Repertory* 46
Kaufman, Barry Neil
    118–119
    Happiness Is a Choice 119
Kaufman, Samahria 119
Keane, Maureen, *Juicing for Life*
    69
Kelder, Peter 171
Kellogg, John Harvey 29
Kenny, Elizabeth 126
Kent, James Tyler 53
khella oil 114
ki **71**. *See also qi (ch'i)*
Kilham, Christopher, *The Five
    Tibetans* 171
kinesiology **71–72**
    in reflex approach 31

King, H. Lawrence 127
Kingsley, Noel 6
Kirlian, Semyon 72
Kirlian, Valentina 72
Kirlian photography **72,** 126
Klinghardt, Dietrich 102
knee douche 59
Kneipp, Sebastian 59
knotweed 139
Korngold, Efrem **18**
  Between Heaven and Earth
    4–5, 18, 133
Korr, I. M. 120
Kraftsow, Gary 171
Krieger, Dolores **72**
  Accepting Your Power to Heal
    72
  Therapeutic Touch
    developed by 72, 73, 150
kripalu yoga **72,** 169
Krishnamacharya, Tirumalai
  166–167, 168, 171
Krishnamurti, Jiddu **72,** 167
Kriyananda, Swami 168
Kriya yoga 168, 169
Kroon, Coen van der 155
ku **72**
Kübler-Ross, Elisabeth **72–73**
  and Myss, Caroline 87
Kuchler, Henriette 53
kundalini **73**
Kundalini yoga 169–170
Kunz, Dora Van Gelder 72, **73,**
  150
Kurtz, Ron 53
Kushi Institute 79

L

labdanum oil 114
labrador tea 114
lactovegetarians 157
Laing, R. D. 10
Lake, Frank 127
Lange, Carl 69
lantana oil 114

Lao Tzu Laozi 149
larch 17
laser therapy, cold 19
laughter 58
lavandin oil 114
lavender, aromatherapy with 9
lavender oil 114
lavender spike oil 114
Law(s)
  of Contraries **75**
  of Cure, Hering's **55**
  of Similars 56, **75**
Lawrence, D. H. xvii
Laya yoga 170
laying on of hands **75**
  in faith healing 43
lay organizations, contact
  information for 177–187
Lazanoff, Gorgi 145
learning disabilities,
  neurolinguistics for 102
lemon balm 115
lemongrass oil 114
lemon oil 114
lemon verbena oil 114
Le Page, Joseph 169
Lewis, Blair **22**
  *Homeopathic Remedies for
    Health Professionals and
    Laypeople* 22
Lewis, Carl 46
Life, David 169
Life After Life (Moody) 86
Life Sciences Institute of Mind-
  Body Health 185
Light on Yoga (Iyengar) 168
light therapy **75–76**
  and color therapy 30, 75
  solar 144
Light Therapy Institute 185
Light Years Ahead (Breiling) 22
lime oil 114
linden blossom oil 115
liniment **76**
Linn, Denise, *Past Lives, Present
  Dreams* 65, 124–125
litsea cubeba oil 115

liver disease, NCCAM on 232
liver flush **76**
living foodists 157
Lomatium dissectum, as herbal
  antibiotic 7
Lomi-Lomi massage 83
longevity medicine **76**
Lourdes (France), waters of
  59
lovage oil 115
lovage root oil 115
Love, Medicine & Miracles (Siegel)
  10, 43, 143
lower trunk douche 59
lymphasizing **77**
lymph drainage, manual 82
lymphedema 82

M

macrobiotics **79–80**
  yin-yang in 163
magnesium therapy, for asthma
  97
magnetic field therapy **80–81**
Magnet Therapy (Kalita et al.)
  80–81
Maharishi Ayur-Veda 151
Maharishi Mahesh Yogi 151
majja (nerve) 34
malaria 56
malas **81**
mambos 142, 158
mamsa (muscle) 34
mandarin oil 115
Mandel, Peter 30
Manners, Peter 32
mansin 142
mantra **81,** 170
Mantra yoga 170
manuka oil 115
maps
  Bagua 45
  body **20**
  foot 136
  tongue 151

Marchant, G. 129–130
Marcus Aurelius 49
marigold oil 115
marjoram oil 115
Markov, M. S. 134
marma **81**
marma puncture **82**
martial arts, in t'ai ch'i 149
Martin, Harvey J., III 130
massage **82–83**
   acupressure **1–2,** 82
   with aromatherapy 83
   Aston-Patterning **11**
   chair 82
   connective tissue 82
   craniosacral 82
   Deep Tissue 82
   effleurage **37**
   Feldenkrais method **44–45,**
     82–83
   intuitive touch **65**
   Lomi-Lomi 83
   lymph drainage 82
   neuromuscular 82
   reflexology 50, 82, 84,
     136–137, 173
   Reiki 11, 83, **137–138,** 144,
     159
   Rolfing 11, **139**
   shiatsu 2, 65, 79–80, 82,
     142
   sports 82
   stone 83
   Swedish 82
   Thai 82, **149**
   Therapeutic Touch 72, 73,
     83, **150**
   Trager Integration **151**
massoia bark oil 115
Matrix, Inc. 185
Matthews-Simonton, Stephanie
  144
Maury, Marguerite 9
Mayr intestinal therapy **83**
Mazzara, Ismael 67
McDowall, Donald, *Psychic
  Surgery* 129

McFadden, Bernarr xxii
McGraw, Phillip C. xix
   Self Matters xix
meda (adipose tissue) 34
medicine men, and sweat
  lodges 148
meditation **83**
   for coronary heart disease
     231–232
   mantra in 81
   transcendental **151–154**
   as yoga 164
MEDLINE 98
melatonin 75, 76, 232, 234
melissa oil 115
Menn, Lise 102–103
mental **83**
mental health, NCCAM on
  233
Mentgen, Janet 150
menthe pouliot oil 115
Menuhin, Yehudi 168
meridians **83–84**
   in acupressure 1, 2
   in acupuncture 2
   as channels 26
Mesmer, Franz Anton 63, 80,
  84
mesmerism **84**
metal, in Five Elements 46
Metamorphic Association
  84–85
Metamorphic Technique
  84–85
miasm **85**
Mifepristone 1
milk 47
milk secretion, breast 49
Milton H. Erickson Foundation
  185
mimosa oil 115
mimulus 17
mind, nonlocal 34, **104**
mind-body connection xviii,
  85
   AMA on 190–191
   NCCAM on 227

The Mind/Body Effect (Benson)
  18
Mind-Body Medical Institute
  185
minority populations
   CAM use in 97
   health disparities in
     97–98
mint 54, 57
Mithal, C. P. 155
molecular nutrition **85–86**
monarda oil 115
Moody, Raymond **86**
   Life After Life 86
Moore, Thomas **86**
   Care of the Soul 46
MORA Concept **86–87**
Morell, Franz, *The MORA
  Concept* 87
Moss, Thelma 126
mother tincture **87**
mouth balancing 19–20
moxa 4, 232
moxibustion 4, **87**
Mozart Effect Resource Center
  185
Muehsam, David J. 134
Muehsam, Patricia A. 134
mugwort 87, 115
Multiple Sclerosis Society, on
  apitherapy 8
muscle testing, in kinesiology
  71–72
musculoskeletal disorders,
  NCCAM on 233–234
Museum of Images from the
  Unconscious (Rio de Janeiro)
  10
music therapy **87,** 144–145
mustard 17
myotherapy **87**
myrrh oil 115–116
myrtle oil 116
Myss, Caroline **87**
   Anatomy of the Spirit 87
   *Why People Don't Heal and
    How They Can* 87

N

Nadi 131
Nakagawa, Kyoichi 81
narcissus oil 116
Naropa Institute 185
nasal douche 35
nasya **89**
National Academies 205
National Acupuncture
  Detoxification Association
  186
National Association for Holistic
  Aromatherapy 185
National Cancer Institute (NCI),
  on Hoxsey therapy 57–58
National Center for
  Complementary and
  Alternative Medicine
  (NCCAM) **89–99**
    contact information for 92
    establishment of xx, 214,
      217
    events in history of
      228–230
    evidence-based reviews in
      240–241
    fact sheet on CAM by
      89–99
    interventions by,
      mechanisms of 93
    members of 241–244
    objectives of xx–xxi, 89, 93,
      217–218
    priorities of 93–98
    research centers of 235–238
    strategic plan of, text of
      213–244
    and Therapeutic Touch 150
National Center for
  Homeopathy 186
National Commission for the
  Certification of Acupuncturists
  186
National Council against Health
  Fraud (NCAHF) 130–131, 186
National Guild of Hypnotists
  186

National Institute of Ayurvedic
  Medicine (NIAM) 13
National Institute of Endocrine
  Research 186
National Institute of Nutrition
  186
National Institutes of Health
  (NIH)
    on acupuncture 3, 4
    consensus conferences at
      241
    naturopathy and 101
    new study by 205–206
National Qigong Association
  (NQA) 134, 186
National Stress Institute 142
Native American healing
  practices **99–100**
    sweat lodge in 147–148
Natrum mur 24
Natrum muriaticum 24
Natural Medicine Clinic 101
naturopath **100**
naturopathy **100–101**
    AMA on 197
    fasting in 44
    NCCAM on 227
Navarra, Tom 142–144
NCAHF. *See* National Council
  against Health Fraud
NCCAM. *See* National Center
  for Complementary and
  Alternative Medicine
NCI. *See* National Cancer
  Institute
near-death experience 86, **101**
neck douches 60
neck pain, acupuncture for 3
negative energy **101–102**
Nelson, Mildred 58
Nelson Bach USA 186
neroli oil 116
nervous system 12. *See also*
  autonomic nervous system
neural therapy 19, **102**
Neuro-Linguistic Programming
  (NLP) 102

neurolinguistics **102–103**
neurological disorders, NCCAM
  on 234
neuromuscular massage 82
neuropeptides 85
neuroprotective agents 234
Neurostructural Integration
  Technique (NST) 22
NH-PAI. *See* Nurse Healers-
  Professional Associates
  International Inc.
NIAM. *See* National Institute of
  Ayurvedic Medicine
Niaouli oil 116
Niehans, Paul 25
Nightingale, Florence **103–104**
    on mind-body connection
      xviii
    Notes on Nursing 103–104
NIH. *See* National Institutes of
  Health
Nixon-Levy, Michael 22
niyama 164, 165
NLP. *See* Neuro-Linguistic
  Programming
Nogier, Paul 4
nonlocal mind 34, **104**
North American Vegetarian
  Society 186
nosode 15, **104**
Notes on Nursing (Nightingale)
  103–104
NQA. *See* National Qigong
  Association
NST. *See* Neurostructural
  Integration Technique
Nurse Healers-Professional
  Associates International Inc.
  (NH-PAI) 150, 186
nursing
    holistic **104**
    and Nightingale, Florence
      103–104
nutmeg oil 116
nutrition
    in *ahara rasa* 5
    AMA on 191

in green superfoods 50
    molecular **85–86**
nutritional therapy **104–105**
    Gerson therapy **49–50**
    juice therapy **69–70**

O

oak 17
OAM. *See* Office of Alternative
    Medicine
obeah **107**
Office of Alternative Medicine
    (OAM) 197–198. *See also*
    National Center for
    Complementary and
    Alternative Medicine
office yoga 170
Offner, Yonah 170
oils, essential **107–118**
    aromatherapy with **9–10**
oja **118**
olive 17
omega-3 fatty acids 233
Omura, Y. 129
*The One Spirit Encyclopedia of
    Complementary Health* 2
Options Institute **118–119**
O'Quinn, John F. 155
oral acupuncture 19
orange oil 116
oranges 47
oregano oil 116
organizations, contact
    information for 177–187
Organon (Hahnemann) 53
organ remedies **119**
Orloff, Judith **119**
Ornish, Dean **119**
    on vegetarianism 157
orris root oil 116
orthomolecular medicine
    119–120
osha, as herbal antibiotic 7
Osler, William xiii
osmanthus oil 116

osteoarthritis, NCCAM on 96
osteopathy **120–121,** 146
    AMA on 193
Our NET Effect (ONE)
    Foundation 186
out-of-body experience 86. *See
    also* near-death experience
overheating therapy. *See*
    hyperthermia; Issels's fever
    therapy
ovolactovegetarians 157
Oxford Health Plan 198
oxidative cell injury 233

P

pacemakers, Reiki and 138
Pacific Institute of
    Aromatherapy 186
packs
    herbal vaginal **157**
    hot 61
pain
    acupuncture for 3, 4, 232,
        233
    back 234
    Bonnie Prudden
        Myotherapy for 21
    dental 232
    neck 3
    transcutaneous electrical
        nerve stimulation for 39
palmarosa oil 116
Palmer, Bartlett J. 123
Palmer, Daniel David 27, 28,
    123–124
palmistry **124**
panchakarma **124**
papaya 47
Paracelsus **124**
    on magnets 80
    and organ remedies 119
paraffin wax, in hyperthermia
    61–62
Paramananda, Swami 165,
    166

parasympathetic nervous
    system 12
Parkinson's disease 234
parsley 57
parsley seed oil 116
particulars **124**
passive volition 19
Pasteur, Louis 80
past-life regression therapy
    124–125
Past Lives, Present Dreams (Linn)
    65, 124–125
Patanjali 164, 166, 168
patchouli oil 116
Pauling, Linus 119, 120
*PDR Family Guide to Natural
    Medicines & Healing Therapies,*
    on apitherapy 8
Peale, Norman Vincent **125**
    The Power of Positive Thinking
        125
Peale, Ruth Stafford 125
peculiars **125**
Peczeley, Ignatz von 66
penicillamine 26
Pennsylvania, University of,
    cancer research at 93–94
The People's Repertory (De
    Schepper) 56
pepper, black 109
peppermint oil 116–117
peridot 32
Perls, Fritz 102
personality profiles 35
*Personality Profiles of the Major
    Constitutional Remedies* (Baily)
    17
Pert, Candace 85
pet(s). *See also* animal(s)
    naturopathy for 101
    therapy for **125–126**
petitgrain oil 117
Pew, J. Howard 125
Philippine Medical Association
    (PMA) 129–130
Philippines, psychic surgery in
    128–131

Philpott, William H., *Magnet Therapy* 80–81
phlegm, as humor 58
Phoenix Rising yoga 170
photography, Kirlian **72,** 126
physical therapy **126**
physicians. *See also specific types*
   botanic **21**
   conventional
      as triage officer xx
      views on alternative medicine 200
phytotherapy **126.** *See also* herbalism
Pilates **126**
Pilates, Joseph H. 126
Pilla, Arthur A. 134
pine 17
pine oil 117
pitta 34, **126,** 154
   refrigerants for 137
   in urine therapy 155–156
placebo **126**
placebo effect 126
   NCCAM on 95–96
   spontaneous healing as 146
placebo surgery 130
plant-spirit healing **126**
Plants Used Against Cancer (Hartwell) 58
PMA. *See* Philippine Medical Association
PMRI. *See* Preventive Medicine Research Institute
polarity therapy **126–127**
polypeptides 38
pools, heated, in aquasonics 8
positive thinking 125
posture training. *See* Alexander Technique
potassium chloride 24
potassium phosphate 24
potassium sulfate 24
poultice, herbal **127**
PowerBreathing 170
The Power of Positive Thinking (Peale) 125

The Power to Heal: Ancient Arts & Modern Medicine xxi, xxii
   on art therapy 10
Power yoga 170
A Practical Guide to Vibrational Medicine (Gerber) xviii, 47
   on magnetism 80
   on radionics 135
pragmatism 69
prakruti **127**
pranayama **127,** 164, 166
pranic bath 161
pranic healing **127**
pratyahara 164
prayer, power of 34, **127**
pregnancy, depression during, acupuncture for 235
Prescription for Nutritional Healing (Balch and Balch) 17
Preventive Medicine Research Institute (PMRI) 119
Priessnitz, Vincenz 59
primal integration 127–128
primal scream therapy **127–128**
primitive medicine 245
professional organizations, contact information for 177–187
prostatic hyperplasia, benign (BPH) 234–235
protease 40
Prudden, Bonnie 21
psoric miasm 85
psychiatry, consultation-liaison 35, 36
psychic surgery **128–131**
Psychic Surgery (McDowall) 129
psychoimmunology xxii
The Psychology of the Unconscious (Jung) 70
psychosomatic disease **131**
psychosomatic medicine
   and behavioral medicine 18
   definition of 18
   Dunbar's work in 35, 36
PubMed 90, 98

pulse analysis **131**
Punctoscope 4
purvakarma **131**
Pyrifer 67

Q

qi (ch'i) **133**
   in acupressure 1, 2
   in acupuncture 2–3
qigong **133–134**
   internal 133
   medical 133
Qigong Institute 134, 186
qi ni **134**
qi xian **134**
qi zhi **134**
Quackwatch 146
quartz 32

R

radical healing xviii, **135**
Radical Healing (Ballentine) xviii, 135
   on allopathy 6
   on flower remedies 15–16
   on Hering's Law of Cure 55
   on sweat lodges 147–148
radiesthesia, medical 35
radionics **135–136**
Raj, Maharishi Ayur-Veda Health Institute 186
rajas 50, 136
rajasic **136**
Raja yoga 164
rakta (blood) 34
rakta moksha **136**
Ramakrishna Order 166
Ramakrishna Paramhansa 165, 166
Ramdas, Papa 167
rapeseed oil 109
rasa (plasma) 34, **136**
rasayana **136**

Rauch, Erich, *Health Through Inner Body Cleansing* 83
Ravensara anisata 117
Ravensara aromatica 117
Ray, Kali 169
rebirthing **136**
reconstructive therapy **136**
rectal. *See* colonic irrigation
Rector-Page, Linda G., *Healthy Healing*
    on anxiety treatments 7–8
    on ascorbic acid flush 10–11
red chestnut 17
reflex approach 31
reflexology 82, **136–137,** 173
    Grinberg Method of **50**
    in Metamorphic Technique 84
refrigerant **137**
regression therapy, past-life **124–125**
Reich, Wilhelm **137**
Reichian therapy 137
Reichmanis, Maria 3
Reiki 83, **137–138**
    attunement (initiation) in 11
    solar plexus in 144
    White Light 138, **159**
Reinventing Medicine (Dossey) 40, 104, 133–134
rejuvenation therapy **138**
relaxant **138**
relaxation 138
    autogenic training for **12–13**
    biofeedback for **19**
    breathing techniques for **22**
    floatation therapy for 46
Relaxation Response **138**
remedy picture **138–139**
remission **139**
    spontaneous 139, **145–146**
        Siegel on 143
ren **139**
Renner, John 190, 194
rennin 39
Rescue Remedy 17
Reston, James 216

restorative **139**
rice 47
Rich, Tracey 171
Rickey, Branch 125
Rig-Veda 165
Rimland, Bernard 120
Rio de Janeiro, Museum of Images from the Unconscious in 10
Rishis **139**
Ritacco, Barbara 46
rituals, Native American 99
rock rose 17
rock water 17
Rolf, Ida P. 139
Rolfing **139**
    Aston-Patterning and 11
root (sexual) chakra 25, **139, 142**
rose
    rock 17
    Sturt Desert 12
    wild 17
rosemary oil 117
Rosen, Marion **139**
Rosen method 139, 187
rose oil 117
rosewood oil 117
Rovesti, Paolo 9
Rowan, John 127–128
Roy, Ram Mohun 165
royal jelly 8
RU486 1
rubefacient **139**
Rubenfeld, Ilana 139
Rubenfeld Synergy Center 139, 187
Rubenfeld Synergy Method **139–140**

S

Sacred Plant Medicine (Buhner) 22
Sacro-Occipital Research Society International 187

Sacro-Occipital Technique (S.O.T.) 31
SAD. *See* seasonal affective disorder
Sagan, Carl 201
sage oil 117
St. John, Robert 84
St. John's wort
    AMA on 192
    as essential oil 117–118
    NCCAM on 96, 217*f,* 233
Saint-Pierre, Gaston 84
salve **141**
samadhi 164
samagni **141**
Sama-Veda 165
Samkara 165
Samkhya philosophy 50–51
SAMONAS. *See* Spectral Activated Music of Optimal Natural Structure
Sampson, Wallace 200–201
sandalwood oil 117
sangomas **141**
Sanskrit 164
Satchidananda, Sri Swami 168
Satir, Virginia 102
satva 50
saunas
    in hydrotherapy 60
    sweat lodges as 147–148
savoy cabbage 47
saw palmetto 7, 234–235
scent. *See* aromatherapy
Scheel, John 197
Schizophrenia (journal) 120
Schuessler, W. H. 21, 24
    An Abridged Therapy Manual for the Biochemical Treatment of Disease 24
Schultz, Johannes H. 12
Schweitzer, Albert 49
The Science of Mind (Holmes) 43, 56
scleranthus 17
scream therapy, primal **127–128**

scutellaria 27

seasonal affective disorder (SAD) 75–76, 144

The Seat of the Soul (Zukav) 173

Self Matters: Creating Your Life from the Inside Out (McGraw) xix

Selye, Hans **141–142**

Semicarpus anacardium 13

Senate, U.S., hearing on alternative medicine in xviii

SER. *See* SomatoEmotional Release

sexual (root) chakra 25, **139, 142**

shad rasa **142**

shaking 147

shaman(s) 99, **142**
 psychic surgery by 128–131
 sangoma **141**
 women as 142

Shamanism 142

Shankara 165

shark cartilage 94, 231

Sharp Institute for Human Potential and Mind-Body Medicine 187

Shealy, C. Norman **142**
 American Holistic Medical Association founded by xxi, 142
 on triage by physicians xx

Shealy Institute 142

Sheddon, Peter 120–121

shen **142**

Shen, Ronger 133–134

Shen Nung 27

She Oak 12

shiatsu 65, 82, **142**
 macrobiotic 79–80
 vs. acupressure 2

Shiva (Hindu god) 155, 165

shivananda yoga **142**

shukra (reproductive tissue) 34

Siegel, Bernie S. xviii, **142–144**
 interview with 142–144
 Love, Medicine & Miracles 10, 43, 143

Siegler Center for Integrative Medicine xi

Sieglinger, Frank 33

Signorini, Andrea **18–19**
 Homeopathy, a Frontier in Medical Science 18–19

silicic acid 24

silver 32

Similars, Law of 56, **75**

Simonton, O. Carl **144**
 guided imagery used by 50

Simonton Cancer Center 187

Sinatra, Frank xviii

sitz bath 60

Sivananda, Swami 167–168, 170

Sivananda yoga 170

six stage patterns **144**

The Skeptic's Dictionary (Carroll) 81

skin, applications applied to **8**

sleep disorders 76, 234

Smallwood, William L., *The West Point Candidate Book* xix

smartweed 139

smell. *See* aromatherapy

Smith, Fritz 173

smoking cessation, for anxiety 8

smudging 99

Soaring Crane *qigong* 133

Society for Light Treatment and Biological Rhythms 187

Society for Orthomolecular Health Medicine 187

sodium chloride 24

sodium phosphate 24

sodium sulfate 24

solar plexus **144**
 as third chakra 25, 144

solar therapy **144**. *See also* light therapy

SomatoEmotional Release (SER) 31

S.O.T. *See* Sacro-Occipital Technique

soul therapy. *See* flower remedies

Sound, Listening and Learning Center 187

Sound Healers Association 187

Sound Health Research Institute 187

sound therapy **144–145**
 cymatics **32**
 aquasonics in 8, 32
 music in **87**, 144–145

Southwest, *curanderismo* in 32

soy supplements 96–97

spearmint oil 117

specificity hypothesis 35–36

Spectral Activated Music of Optimal Natural Structure (SAMONAS) 145

spikenard oil 117

spinal manipulation, NCCAM on 95

spinal reflexes, in Metamorphic Technique 84

Spinifex 12

spiritual healing. *See* faith healing

spirulina 50

spontaneous healing (remission) 139, 143, **145–146**

sports massage 82

Srinivasan 171

star of bethlehem 17

Stead, Eugene A., Jr. xx

steam baths, in hydrotherapy 60

Steinbach, Ingo 145

Steiner, Rudolf 21, **146**

Still, Andrew Taylor 120, 121, **146,** 193

Stillpoint Publishing Company 87

stimulant **146**

stomach wash **146**
Stone, Randolph 127
stone massage 83
Straus, Stephen E. 214, 230
stress **146–147**
  reduction of, Alexander
    Technique for **5–6**
  Selye's theory of (general
    adaptation syndrome)
    141–142
stressors 147
Stress Reduction and Relaxation
  Program 187
structural integration. *See* Trager
  Integration
Study of Women's Health
  Across the Nation (SWAN)
  235
Sturt Desert Pea 12
Sturt Desert Rose 12
styrax 118
subclinical symptoms **147**
succussion **147**
Sufi Healing Order 66–67
Sufi healing practices, Islamic
  66–67
  Zikr in **173**
superfoods, green **50**
surgery
  placebo 130
  psychic **128–131**
Sutherland, William Garner
  31
Sutra 164
Svaroopa yoga 170–171
Svatmarama, Yogindra 166
SWAN. *See* Study of Women's
  Health Across the Nation
Swartley, Bill 127
sweat lodge **147–148**
Swedish massage 82
sweet birch 108
sweet chestnut 17
sweet flag 109
sycotic miasm 85
sympathetic nervous system
  12

symptoms
  in remedy picture 138–139
  subclinical **147**
Synergy Method, Rubenfeld
  139–140
syphilitic miasm 85

T

*Taber's Cyclopedic Medical
  Dictionary* xvii, 6
t'ai ch'i (t'ai ch'i chuan) **149**
  yin-yang in 163
tamas 50
tangerine oil 118
Tantra yoga 171
Tantric tradition, Five Elements
  in 46
Taoism 149
Tao Te Ching 149
tarragon oil 118
taste
  in Ayurveda 46, 136, 142
  in Chinese medicine 161
taste testing 46
tea
  herbal **149**
  as infusion 65
tea tree oil 118
TENS. *See* transcutaneous
  electrical nerve stimulation
*Textbook of Dr. Vodder's Manual
  Lymph Drainage* (Wittlinger
  and Wittlinger) 77
Thacher, C. J. 80
Thai massage 82, **149**
theophylline 27
Therapeutic Astrology (Bogart)
  21
Therapeutic Touch (TT) 83,
  150
  development of 72, 73, 150
thiamine 157
thigh douche 59
Thomson, Samuel 21,
  150–151

Thornburg, Raymond 125
throat chakra 26
thrombin 39
thyme oil 118
Tibb medicine 66
Tibetan yoga 171
*Timeless Healing: The Power and
  Biology of Belief* (Benson) xx
  on acupuncture 4
  on faith healing 43
tinctures **151**
  flower 15
  mother **87**
tissue remedies. *See* cell salts
tissue salts. *See* cell salts
TM. *See* transcendental
  meditation
Toffler, Alvin 141
Tomatis, Alfred A. 144
tongue analysis **151**
tongue maps 20
tonics
  blood 20
  hot 22, **151**
  purpose of 22
tonification **151**
toning 145
touch
  Healing 150
  intuitive **65**
  Therapeutic 72, 73, 83,
    150
tourmaline, clear 32
toxins, as *ama* 6
Trager, Milton 151
Trager Institute 187
Trager Integration **151**
Transcendental Meditation
  (TM) **151–154**
transcutaneous electrical nerve
  stimulation (TENS) 39
trauma remedies **154**
tribal healing practices. *See*
  Native American healing
  practices
tridoshas 34, **154**. *See also doshas*
trigger points. *See* acupoints

trunk douche 59–60
TT. *See* Therapeutic Touch
tui na 2
turquoise 32
The Twelve Healers and Other Remedies (Bach) 15
The Twelve Tissue Remedies of Schuessler (Boericke and Dewey) 21

U

ulcers, Chinese herbs for 27
ultrasound, hyperthermia with 61, 62
Upanishads 165
Upledger, John E. 31
upper trunk douche 59–60
urinalysis 155
urinary tract infections 97
urine therapy **155–156**
urological disorders, NCCAM on 234–235
usnea 7
Usui, Mikao 137, 159

V

Vacaspati Mishra 164
vaccines
    as homeopathy 56
    Law of Similars in 75
vaginal douche, herbal 35
vaginal pack, herbal **157**
vaginitis 157
Valnet, Jean 9
vaman 146
vamankarm 146
vanilla oil 118
vata 34, 154, 155, **157**
Vedanta 165, 166
Vedas 13, 165
veganism 157
Vegetarian Education Network 187

vegetarianism **157**
    in macrobiotic diet 79–80
Verus, Lucius Aurelius 49
vervain 17
veterinary medicine. *See* pet(s)
vetivert oil 118
vibrational medicine **157**. *See also specific types*
    definition of xviii
    effects of depression in 33–34
    Gerber on xviii
    radionics in 135–136
Vilayat Khan, Pir 67
vine 17
Viniyoga 171
violet
    Fringed 12
    water 17
violet leaf oil 118
Vishnu (Hindu god) 139
Vishnu-devananda, Swami 170
vision, Bates Method for Improving **18**
visualization
    in guided imagery 50
    in Imaginal Therapy 67
vital force **157**
vitalism **157**
vitamin(s) **157–158**
vitamin A 157
vitamin B 158
vitamin B$_1$ 157
vitamin C 119, 158
vitamin D 158
vitamin E 231
vitamin K 157
Vithoulkas, George 57
Vivekananda, Swami 165–166
voice, in sound therapy 145
vomiting, therapeutic 146
Voodoo (Vodun) 142, **158**

W

walnut 17
Walters, J. Donald 168

water
    in Five Elements 46
    in flotation therapy **46**
    in hydrotherapy **58–61**
watercress 47
water violet 17
wax, paraffin, in hyperthermia 61–62
Weil, Andrew **159,** 201
wei qi 133
Weiss, Brian L. 124, **159**
West, C. Samuel, *The Golden Seven Plus One* 77
The West Point Candidate Book (Smallwood) xix
wheat grass 50
White, Ganga 171
White, Ian 12
white birch 109
white chestnut 17
White Light Reiki 138, **159**
White Lotus yoga 171
WHO. *See* World Health Organization
Wholeness and the Implicate Order (Bohm) 21
Why People Don't Heal and How They Can (Myss) 87
Wilde, Stuart, *Affirmations* 5
wild oat 17
wild rose 17
willow 17, 148
wintergreen oil 118
Wittlinger, H. and G., *Textbook of Dr. Vodder's Manual Lymph Drainage* 77
women's health, NCCAM on 235
Woods, Bobby 148
World Chiropractic Alliance 187
World Health Organization (WHO)
    on acupuncture 3
    Constitution of, on health xvii
    on homeopathy 57

Worrall, Olga 126
wraps
    herbal 8, **55,** 61
    in hydrotherapy 60–61
Wright, Carol 130
Wright, Donald F. 130

X

xenobiotics **161**
xian **161**
xin **161**
X rays, chiropractic **161**
xu **161**

Y

Yajur-Veda 165
yama 164, 165
Yamamoto, Shizuko 79
yang 163

yarrow oil 118
yeast infections 157
yellow bile 58
yellow fever 57
yin 163
yin-yang **163**
Yi Wu 133–134
ylang ylang oil 118
yoga **164–172**. *See also specific types*
    branches of 168–172
    definition of 164
    history of 164–165
    important figures in
        164–168
    writings on 164–165
YogaDance 171–172
Yoga Makarandam
    (Krishnamacharya) 167
Yogananda, Paramhansa 167,
    168, 169
Yoga-Sutra 164, 165, 166
Yoga Zone Studios 169

yogi 164
yogurt 47
You Don't Have to Die (Hoxsey)
    58

Z

Zak, Victor 23–24
zanfu zhi qi **173**
zang 163
zang fu **173**
zanthoxylum oil 118
zero balancing **173**
zheng qi 133, **173**
Zikr **173**
zone therapy **173**. *See also*
    reflexology
zong qi 133, **173**
Zukav, Gary **173**
Zulu culture 141